VIDEO WEB SITE PASSCODE

Here is your passcode for *Phaco Chop and Advanced Phaco Techniques: Strategies for Complicated Cataracts Second Edition* Web Site. In order to view the videos, you will have to complete the registration process at the Web site. The unique passcode provided below is required to complete registration. At this time you will then be able to create a new password. Do not share your password with anyone.

To register, go to the following site:
www.healio.com/phacochopvideos

The unique passcode is located under the scratch-off below. Questions can be sent to **techsupport@slackinc.com**.

By scratching off this sticker, you accept the following Terms and Conditions: This passcode is for the original purchaser only and cannot be downloaded, posted online, or reprinted in any way. The passcode is for the original purchaser only and not for institutional use.

059PC780956

Second Edition

Phaco Chop and Advanced Phaco Techniques

Strategies for Complicated Cataracts

Second Edition

Phaco Chop and Advanced Phaco Techniques

Strategies for Complicated Cataracts

David F. Chang, MD

Clinical Professor of Ophthalmology
University of California, San Francisco
San Francisco, California

Altos Eye Physicians
Los Altos, California

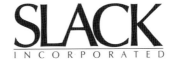

SLACK
INCORPORATED

Published by: SLACK Incorporated
                  6900 Grove Road
                  Thorofare, NJ 08086 USA
                  Telephone: 856-848-1000
                  Fax: 856-848-6091
                  www.Healio.com/books

Contact SLACK Incorporated for more information about other books in this field or about the availability of our books from distributors outside the United States.

Library of Congress Cataloging-in-Publication Data

Phaco chop and advanced phaco techniques : strategies for complicated cataracts / [edited by] David F. Chang. -- 2nd ed.
    p. ; cm.
  Rev. ed. of: Phaco chop / [edited by] David F. Chang. c2004.
  Includes bibliographical references and index.
  ISBN 978-1-61711-075-7 (alk. paper)
  I. Chang, David F., 1954- II. Phaco chop.
  [DNLM: 1. Phacoemulsification--methods. WW 260]

617.7'42059--dc23
                          2012040295

For permission to reprint material in another publication, contact SLACK Incorporated. Authorization to photocopy items for internal, personal, or academic use is granted by SLACK Incorporated provided that the appropriate fee is paid directly to Copyright Clearance Center. Prior to photocopying items, please contact the Copyright Clearance Center at 222 Rosewood Drive, Danvers, MA 01923 USA; phone: 978-750-8400; website: www.copyright.com; email: info@copyright.com

Printed in the United States of America.

Last digit is print number: 10   9   8   7   6   5   4   3   2   1

DEDICATION

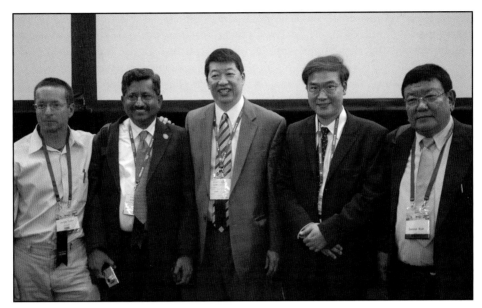

Beijing, 2010. (From left to right) Geoff Tabin, R.D. Ravindran, David Chang, Dennis Lam, and Sanduk Ruit.

During the 45 years since Charlie Kelman first attempted phaco in a human eye, we have seen continual improvement in phaco technology and techniques. Now, cataract surgery is becoming even more high-tech with the development of adjunct femtosecond laser automation. However, the tragic irony is that more than 20 million patients, mostly in the developing world, have no access to surgery and remain blind from bilateral cataracts. This growing backlog of cataract blindness, which will multiply with the aging of populations worldwide, remains the single greatest challenge in cataract surgery for us and for future generations of ophthalmologists.

Fortunately, there is hope if we follow the cost effective and scalable blueprints being successfully implemented by several pioneering groups. In densely populated cities throughout Southern India, the Aravind Eye Hospital System is solving the burden of cataract blindness without government financial support through its self-sustaining cost recovery system. The free surgery provided to 70% of their patients is subsidized by revenue from the 30% who pay. In China, which has one of the lowest per capita cataract surgery rates in the world, the problem is less economic than it is a dire shortage of surgeons and surgical training. Project Vision, a Hong Kong-based NGO, is succeeding with a bold initiative to train hundreds of new Chinese cataract surgeons to work in underserved rural areas. Finally, the Tilganga Eye Center in Nepal is flourishing proof that outside seed investment can spawn a financially sustainable center of excellence in a very poor society—a program dedicated to charity eye care and to training doctors from other poor countries to do the same.

Underlying the promising success of these 3 remarkable model programs are several common key elements. All promote and excel at efficient, high-volume cataract surgery in which the productivity of the scarcest resource—the surgeon—is maximized by a well-trained and choreographed support staff. Quality outcomes are achieved at lower cost by combining a low-tech method of ECCE—manual sutureless, small incision cataract surgery (M-SICS)—and inexpensive IOLs, manufactured locally or in-house. M-SICS is not only more affordable, but it is easier and safer for inexperienced surgeons to learn, particularly with the advanced mature cataracts so prevalent in poor populations. Finally, surgeons in all 3 of these systems eventually learn phaco after mastering M-SICS. This allows the surgeon's clinic to attract private paying patients, whose care can subsidize services for the poor. Visit www.globalsight.org to learn more about M-SICS and to view the video presentation, *Our Greatest Challenge in Cataract Surgery,* that describes and compares these 3 model programs.

It is for these reasons that I believe the most important cataract surgeons in the world today are the visionary leaders guiding these innovative training programs of excellence. Long recognized as one of the best surgeons, teachers, and administrators in their system, R. D. Ravindran is chairman of the Aravind Eye Hospital System. Ravi's exceptional leadership has been pivotal in the growth and expansion of Aravind, and he was brought in to serve as the first chief when each of their last 3 regional eye hospitals was opened. The 2011 book, *Infinite Vision*, is a wonderful narrative describing the genesis and evolution of Aravind, one of the most inspirational success stories in all of medicine.

As one of Asia's top academic ophthalmologists, Dennis Lam has directed 2 of the most prestigious ophthalmology departments (Chinese University in Hong Kong and the Zhongshan Ophthalmic Center, Sun Yat-sen University in Guangzhou) and is the CEO and secretary general of the Asia-Pacific Academy of Ophthalmology. On top of these responsibilities, Dennis launched and directs Project Vision—an ambitious initiative to establish 100 charity eye centers throughout underserved areas in rural China. The encouraging progress and potential of Project Vision can be ascribed to Dennis' unique combination of surgical and teaching skills, administrative expertise, academic prominence, and political stature as an elected Hong Kong representative to the Chinese National Peoples' Congress.

Born in a remote mountainous village with no school on the Tibetan plateau, Sanduk Ruit founded Tilganga Eye Center in Kathmandu and transformed ophthalmic care throughout Nepal. In 2006 he received the Magsaysay Award (considered Asia's Nobel Prize) for his Herculean efforts to fight cataract blindness in the poorest countries in Asia. The remarkable international outreach efforts of Dr. Ruit and his team combine high volume surgical camps with training and equipping local surgeons to perform M-SICS.

The University of Utah's Geoff Tabin was one of the world's top alpine mountaineers (he was the fourth individual to summit the highest peak on all 7 continents) before becoming an academic cornea specialist. He partnered with Sanduk Ruit to form Himalayan Cataract Project in 1995 and, by virtue of a career dedicated to teaching surgeons in the developing world, Geoff is probably the leading Western authority on cataract blindness. The United Nations Millennium Project recruited Geoff to lead its eye care interventions in Sub-Saharan Africa. Published in 2013, *Second Suns* by David Relin (coauthor of the *New York Times* bestseller, *Three Cups of Tea*) chronicles the remarkable lives and partnership of Ruit and Tabin, and should be read by every ophthalmologist.

I am indebted to each of these individuals for teaching me so much about the challenges and the potential solutions for overcoming cataract blindness worldwide. Through our friendships I have been inspired first-hand by their surgical talent, their creative problem solving ability, their superhuman energy and drive, and their compassion and selflessness. Most of all, I marvel at the determination and resolve needed to continually confront challenges that would vanquish anyone less courageous. I dedicate this textbook, which highlights our quest to master cataract surgery, to Drs. Ravindran, Lam, Ruit, and Tabin. These 4 individuals, and the many dedicated colleagues working under their leadership, are the greatest heroes in our field and I hope that cataract surgeons reading this textbook will support, follow, and celebrate their work.

Dr. Chang donates all textbook royalties to the Himalayan Cataract Project and Project Vision through the American Society of Cataract and Refractive Surgery (ASCRS) Foundation.

CONTENTS

ACKNOWLEDGMENTS

In my 2012 inauguration speech as the American Society of Cataract and Refractive Surgery (ASCRS) president, I highlighted our remarkable willingness to teach and help one other:

> For busy clinicians, our personal time is precious. And yet I know of no other profession where so many of its members regularly volunteer so much of their time to teach others the skills to become as good as the teacher. The expression "pay it forward" describes the unselfish concept of having someone repay your good deed not to you, but rather to a future stranger. We teach residents and colleagues not because of obligation or compensation, but out of appreciation for those who so generously taught and mentored us.

This tradition is indeed a big part of what makes our profession special. I remain indebted to so many individuals who taught me the clinical, surgical, and professional practice skills that have made my career performing cataract surgery so rewarding. Along with my coauthors, I am fortunate to now have the opportunity to share this knowledge with others through this textbook. Randy Olson, Skip Nichamin, and Barry Seibel are gifted teachers who have collaborated with me on our phaco chop course at every American Academy of Ophthalmology (AAO) and ASCRS meeting since 1998. I want to thank them along with each of the other talented friends who contributed chapters to this edition.

I am grateful to have a wonderful relationship with the entire SLACK publishing team that has produced this, our fifth major book together. My good friend John Bond has shepherded me through each of these projects and has always provided the resources and support that I have needed. The production quality of this new edition was made possible through the hard work of April Billick, Cara Hvisdas, and the proficient editing of Stephanie Wieland. Thank you all for being simultaneously patient, flexible, professional, and cheerful in what is always a strenuous process. By pioneering 3D surgical video technology, TrueVision of Santa Barbara, California has provided us with an amazing tool for eye surgical education. I want to thank Forrest Fleming and his team for all of their support in my efforts to use 3D video to teach surgical techniques. Special thanks go to Burton Tripathi for his expert technical help in producing the companion 3D videos for this textbook.

I want to thank my family—Courtney, Alex, and my wife of 33 years, Victoria—for tolerating and supporting my time consuming "hobby" of learning, teaching, performing, and studying cataract surgery. And finally, I want to thank my nonagenarian father who, by overcoming the many hurdles facing a foreign medical graduate from China in the early 1950s to become an accomplished anesthesiologist, taught me the value of hard work and inspired my career in medicine.

ABOUT THE AUTHOR

David F. Chang, MD is a Summa Cum Laude graduate of Harvard College and Harvard Medical School. He completed his ophthalmology residency at the University of California, San Francisco (UCSF) where he is now a clinical professor. Having chaired the American Society of Cataract and Refractive Surgery (ASCRS) Cataract Clinical Committee, Dr. Chang joined the ASCRS Executive Committee in 2009, serving as president in 2012-2013. He is also chairman of the American Academy of Ophthalmology (AAO) Cataract Preferred Practice Pattern Panel, immediate past chair of the AAO Practicing Ophthalmologist Curriculum Panel for Cataract/Anterior Segment, and in 2009 completed his 5-year term as chair of the AAO Annual Meeting program committee. Dr. Chang is a board member of the ASCRS Foundation and serves on the medical advisory board of 2 global humanitarian organizations (Himalayan Cataract Project and Project Vision). He is also an adjunct clinical professor of ophthalmology at the Chinese University in Hong Kong and honorary professor for the Zhongshan Ophthalmic Center of Sun Yat-Sen University in China.

In 2006, Dr. Chang became only the third ophthalmologist to ever receive the Charlotte Baer Award honoring the outstanding clinical faculty member at the UCSF Medical School. He has received the highest honor for cataract surgery from the ASCRS (Binkhorst Medal), the AAO (Kelman Lecture), the Asia Pacific Association of Cataract and Refractive Surgery (Lim Medal), the United Kingdom and Ireland Society of Cataract & Refractive Surgery (Rayner Medal), the Canadian Society of Cataract and Refractive Surgery (Award of Excellence/Stein Lecture), the Indian Intraocular Implant and Refractive Society (Gold Medal), the Italian Ophthalmological Society (Strampelli Medal), and the Royal Australia and the New Zealand College of Ophthalmologists (Gregg Medal). He has also been asked to give the Keynote Lecture for the Asia Pacific Academy of Ophthalmology Annual Meeting.

Dr. Chang has been selected to deliver the following additional named lectures: Transamerica Lecture (UCSF), Wolfe Lecture (University of Iowa), DeVoe Lecture (Columbia-Harkness), Gettes Lecture (Wills Eye Hospital), Helen Keller Lecture (University of Alabama), Williams Lecture (UCSF), Kayes Lecture (University of Washington, St. Louis), Thorpe Lecture (Pittsburgh Ophthalmology Society), Schutz Lecture (New York University Medical Center), Wallace-Evan Lecture (Casey Eye, Oregon), Kambara Lecture (Loma Linda), Boyaner Lecture (McGill), Herbert Lecture (UC Irvine), Rodriguez Lecture (Univ Arizona), Jules Stein Lecture (UCLA-Jules Stein), Paton Medal Lecture (Baylor/Cullen Eye), Weinstock Lecture (Wills Eye Hospital), and the Proctor Lecture (UCSF/Proctor Foundation). In addition to the AAO Achievement and Senior Achievement awards, Dr. Chang is also a 6-time AAO Secretariat Award recipient. He was the inaugural recipient of the UCSF Department of Ophthalmology's Distinguished Alumni Award (2005).

Dr. Chang is the chief medical editor of *EyeWorld*, associate international editor for the *Asia-Pacific Journal of Ophthalmology,* and served for 5 years as co-chief medical editor for *Cataract and Refractive Surgery Today*. He was the textbook editor of *Cataract Surgery Today* (CRST 2009), *Mastering Refractive IOLs—The Art and Science* (SLACK Incorporated 2008) and *Curbside Consultation in Cataract Surgery* (SLACK Incorporated 2007), the series editor for the 8 SLACK Incorporated *Curbside Consultation* ophthalmology textbooks, and the principal author of *Phaco Chop* (SLACK Incorporated 2004).

CONTRIBUTING AUTHORS

Takayuki Akahoshi, MD (Chapter 6)
Director of Ophthalmology
Mitsui Memorial Hospital
Tokyo, Japan

Lisa B. Arbisser, MD (Chapters 20 and 29)
Eye Surgeons Associates
Bettendorf, Iowa

Robert J. Cionni, MD (Chapter 13)
Cincinnati Eye Institute
Cincinnati, Ohio

Alan S. Crandall, MD (Chapter 10 Sidebar)
John A. Moran Eye Center
University of Utah
Salt Lake City, Utah

Louis D. "Skip" Nichamin, MD (Chapters 3, 12, 14, and 30)
Laurel Eye Clinic
Brookville, Pennsylvania

Randall J. Olson, MD (Chapter 2)
John A. Moran Eye Center
Salt Lake City, Utah

Robert H. Osher, MD (Foreword)
Professor of Ophthalmology
University of Cincinnati
College of Medicine
Medical Director Emeritus
Cincinnati Eye Institute
Cincinnati, Ohio

Mark Packer, MD, FACS, CPI (Chapter 7)
Clinical Associate Professor
Oregon Health & Science University
Portland, Oregon

Barry S. Seibel, MD (Chapters 8, 10, and 15)
Clinical Assistant Professor of Ophthalmology
University of California, Los Angeles
Geffen School of Medicine
Seibel Vision Surgery
Los Angeles, California

FOREWORD

To write a good foreword, it may be helpful to begin by looking backward. I first met David F. Chang, MD in the late 1980s when I was drawn into a cataract lecture where a young ophthalmologist had the standing-room crowd in the "palm of his hand." It was immediately obvious why so many had converged to hear this speaker. His words were carefully prepared, full of wisdom, and delivered with humor and enthusiasm.

Over the next 2 decades, few have experienced such a meteoric rise, developing a reputation as one of the finest teachers and surgeons on the planet. Armed with a prodigious work ethic and boundless energy, ophthalmologists around the world were treated to one brilliant lecture after another, chapter after chapter, and book after book. All were accomplished with humility and integrity.

Major organizations quickly recognized Dr. Chang's contribution and he was drafted into the leadership of the American Academy of Ophthalmology (AAO) and American Society of Cataract and Refractive Surgery (ASCRS). Industry identified his credibility and he was sought after for his thoughtful and innovative advice. Even other disciplines in medicine, such as urologists, were impacted by his observations.

Among his recent accomplishments, Dr. Chang is the perennial organizer of the AAO Spotlight Session and he serves as the Editor of the ASCRS publication, *Eye World*. He has delivered the most prestigious named lectures including the Binkhorst and the Kelman lectures. He is currently serving as the president of ASCRS.

I was delighted when my dear friend David invited me to write the foreword to his Second Edition of *Phaco Chop*. I could strongly support the importance of phaco chop while complimenting the other authors whose chapters are filled with essential information. I knew I could also say loud and clear what we all know to be true: Dr. David Chang is a gifted surgeon, a gifted teacher, and a gift to ophthalmology.

Robert H. Osher, MD
Professor of Ophthalmology
University of Cincinnati
College of Medicine
Medical Director Emeritus
Cincinnati Eye Institute
Cincinnati, Ohio

INTRODUCTION

Like most surgeons, ophthalmologists need a good reason to alter something that they are already comfortable with and which works very well for them. According to the latest Leaming surveys, roughly half of all cataract surgeons still rely on some form of divide-and-conquer technique, because it is both reliable and effective for the majority of their cases.[1] However, since Dr. Kunihiro Nagahara[2] first introduced the concept to us in 1993, I've been a strong proponent of phaco chop. In performing this technique exclusively for nearly 20 years, I have found that it is not only more efficient for routine cataracts, but is particularly effective for complicated cases, such as those with small pupils, loose zonules, brunescent nuclei, or mature white lenses. It is during stressful surgical situations such as these, that we always wonder if there is a better and safer way. In this textbook, my coauthors and I will review why we believe that phaco chop is the better and safer way, and how it can help us avoid complications in these high-risk cases. Of course, in order to reap the benefits of phaco chop for difficult cataracts, one needs to have first mastered this technique in routine eyes.

The first section of this textbook will discuss the mechanics of chopping. We will describe and compare the 2 basic techniques—horizontal and vertical chopping—and discuss where each is most effective. We will discuss the universal advantages of chopping and how to maximize these benefits. Finally, compared to divide-and-conquer, the technique of phaco chop is harder to master because many of the most difficult maneuvers are performed with the non-dominant hand. This is one of the reasons why the learning curve may be more difficult than ophthalmologists initially anticipate. We will attempt to guide you through the learning curve by discussing pearls for transitioning to chop from divide-and-conquer based upon our collective experience in teaching residents and transitioning surgeons.

The second section will address the phacodynamics of chopping. More than any other operative technique, phaco chop has benefited from continual innovation and advances in phaco technology. While this is a complicated and evolving topic, understanding the principles of configuring the phaco machine for chopping is necessary if one is to maximize success with this technique. The newest technology to impact chopping is of course the femtosecond laser, which can image and then fragment the nucleus in situ using a variety of prechop patterns. We provide information on nuclear softening and fragmentation strategies from the 3 femtosecond laser manufacturers that are farthest along in the development of this technology.

The third section will discuss the avoidance and management of complications. Because a capsulorrhexis and the hydro steps are prerequisites to safe chopping, we will discuss how to avoid problems with these maneuvers. We will discuss the overall approach to complicated cataracts, and the ways in which phaco chop can help. Finally, we will discuss how to manage complications of chopping. Posterior capsule rupture, vitreous loss, and descending nuclei can complicate any phaco technique and are discussed in detail.

Much of the core material in this textbook is based upon a phaco chop instruction course that, since 1998, has been attended annually by hundreds of surgeons at both the American Academy of Ophthalmology (AAO) and the American Society of Cataract and Refractive Surgery (ASCRS) meetings. The course continually ranks among the highest attended instruction courses at both meetings, demonstrating high interest in this subject. The authors include the four faculty members of the chop course, along with additional invited experts in specific methods of chopping. Because of time limitations, we are unable to cover many important topics in sufficient detail in a 2-hour long course curriculum at these meetings. This book provides us with an opportunity to expand upon these areas.

Several topics are covered by more than one author, which provides some intentional overlap. Many would argue that teaching and performing cataract surgery is as much art as science. Thus, while the lead author has sought to provide a unifying style and approach throughout the book, the opportunity to read differing perspectives, opinions, and approaches is also invaluable. With this in mind, exposure to our collective teaching and surgical experience will hopefully enhance rather than confuse the educational process.

Finally, it is difficult to teach ophthalmic microsurgical techniques without the use of video. It is equally difficult to provide enough background detail and explanation in a video presentation alone. For this reason, a companion DVD with footage on phaco chop, complications, and complex cases has been produced. The first edition of this book was the first instance in which a companion DVD was paired with an ophthalmic surgical textbook.

David F. Chang, MD

REFERENCES

1. Leaming DV. Practice styles and preferences of ASCRS members—2011 survey. Analeyz Inc. http://www.analeyz.com/AnaleyzASCRS2011.htm
2. Nagahara K. "Phaco Chop" film International Congress on Cataract, IOL, and Refractive Surgery; May 1993; Seattle, WA.

SECTION I

Phaco Chop Technique

1

Why Learn Chopping?

David F. Chang, MD

All modern phaco methods rely on the principle of lens "disassembly," in which the firm nucleus is divided into smaller, maneuverable pieces.[1-9] This strategy of disassembly achieves 2 advantages. First, the 10-mm wide nucleus can be removed through a 5-mm diameter capsulorrhexis. Second, the majority of the nuclear material is emulsified near the center of the pupil at a safe distance from the iris, posterior capsule, and corneal endothelium.

A capsulorrhexis is imperative because it preserves the bag-like anatomy and function of the capsule (Figure 1-1A). Not only does this provide the most secure fixation and centration of the intraocular lens (IOL), but its continuous edge renders the entire capsular bag much more resistant to tearing during nuclear emulsification (Figure 1-1B).[10-13]

The "hydro" steps are equally important. Because there is only one fixed phaco incision, rotation of the large diameter nucleus is vital for maximum safety. Hydrodissection separates the nucleus (both endonucleus and epinucleus) from the capsule so that it can spin within the capsular bag.[14] It also loosens the capsular-cortical attachments, which facilitates subsequent cortical clean-up (Figure 1-2).[15]

Although optional, the hydrodelineation wave cleaves a thin epinuclear shell apart from the firm endonucleus. Because the epinucleus is soft enough to be aspirated, this method of disassembling the lens into 2 separate nuclear components reduces the dimensions of the central mass that must be chopped, fragmented, and emulsified. In addition, because it has some bulk and stiffness, the epinuclear shell blocks the tendency of the exposed posterior capsule to trampoline toward the phaco tip as the final pieces of endonucleus are emulsified.

NUCLEOFRACTIS PRINCIPLES

If one imagines a wooden log, there are 2 very dissimilar approaches to splitting it. After laying it horizontally on the ground, one could saw through most of the diameter until the last connecting bridge is weak enough to be cracked or snapped apart. Alternatively, one could place the log upright and use an axe to chop it. As long as the initial split travels more than 50% of the distance, the cleavage plane can be extended through the remainder of the log by manually prying the 2 sections apart.

This analogy conveys the conceptual difference between the 2 most popular nucleofractis strategies: divide-and-conquer and chopping.[6] With divide-and-conquer, a deep groove must be cut across the central diameter of the nucleus. In thick, brunescent nuclei without an epinucleus, the groove must extend much deeper and closer to the posterior capsule. At that point, manually separating the segments will crack the remaining posterior bridge of tissue

Chang DF.
Phaco Chop and Advanced Phaco Techniques: Strategies for Complicated Cataracts, Second Edition (pp 3-9).
© 2013 SLACK Incorporated.

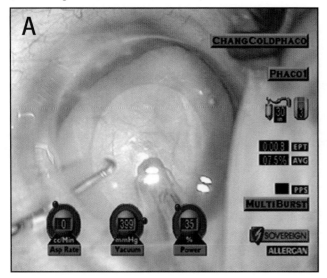
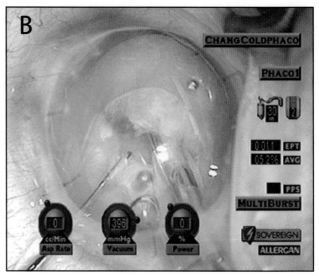

Figure 1-1. Vertical chop of a mature white cataract with trypan blue dye staining of the anterior capsule. (A) Nucleus is impaled with high vacuum and burst mode. (B) Hemisections are separated following initial vertical chop. The capsulorrhexis stretches without tearing.

apart. Like sawing through a log against the grain, significant energy and multiple sculpting passes are required. The same steps are repeated in order to subdivide each heminucleus.

Phaco chop would be analogous to placing the log upright on one end and chopping it with an axe. As Nagahara reasoned, the crystalline lens fibers are arranged in lamellae oriented much like the grain within wood. Because the chopping force is oriented parallel to these lamellae, or "with the grain," a natural fracture plane is exploited and the nucleus can be split with surprisingly little manual force. Again, once more than half of the log is split, prying the 2 sections apart propagates the fracture until the remaining wood is cleaved.

As with an axe, all chopping techniques utilize manual instrument forces to segment the nucleus, thereby replacing the ultrasound power otherwise needed to sculpt grooves. Such energy efficiency is possible because the lamellar orientation of the lens fibers creates natural fracture planes within the hardened nucleus that the chopping maneuver takes advantage of.

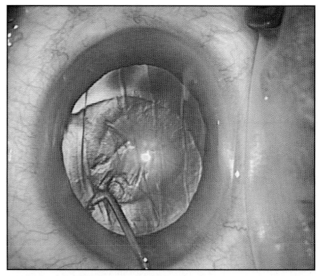

Figure 1-2. Hydrodissection wave moving toward the contraincisional pole of the lens.

CLASSIFICATION: HORIZONTAL VERSUS VERTICAL CHOP

Since Nagahara first introduced the concept of phaco chop at the 1993 American Society of Cataract and Refractive Surgery (ASCRS) meeting, many different chopping variations have evolved. The various innovators have used an assortment of descriptive names based upon the type of maneuvers involved in their particular technique.[4,6-9] However, this diverse array of slight technique

modifications can be quite confusing to the transitioning surgeon. For simplification, this author first proposed that all chopping methods be conceptually divided into 2 general categories of chopping: horizontal and vertical.[6] Both share the same benefits of being able to fragment the nucleus manually, but they accomplish this objective in different ways.

The classic Nagahara technique is an example of horizontal chopping, because the instrument tips move toward each other in the horizontal plane during the chop (Figure 1-3).[6] In vertical chopping, the 2 instrument tips move toward each other in the vertical plane in order to create the fracture (Figure 1-4). Although David M. Dillman, MD later popularized the name "Phaco Quick Chop," the

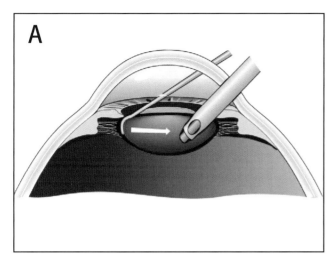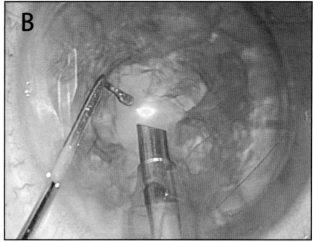

Figure 1-3. Horizontal chop. (A) Initial movement of chopper tip is toward the phaco tip in the horizontal plane. Both instrument tips must be positioned deeply enough in order to maximize the amount of nucleus in the path of the chopper. (B) Horizontal chopper tip (Chang Combination Chopper, Katena Eye Instruments, Denville, NJ) featuring a curved, elongated microfinger design.

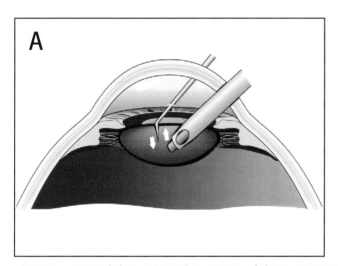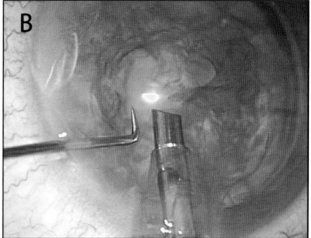

Figure 1-4. Vertical chop. (A) Initial movement of chopper tip is toward the phaco tip in the vertical plane. The phaco tip must be deeply impaled centrally, and the chopper tip incises just anterior to the phaco tip. (B) Vertical chopper tip (Chang Combination Chopper, Katena Eye Instruments) featuring a short, sharpened tip to incise with minimal resistance.

"Phaco Snap and Split" by Hideharu Fukasaku, MD, was the first incarnation of this concept.[16] Horizontal and vertical chop will be detailed in the following 3 chapters.

PHACO PRECHOP

Among the many chopping variations, Takayuki Akahoshi, MD and Jochen P. Kammann, MD have devised instrumentation and techniques for prechopping the nucleus prior to insertion and use of the phaco tip.[17] These prechop techniques constitute a separate special category but incorporate the principles of horizontal chopping. In the case of a denser lens, one manual instrument must generally hook the equator so that the penetrating and

chopping forces are not transmitted directly to the capsular bag and zonules.

Prechopping techniques have many proponents, and a subsequent chapter is devoted to this subject. Others find that devising a way to perform chop without the phaco tip is unnecessary. One potential problem with prechop techniques is that a certain amount of debris is liberated after the initial chop. Without the phaco tip to aspirate it, this may impair visibility for the subsequent steps. Another problem is that most prechop techniques and instrumentation are designed to create 4 nuclear quadrants. While adequate for soft and medium nuclei, it is more difficult to create multiple, smaller pieces with prechopping, as would be desirable for denser and larger nuclei.

A specific challenge to using any prechopper is the ability to judge how deeply it has penetrated into a thicker, firm

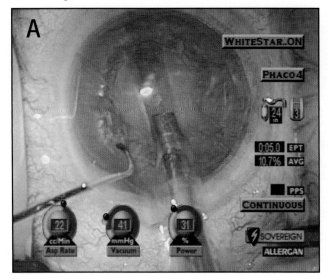

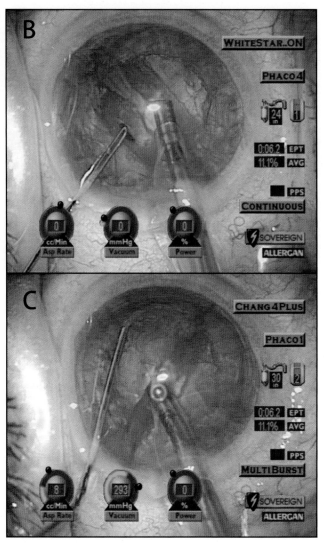

Figure 1-5. Stop and chop technique. (A) As with divide-and-conquer, a deep, central trench is sculpted across the nucleus. The red reflex helps in judging the depth of the sculpting tip. (B) Without vacuum, the 2 instrument tips are used to crack through the posterior connecting plate. (C) Chopping is initiated by first hooking the equator of one hemisection with the chopper. Next, the phaco tip is lowered into the trench and placed against one side of the nuclear hemisection.

nucleus. Adequate depth is necessary before separation is commenced, but over-penetration can be risky for the capsular bag. Finally, prechopping requires additional steps and instrumentation that are avoided when the phaco tip itself is utilized for the chopping technique. This is the same reason that most divide-and-conquer surgeons do not remove the phaco tip to use a manual cracking instrument to separate the heminuclei and quadrants. By prechopping and softening the nucleus, the femtosecond laser further reduces the amount of ultrasound or manual instrument energy needed to remove the lens. As would be expected, the denser the nucleus the greater the reduction in ultrasound energy and time afforded by femtosecond laser nucleotomy is.[18]

STOP AND CHOP

In 1994, Paul S. Koch, MD published his variation of Nagahara's pure chopping technique that he named "stop and chop."[3] Koch felt that an inherent disadvantage of Nagahara's concept was that the chopped fragments would remain tightly wedged within the capsular bag like jigsaw puzzle pieces. He noted that Dr. Howard V. Gimbel's technique of fracturing across a trench first involved sculpting a crater at the center, which provided mobility to subsequently fractured pieces.[2] Seeking to marry the advantages of these 2 techniques, Koch described first dividing the nucleus in half with a traditional groove and cracking step (Figure 1-5A and 1-5B). He then would stop sculpting and chop each heminucleus into 3 pieces using Nagahara's horizontal chop technique (Figure 1-5C).

Stop and chop became popular because it eliminated the difficult first step of chopping the entire nucleus in half without any sculpting. However, the majority of sculpting with divide-and-conquer takes place during the initial groove. Thus, although stop and chop utilizes some chopping, it cannot deliver the full benefits that pure horizontal and vertical chopping techniques can.

ADVANTAGES OF CHOPPING

Virtually without exception, surgeons who are able to master it will continue to prefer chopping. There has been a steady increase in the percentage of surgeons preferring chop during the past 15 years. According to the ASCRS Leaming surveys, this percentage was 11% in 1997, and

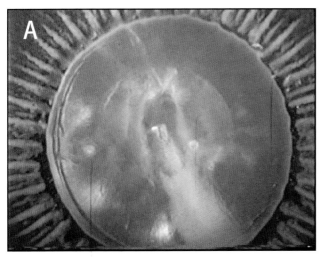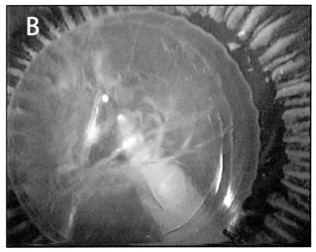

Figure 1-6. (A) Miyake-Apple cadaver eye view of sculpting. In real time, lateral lens movement caused by sculpting is readily appreciated. (B) Miyake-Apple cadaver eye view of vertical chopping. In real time, there is no lateral lens displacement caused by the chop.

increased to 18% by 1998, 24% by 2002, and was 41% in the 2011 survey. The fact that the phaco chop technique is generally more difficult to learn may be an important factor underlying these statistics. The following are 5 important advantages to phaco chop that explain this preference:

1. Reduction in phaco energy
2. Reduction in stress on the zonules and capsular bag
3. Ability to perform supracapsular emulsification
4. Decreased reliance on the red reflex
5. Greater reliance on maneuvering the second instrument than the phaco tip

Reduction in Phaco Energy Delivery

Since pure chopping techniques ultimately eliminate lens sculpting, ultrasound energy is no longer required to divide the nucleus into smaller pieces. Ultrasound is reserved for the phaco-assisted aspiration of the nuclear fragments. A number of studies have shown a reduction in ultrasound energy when employing a phaco chop method compared to divide-and-conquer.[19-27] The correlation of phaco chop with reduced endothelial cell loss is less consistent in the literature.[19,23-26] Part of the variability of the results from these studies undoubtedly relates to the varying density of the nuclei encountered in the study population. For example, Park and coauthors compared phaco chop to stop and chop in a bilateral eye study involving 51 patients.[27] There was no statistical difference in mean effective phaco time (EPT) for moderately dense nuclei; however, with dense nuclei, there was a statistically significant reduction in mean EPT with chopping ($P<.01$). This supports the conclusion that the marked reduction in the phaco power and

energy that is otherwise needed for sculpting is particularly important for brunescent nuclei where the risk of endothelial cell loss and wound burn is much higher.[27]

Reduction in Stress on the Zonules and Capsular Bag

In addition to requiring less phaco power and time, chopping minimizes the stress placed on the zonules and the capsule during nuclear emulsification.[6] During sculpting, the capsular bag immobilizes the nucleus as the phaco tip cuts the groove. Removing a bulky brunescent lens may become problematic for this reason (see Figure 1-5A). Unlike a soft nucleus that absorbs pressure like a pillow, a large firm nucleus moves as one solid unit. It therefore directly transmits any instrument forces—such as those used for sculpting, rotation, and cracking—directly to the capsular bag and zonules. Any lateral displacement of a brunescent nucleus during sculpting will exert significant stress on the zonules. Excessive movement can occur if there is inadequate ultrasound power, too rapid of a phaco stroke, or too deep a path being cut through the nucleus.

In contrast, when chopping a dense lens, it is the phaco tip that is bracing and immobilizing the nucleus against the incoming mechanical force of the chopper (see Figure 1-1). The manual forces generated by one instrument pushing against the other replace the need for ultrasound energy to subdivide the nucleus. In addition, these manual forces are directed centripetally inward, away from the zonules, rather than outward toward the capsule. This significant difference in zonular stress is readily appreciated when both chopping and sculpting are compared from the Miyake-Apple viewpoint in cadaver eyes (Figure 1-6).

The phaco tip secures its purchase by penetrating deeply into the core of the brunescent mass and utilizing high vacuum for holding power so that the nucleus does not become dislodged. In a brunescent lens, using single bursts of phaco avoids the coring away of material around the tip that occurs with continuous mode. The result is improved purchase and a much better seal around the tip, which is a prerequisite for attaining and maintaining high vacuum.

Ability to Perform Supracapsular Emulsification

Chopping shares many of the same advantages of supra-capsular phaco techniques.[5] Virtually all of the emulsi-fication is reserved for phaco-assisted aspiration of the fragments that, because they are small, have been elevated out of the capsular bag. This allows the emulsification to be done centrally in the pupillary plane at a safe distance from the posterior capsule and endothelium. The phaco tip does not need to travel outside the central 2- to 3-mm zone of the pupil, which decreases the chance of incising the iris or capsulorrhexis edge in small pupil cases. However, unlike with other supracapsular techniques, the all-or-none pre-requisite of prolapsing the entire nucleus anteriorly out of the capsular bag and through the capsulorrhexis is avoided. This need to prolapse or flip the nucleus is more risky with a shallow chamber or when the capsulorrhexis is much smaller than the diameter of the endonucleus. Flipping a larger diameter, dense nucleus also risks excessive endothe-lial cell loss.

Decreased Reliance on the Red Reflex

Seeing the appearance of an increasingly brighter red reflex at the base of the trough allows us to judge the depth of the phaco tip during sculpting (see Figure 1-5A). Small pupils complicate this step by diminishing the overall red reflex and limiting how peripherally we can sculpt. With phaco chop, the maneuvers performed with the second instrument are more kinesthetic and tactile and there is much less of a need to visualize the exact depth of the phaco tip. This is why chopping is advantageous with a poor or absent red reflex, as is seen with small pupils and mature nuclear or cortical cataracts (see Figure 1-1).

Greater Reliance on the Chopper Than the Phaco Tip

With phaco chop, it is the chopper that executes the most important maneuvers. The phaco tip remains rela-tively immobile in the center of the pupil, providing an exit conduit for the fragmented lens material. Using a slender and maneuverable chopper instead of the phaco tip to manipulate the nucleus lessens the need to use ultrasound and vacuum near the posterior capsule, or close to the edge of the pupil and capsulorrhexis.

Compared to the phaco tip, the chopper provides much greater maneuverability and freedom of motion. These features are particularly advantageous if the nucleus fails to rotate for any reason. This could be the result of extremely loose zonules, of unsuccessful hydrodissection, or the need to avoid hydrodissection, as with polar cataracts. In these situations, sequential chops can be made without rotating the nucleus by simply repositioning the chopper in different equatorial locations and chopping toward the centrally impaled phaco tip. Using this technique, one may intentionally choose to avoid rotation if there is a tear in the capsulorrhexis or if the zonules are extremely weak. Of all of the phaco steps, it is rotation of the nucleus that exerts the most force on the capsular structures, and is most apt to extend a radial capsulorrhexis tear into the posterior capsule. These same 5 benefits apply to both hori-zontal and vertical chop. In addition to improved surgical efficiency, safety is enhanced by the aforementioned attri-butes of reduced ultrasound power, reduced zonular stress, decreased reliance on the red reflex, and the supracapsular and central location of emulsification. These universal features make chopping the optimal technique for difficult and complicated cases that entail greater risk of posterior capsule rupture or corneal decompensation (see Figure 1-1). The improved ability to handle brunescent nuclei, white cataracts, loose zonules, posterior polar cataracts, crowded anterior chambers, capsulorrhexis tears, and small pupils should be the primary motivation for a divide-and-conquer surgeon to transition to phaco chop.[4,6,27-29]

REFERENCES

1. Shepherd JR. In situ fracture. *J Cataract Refract Surg.* 1990;16:436-440.
2. Gimbel HV. Divide and conquer nucleofractis phacoemulsi-fication: development and variations. *J Cataract Refract Surg.* 1991;17:281-291.
3. Koch PS, Katzen LE. Stop and chop phacoemulsification. *J Cataract Refract Surg.* 1994;20:566-570.
4. Vasavada AR, Desai JP. Stop, chop, chop, and stuff. *J Cataract Refract Surg.* 1996;22:526-529.
5. Maloney WF, Dillman DM, Nichamin LD. Supracapsular phaco-emulsification: a capsule-free posterior chamber approach. *J Cataract Refract Surg.* 1997;23:323-328.
6. Chang DF. Converting to phaco chop: why and how. *Ophthalmic Practice.* 1999;17(4):202-210.
7. Arshinoff SA. Phaco slice and separate. *J Cataract Refract Surg.* 1999;25:474-478.
8. Fine IH, Packer M, Hoffman RS. Use of power modulations in phacoemulsification. Choo-choo chop and flip phacoemulsifica-tion. *J Cataract Refract Surg.* 2001;27:188-197.
9. Vanathi M, Vajpayee RB, Tandon R, Titiyal JS, Gupta V. Crater-and-chop technique for phacoemulsification of hard cataracts. *J Cataract Refract Surg.* 2001;27:659-661.
10. Gimbel HV, Neuhann T. Development, advantages, and methods of the continuous circular capsulorhexis technique. *J Cataract Refract Surg.* 1990;16:31-37.

11. Wasserman D, Apple DJ, Castaneda VE, et al. Anterior capsular tears and loop fixation of posterior chamber intraocular lenses. *Ophthalmology.* 1991;98:425-431.

12. Assia EI, Legler UF, Apple DJ. The capsular bag after short- and long-term fixation of intraocular lenses. *Ophthalmology.* 1995;102:1151-1157.

13. Ram J, Apple DJ, Peng Q, et al. Update on fixation of rigid and foldable posterior chamber intraocular lenses. Part I: elimination of fixation-induced decentration to achieve precise optical correction and visual rehabilitation. *Ophthalmology.* 1999;106:883-890.

14. Fine IH. Cortical cleaving hydrodissection. *J Cataract Refract Surg.* 1992;18:508-512.

15. Vasavada AR, Singh R, Apple DJ, et al. Effect of hydrodissection on intraoperative performance: randomized study. *J Cataract Refract Surg.* 2002;28:1623-1628.

16. Fukasaku H. Snap and split phaco technique safely cracks the nucleus. *Ocular Surgery News International Edition.* 1995;6(8):5.

17. Akahoshi T, Kammann J. Minimal energy chopping has advantages. *Ophthalmology Times.* 1997.

18. Uy HS, Edwards K, Curtis N. Femtosecond phacoemulsification: the business and the medicine. *Curr Opin Ophthalmol.* 2012;23:33-39.

19. Pirazzoli G, D'Eliseo D, Ziosi M, Acciarri R. Effects of phacoemulsification time on the corneal endothelium using phaco-fracture and phaco chop techniques. *J Cataract Refract Surg.* 1996;22:967-969.

20. DeBry P, Olson RJ, Crandall AS. Comparison of energy required for phaco-chop and divide and conquer phacoemulsification. *J Cataract Refract Surg.* 1998;24:689-692.

21. Ram J, Wesendahl TA, Auffarth GU, Apple DJ. Evaluation of in situ fracture versus phaco chop techniques. *J Cataract Refract Surg.* 1998;24:1464-1468.

22. Wong T, Hingorani M, Lee V. Phacoemulsification time and power requirements in phaco chop and divide and conquer nucleofractis techniques. *J Cataract Refract Surg.* 2000;26:1374-1378.

23. Vajpayee RB, Kumar A, Dada T, Titiyal JS, Sharma N, Dada VK. Phaco-chop versus stop-and-chop nucleotomy for phacoemulsification. *J Cataract Refract Surg.* 2000;26:1638-1641.

24. Can I, Takmaz T, Cakici F, Ozgül M. Comparison of Nagahara phaco-chop and stop-and-chop phacoemulsification nucleotomy techniques. *J Cataract Refract Surg.* 2004;30:663-668.

25. Pereira AC, Porfírio F Jr, Freitas LL, Belfort R Jr. Ultrasound energy and endothelial cell loss with stop-and-chop and nuclear preslice phacoemulsification. *J Cataract Refract Surg.* 2006;32:1661-1666.

26. Storr-Paulsen A, Norregaard JC, Ahmed S, Storr-Paulsen T, Pedersen TH. Endothelial cell damage after cataract surgery: divide-and-conquer versus phaco-chop technique. *J Cataract Refract Surg.* 2008;34:996-1000.

27. Park JH, Lee SM, Kwon JW, et al. Ultrasound energy in phacoemulsification: a comparative analysis of phaco-chop and stop-and-chop techniques according to the degree of nuclear density. *Ophthalmic Surg Lasers Imaging.* 2010;41:236-241.

28. Chang DF. Prevention pearls and damage control. In: Fishkind W, ed. *Complications in Phacoemulsification: Avoidance, Recognition, and Management.* New York, NY: Thieme; 2002: Chapter 31, 271-279.

29. Chang DF. Mature cataracts—capsular dye and phaco chop. In: Agarwal S, Agarwal A, Agarwal A, eds. *Phako, Phakonit and Laser Phako: A Quest for the Best. Highlights of Ophthalmology.* Panama City, Panama: Jaypee Highlights Medical Publishers Inc; 2002: Chapter 17, 173-178.

Please see companion narrated videos on the accompanying Web site at
www.Healio.com/phacochopvideos

2

Horizontal Chopping
Principles and Pearls

Randall J. Olson, MD

The history of phacoemulsification is fascinating when considering phaco chop. Due to concerns about the capsule and zonules, originally the entire nucleus was brought up into the anterior chamber. This often caused significant corneal damage and delayed acceptance of the procedure until the iris plane carousel technique was developed.[1] This development was rapidly followed by nuclear segmentation techniques such as divide-and-conquer. There are adherents today to both the carousel and particularly to nuclear segmentation techniques; however, nuclear segmentation remains the most popular ophthalmic technique in the United States today. Cutting a typical cross and splitting the nucleus in 4 pieces is very successful. However, the ultrasound tip is often operated near the capsule and iris so that punching through the posterior plate and creating a capsular break or grabbing and tearing the iris—especially in cases of intraocular floppy iris syndrome—is something all segmentation surgeons have experienced. The amount of ultrasound energy necessary to score a cross in a very hard cataract can be substantial and may result in profound corneal edema. Furthermore, trying to hold onto an intumescent nucleus in order to make the scoring grooves can be difficult to almost impossible, considering how the intumescent nucleus simply bounces and floats inside of the capsular bag. Some element of modification certainly seem in order.

Kunihiro B. Nagahara, MD has earned his place in cataract surgery history by first presenting horizontal chop, which to this day often has his name associated with this approach.[2] Dr. Nagahara suggested emphasizing mechanical forces and splitting the nucleus in half without first scoring it, and then mechanically splitting the nucleus into bite-sized chunks, thereby eliminating all of the ultrasound energy used to score the nucleus. Ultrasound is only used sparingly and well away from the capsule, iris, or cornea. Efficiency and improved safety were considered potential benefits. The approach of using mechanical forces was not new; segmentation surgeons, after the grooves were made, would split the nucleus mechanically. Lately, improved fluidics allow higher aspiration levels to aspirate ever larger and harder chunks of nucleus, often without any ultrasonic energy. When ultrasound is needed, there are efficient and nonrepulsive modalities to choose from.

Like many surgeons in the United States, the author was enthralled by Nagahara's approach and assumed that basically any instrument was capable of producing the segmentation without grooving that Nagahara so beautifully displayed. He started with a Sinskey hook, as it was the only instrument available. Even though this worked with softer nuclei, it did not effectively cut the nucleus in half with harder nuclei. Furthermore, the author was quite nervous about placing this underneath the iris, thereby creating

- 11 -

Chang DF.
Phaco Chop and Advanced Phaco Techniques: Strategies for Complicated Cataracts, Second Edition (pp 11-19).
© 2013 SLACK Incorporated.

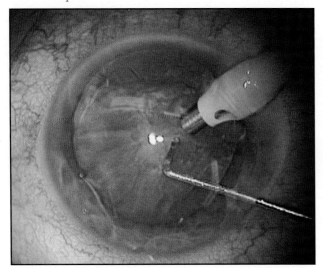

Figure 2-1. A chopper modified with a large rounded tip and 2.0-mm cutting edge for brunescent cataracts.

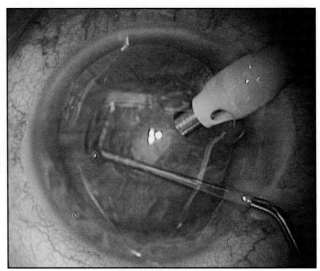

Figure 2-2. The chopper is seen sliding under the anterior capsule. This is guaranteed by starting centrally against the capsule and sliding peripherally with gentle posterior pressure. With the long chopper shown, it is angled to the side to facilitate its placement under the capsule.

nucleus segmentation sight unseen. This seemed to violate many of the core principles of phacoemulsification with which he had been raised. The author tried again with the first Nagahara specialized chopper—which was longer and stouter with a smooth bottom for protecting the capsule—and was very successful. In late 1994, he left divide-and-conquer segmentation surgery behind, never to look back. It was a technique that dramatically decreased the energy needed to remove the nucleus and, by utilizing ultrasound only in a safe area of the eye well away from the capsule and iris, made capsular breakage a rare event.

In the summer of 1995 the author made a trip to India to discuss phaco chop and perform live surgery in Delhi, Bombay, and Madras. While the author had chopped hard nuclei using this technique, some of the cataracts in India were almost impervious to the mechanical efforts of segmentation. An irregular posterior plate would often resist removal of the first segment and sometimes would leave a thin, irregular posterior plate, which would be very tricky to chop. Although the author successfully chopped over 20 very hard nuclei with one capsular breakage while removing one of the last fragments in a single case, it was obvious that for hard cases a slightly different chopping instrument may be helpful. This resulted in a chopper (Figure 2-1) that has a relatively large, flat end for safety near the capsule and a 2.0-mm long cutting edge. It can be used to retract the anterior capsular edge and iris. It chops the posterior plate cleanly, particularly in brunescent cataracts which often have woody connections that, after chopping, can still hold cut fragments together. This new chopper, although a bit long for some, has successfully served for even the hardest of cataracts.

Because horizontal choppers are often used under the iris and placed deep in the capsule to successfully cleave the posterior plate, they must be designed to be safe in case they come in contact with the capsule. In actual fact, the nucleus is much thicker than most surgeons realize and contact with the capsule is uncommon in any of the unvisualized initial maneuvers. There are a multitude of chopping instruments now available and any that are not blunt or rounded on the tip are generally not safe for initial horizontal chopping. After chopping thousands of cataracts, the author has never seen either the original Nagahara chopper or his modification of that instrument ever break the capsule. This speaks well of having a very safe tip.

The biggest danger in horizontal chopping is not breaking the posterior capsule but tearing zonules when initiating the first chop, due to the fact that the chopper is sometimes placed on top of the anterior capsule. Avoiding this requires discipline on the part of the surgeon to always visualize the chopper going under the anterior capsule. With nuclear and cortical debris in the anterior chamber, however, this is not always possible. Therefore, the chopper must start centrally and be in constant contact with the nucleus before the surgeon slides the chopper out into the periphery, in which case the anterior capsule will always come on top of the chopper, thereby avoiding tearing the zonules (Figure 2-2). With the very long design of the Olson chopper, if there is still a significant amount of nuclear material remaining, the author starts the chopper almost parallel to the surface of the nucleus and pushes gently against the nucleus to be certain the instrument goes under the anterior capsule without tearing it. This concern is only of significance early on when the majority of the nucleus is in place. As soon as the nucleus is debulked, then the remaining nucleus can be moved around in such a way that zonular breakage is no longer a concern. Tearing several clock hours of zonules has

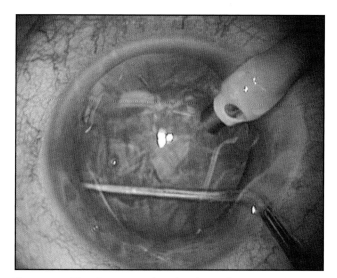

Figure 2-3. The chopper is placed in the "golden ring" of hydrodelineation prior to initiating the first chop. Note how deep the tip is in the capsular bag.

been one of the most common reasons those very experienced in the art of cataract surgery have given for why they soured on horizontal chop. It is a severe and easy complication to induce, but completely preventable.

Horizontal chop starts with either the chopper placement or nucleus impalement. Early on the author started with nucleus impalement because one must be absolutely certain that the chopper stays in position after its placement. Now, however, the author is convinced that placing the chopper first is a bit easier with the nucleus intact. As in all surgical techniques, all the steps for surgical success must be in place; this is no less true for phaco chopping. An intact, continuous curvilinear capsulorrhexis with hydrodissection, hydrodelineation, and good nucleus rotation are all important steps for both the safety and successful completion of the case. A capsular tear is a complication that must be avoided, as undue traction on the anterior capsule can cause a single tear to extend. A tear in the capsulorrhexis is considered a partial contraindication to horizontal chop; however, the procedure has certainly been successfully carried out many times as long as the surgeon is cautious. As a personal preference, the author now switches to vertical chopping if the capsulorrhexis edge is not intact. The chopper itself is placed in the "golden ring" of hydrodelineation and this can often be visualized in a widely dilated pupil. However, with a little experience, this can easily be done by feel—a small pupil is of minimal concern. The author has also found that aspirating a little cortex off the surface of the nucleus may help visualization. However, that is not a necessary step for more experienced surgeons.

Because initial placement of the chopper is such an important maneuver—a valuable maneuver in complicated cases—it is important to feel where the chopper should sit. Start well inside the capsulorrhexis edge with direct gentle

pressure against the nucleus (the chopper angled with the surgeon's chopper) and slide peripherally under the capsulorrhexis (see Figure 2-2). If the chopping tip becomes invisible due to the iris, there is a kinesthetic feeling of the chopper slipping around the nucleus into the golden ring of hydrodelineation. This sense of slipping into the appropriate position is the single most important learning curve issue in this approach to cataract surgery (Figure 2-3). All too often surgeons are concerned that the chopper has already gone out too far; if the chopper itself is not completely around the edge of the nucleus then a superficial chop will result. Furthermore, once the surgeon has this sense of appropriate placement, a small pupil or a hazy peripheral cornea is no longer an impediment to successfully segmenting a cataract. Complete confidence can be generated by doing this without visualization and with a sense of complete safety in the procedure.

Impalement, which is the second important step, is quite simple. The sleeve, however, should be rotated back so that at least 1 mm of the tip is exposed (the author's preferred length generally measures 1.2 mm from the outside tip of the phacoemulsification needle to the sleeve). The tip itself can be almost any configuration. In order to ensure the tip is completely encased in nucleus material and to guarantee this is done with minimal risk of the tip ever coming near the posterior capsule, small tip angulation is preferable, usually 30 degrees and many surgeons like 0-degree tips. With so much mechanical work being done by the chopping instrument, tip designs that do not easily impale a tight round hole, such as a Kelman tip, or ultrasound energy that tends to enlarge the hole, such as OZil (Alcon Laboratories, Fort Worth, TX) or the Ellips (Abbott Medical Optics [AMO], Santa Ana, CA) into the nucleus may have a disadvantage in fixating the nucleus by the vacuum of the machine. That being said, an experienced surgeon can use basically any tip design or ultrasound modality with great success.

The author prefers impaling the nucleus very near the wound, pointing it almost to the optic nerve head and burying it right up to the sleeve (Figure 2-4). This is very safe in the thick part of the nucleus and enhances the complete separation of the nucleus with the first chop. Placement of the bevel is not an issue with a 0-degree tip; however, with a 30-degree tip it is best done bevel down with occlusion occurring with maximum vacuum to assist in maintaining control the nucleus. A machine with the ability to safely use high vacuum levels without postocclusion surge clearly enhances this holding of the nucleus, particularly in the early stages of learning phaco chop. Experienced surgeons, however, can place a chopper and complete the chop with no vacuum at all.

Basic movement in horizontal chop is the chopper being drawn toward the phaco tip with some posterior pressure to make sure the posterior plate is fully cleaved. The sense of how much posterior pressure is the second biggest problem

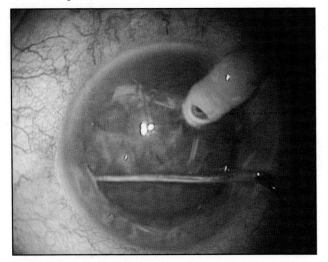

Figure 2-4. Impale the nucleus with the phaco tip up to the sleeve. Point the tip toward the optic nerve and impale as close to the incision as possible.

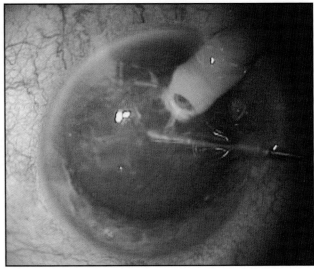

Figure 2-5. The initial chop is started by drawing the chopper toward the phaco tip. Note the deep position of the chopper.

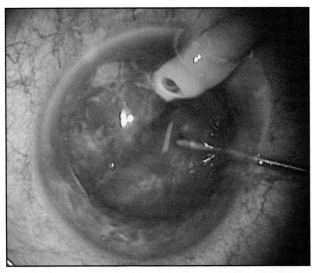

Figure 2-6. The nucleus is separated into 2 pieces as seen by the red reflex. This is guaranteed by moving the chopper to the left and the phaco tip to the right as the chopper nears the phaco tip (if the surgeon is right handed).

The first nucleus split is routinely completed with a little experience (Figure 2-5). The mass of the nucleus can clearly be felt, and as this split starts approaching the phaco needle, the chopping instrument—if in the left hand—is pulled slightly to the left and the phaco needle is pulled slightly to the right to complete the split all the way through the nucleus, separating it into 2 complete halves (Figure 2-6). In very hard nuclei, the separation may not be complete all the way through the nucleus. It is not necessary to get the first chop to completely split the nucleus in half. As long as the posterior plate is cleaved, complete separation certainly makes removal of the first piece easier.

With a little experience, doing this in routine cases becomes quite easy. Very hard nuclei, especially the black/brown brunescent type, can be a challenge to any surgeon and often requires separation of all the woody connections between the segments before segments can be removed (Figure 2-7). Chopping instruments that are short can leave a very irregular split in the posterior plate in hard cataracts that can resist further removal of the nuclear segments. Reinsert the chopper and the phaco tip in the groove to more clearly separate this posterior plate and allow both instruments to probe deeper in the original groove to facilitate removal.

Although completely splitting the nucleus is the hardest step to learn, removing the first nuclear fragment becomes the next important maneuver and the second most difficult step. Place the chopper tip on the central nucleus and move out to the golden ring to remove a segment of a heminucleus. This first piece should be no more than one-third of the heminucleus; a larger piece is harder to free from the capsule. Once the chopper is in place to segment approximately one-third of the heminucleus, the phaco needle itself is placed inside of the initial split and the phaco

for beginners who are usually concerned that they may push through the capsule; beginners usually pull up and create a chop that scratches the surface. This is so uniformly the case that it is helpful to have someone experienced watch this maneuver and comment on the chopper depth. If the chop is superficial, which is quite apparent if the nucleus is intact and no red reflex is visible, then repeat the same maneuver, moving the chopper deeper. If the phaco tip on the second try breaks out toward the chopping instrument, then rotate the nucleus 90 degrees and try again. If all else fails, score out the superficial breaks made and perform a stop and chop or a divide-and-conquer nucleus removal.

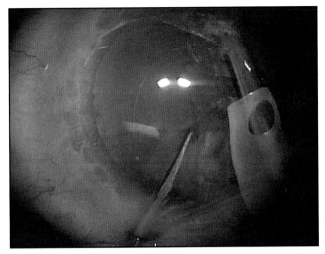

Figure 2-7. Brunescent cataracts often need separation of the "woody connections" between the segments after the initial chop.

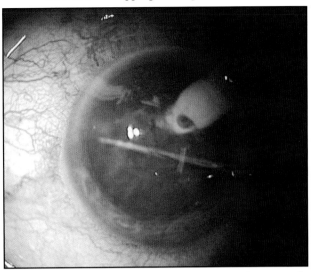

Figure 2-8. The chopper is in place and the phaco needle has engaged the heminucleus so that the first piece can be removed. For the first piece, remove no more than one-third of the heminucleus.

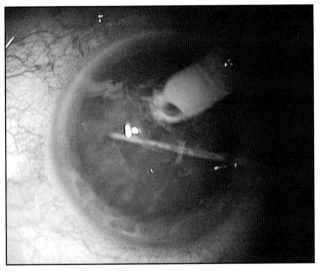

Figure 2-9. Advancing the chopper separates the first fragment from the heminucleus.

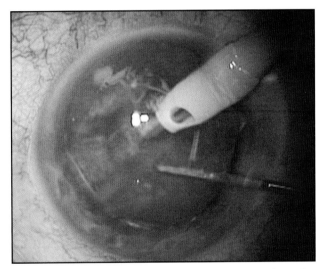

Figure 2-10. By pushing the phaco needle to the right (right-handed surgeon) the chopper is advanced through the apex of the segment to guarantee complete separation.

needle with ultrasound is used to skewer this heminucleus with the needle directed toward the chopping instrument (Figure 2-8). The heminucleus is then held with aspiration and the chopper brought toward the phaco tip to completely separate this segment. Again, with the chopper in the left hand, sweep it slightly to the left and move the phaco needle to the right to complete the chop (Figure 2-9).

An early problem at this stage is that the chopper is not brought all the way through the apex of the pie segment and the piece gets stuck. As a right-handed surgeon, the author makes it a point (after confirming separation) to use the phaco needle to push the bulk of the heminucleus to the right and then bring the chopping instrument all the way through the apex to make sure that every piece of the apex

is separated (Figure 2-10). For a left-handed surgeon, the bulk of the heminucleus will be pushed to the left. Taking this extra step will ensure easy removal of the first nuclear fragment.

With the pie-shaped fragment now completely separated, the apex of the pie-shaped fragment is aspirated and the tip occluded with a small burst of ultrasound. This step is easier with a straight phaco needle and regular pulsed longitudinal ultrasound; however, experience allows the use of all needle configurations and ultrasound variations. The tip should be firmly and completely buried in the nuclear fragment and the vacuum allowed to build so there is a firm hold on this nuclear piece (Figure 2-11).

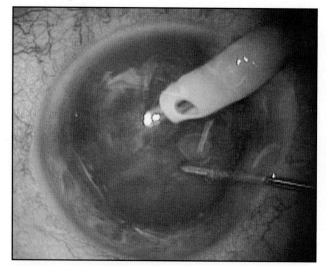

Figure 2-11. The phaco tip is imbedded in the apex of this first piece with a short burst of ultrasound and the vacuum allowed to build.

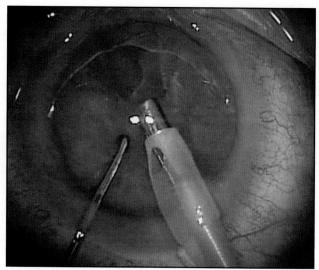

Figure 2-12. With the phaco tip, the first piece is lifted up and centrally out of the capsular bag.

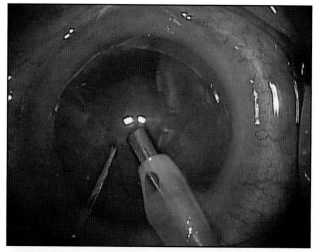

Figure 2-13. The first piece is free and emulsified at the iris plane.

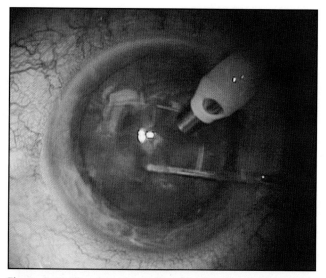

Figure 2-14. The chopper can be placed in the capsular bag to dislodge this first piece into the anterior chamber. This fall-back maneuver guarantees easy removal of the first nuclear piece.

With the resurgence of venturi vacuum phacoemulsification machines that have tamed the vacuum/flow curves and thereby greatly improved postocclusion surge, there is no lag time for full vacuum effect. Peristaltic vacuum has also been modified; the lag time for vacuum to build can be programmed to be very brief. This particular maneuver is achieved with good machine fluidics and a high aspiration level so the fragment is firmly engaged. Once the maximum vacuum is reached, this pie-shaped fragment is removed from the capsular bag by lifting the apex slightly and sliding the fragment out (Figure 2-12). With modern fluidics and a high aspiration level, this is usually a simple step (Figure 2-13). However, learning the fall-back technique will guarantee that this maneuver is not a frustrating one.

In the case of a recalcitrant pie segment that simply will not come out of the capsular bag, impale this segment with the phaco tip and let the chopper run along the segment under the anterior capsule, centered on this pie-shaped segment to engage the outside of the segment. Using the 2 instruments, mechanically pull this piece out of the bag (Figure 2-14). With a little experience this simple maneuver takes a matter of seconds and can absolutely guarantee that the first segment easily comes out of the capsular bag. The author recommends that beginners to chopping should not always rely on aspiration to remove the first segment. After the apex is impaled, surgeons can use the chopper as outlined to help remove this segment so that he or she never has to worry about a stuck first segment.

With this pie segment now at the iris plane, take the chopping instrument and mechanically push this segment

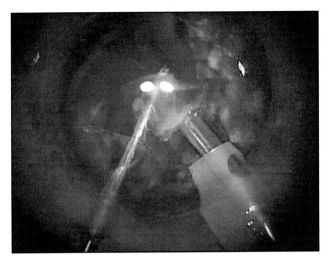

Figure 2-15. The chopper is used to mash nuclear fragment into the phaco needle to minimize the need for ultrasound energy.

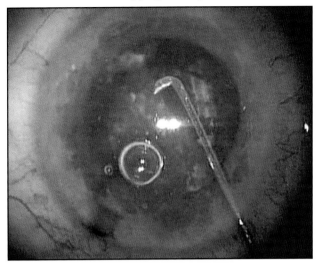

Figure 2-16. The Chang Cannula has an angled tip to guarantee nucleus rotation during hydrodissection.

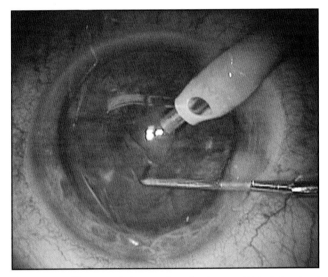

Figure 2-17. The remaining nucleus is chopped into bite-sized pieces. The harder the nucleus the more pieces there are.

into the phaco instrument in order to minimize ultrasound energy. This is particularly effective with a 0-degree tip to mechanically break up the nuclear segment. It allows for cataract removal with a minimal amount of ultrasound. The author calls this the mashing step (Figure 2-15), and with modern fluidics the whole nuclear segment often disappears with no ultrasound necessary. Ultrasound should only be used to assist in aspiration. Micropulsed and horizontal ultrasound (OZil and Ellips) aid the efficient and minimally repulsive removal of each fragment.

Once the nucleus is cleaved and the first fragment removed, the rest of the procedure is very straightforward. The only difficulty the author has encountered at this point is due to lack of rotation of the nuclear segments. So make certain after hydrodelineation that the nucleus rotates! The author has been particularly pleased with the Chang

Cannula (Katena Eye Instruments, Denville, NJ; Figure 2-16), which has an angled tip that can impale the nucleus, providing mechanical force to guarantee that the nucleus rotates easily. With this instrument and minimal hydrodissection, nucleus rotation should be easily accomplished unless encountering very loose or extremely damaged zonules.

After the first segment is removed, the remaining part of the heminucleus is then rotated and usually chopped in half for routine cases. In more difficult cases, chop into bite-size fragments that can easily be removed (Figure 2-17). The general rule is that the harder the nucleus, the more the chopper is used to segment nuclear fragments into smaller pieces. By mashing into small enough pieces, ultrasound can be kept to a minimum even in rock-hard brunescent cataracts. The result is very clear on the first postoperative day with corneas that are as clear as one expects in minimal cataracts.

After removing one heminucleus, the second is rotated and the flat side of the heminucleus is impaled (Figure 2-18). This is a good time to see just how thick the nucleus actually is. This should lend assurance that the ultrasound tip and chopper were never near the posterior capsule. Because there is plenty of room, the last heminucleus is easily segmented into 3 or 4 pieces and removed in exactly the same fashion as the first.

In very hard cataracts with an irregular nucleus, 180-degree rotation may be difficult and is not always necessary. By pushing the nucleus slightly to the opposite side and not rotating it, the nucleus can be impaled on the outside edge and the chopper placed on the flattened side to complete the chop. This is a slightly more advanced technique that can be very handy in some difficult cases. Nonrotation is also convenient in cases with an anterior capsular tear where the surgeon wants to work well away

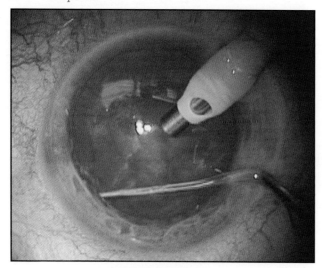

Figure 2-18. The remaining heminucleus is rotated and easily chopped.

from the torn capsulorrhexis edge. For most heminuclei, rotating and impaling in the flat central face is the simplest and easiest approach.

The epinucleus is removed in the usual fashion. If good cortical cleaving hydrodissection has been carried out by aspirating over the edge of the epinucleus and rotating the epinucleus so that aspiration occurs over all 4 quadrants, then the entire cortex is often removed.

There are constantly barriers encountered when learning horizontal chop. Foremost is scratching the surface with the initial chop. The beginner rarely goes deep enough. With a few attempts this barrier is easily overcome. After 2 unsuccessful attempts to split the nucleus, switch to the divide-and-conquer technique. Take every opportunity to chop a quadrant or a heminucleus to gain experience. Many find stop and chop (groove the nucleus, split and chop the heminuclei) a great intermediate technique. The groove creates enough room so that removing the first piece is usually easy.

Getting above the capsule with the chopper and breaking the zonules is an important enough complication that it requires absolute discipline to always place the horizontal chopper on the nucleus centrally then slide peripherally to be certain one is never above the capsule. Fortunately this becomes second nature with time. In the beginning, however, it is best to be careful, consistent, and slow.

The third barrier is freeing the first piece, so use the chopping instrument to mechanically free the first segment. Once this technique is mastered concern evaporates. If the posterior plate is completely separated, there is never a reason why the first piece cannot be removed. With a little experience no aspiration is necessary to get this first piece out.

Horizontal chop is a perfect mate for vertical chop, and vertical choppers usually resort to horizontal chop to do both the mashing maneuver and to split the segments into smaller pieces. Horizontal chop is an excellent small pupil technique because it is kinesthetic and the core elements of splitting the nucleus are often done behind the pupil. Although those experienced in the art will argue whether a hard brunescent cataract is more easily split completely by vertical chopping or horizontal chopping, efficient splitting of the posterior plate with horizontal chopping is guaranteed with the appropriate chopping instrument. In this author's opinion, splitting the woody connections is safer and easier with a horizontal chopper because of how close the work is to the posterior capsule. Certainly, segmenting a very hard cataract into 25 to 30 pieces, which makes removal efficient, requires a significant amount of horizontal chopping even if the initial segmentation occurred with vertical chopping.

Horizontal chop is extremely safe where there is zonular weakness, either due to trauma or pseudoexfoliation syndrome, because very little stress is placed on the zonules and one can perform chopping with very little anterior or posterior movement. This has been clearly documented using Miyake-Apple views during surgery. It has been the author's experience that removing the nucleus in marked zonular weakness is not that hard. The zonules typically break during irrigation and aspiration (I/A) of any cortex, though there have been several cases where nucleus removal caused no zonular breakage despite the fact that the zonules were so weak that the author had to remove the capsule during I/A, creating a very small incision intracap with an intact vitreous face. With capsular tension rings, capsular bag supporting hooks, and artificial zonular support (a Cionni ring or Ahmed capsular segments), the capsule can usually be salvaged in even the most difficult cases.

The author also finds horizontal chopping very effective in cases of decreased endothelial cell counts such as in cases of blunt trauma, previous corneal transplantation, or in primary endotheliopathy such as Fuchs' corneal dystrophy. In these cases, the author uses a dispersive viscoelastic such as sodium chondroitin sulfate (Viscoat), which is reapplied if there is not enough endothelial coverage. The author often turns the ultrasound off (or at the least uses as little ultrasound as possible) and uses mechanical forces. The cornea is amazingly clear on the first postoperative day, and the author prefers a scleral tunnel incision in such cases to minimize endothelial damage around the incision. The endothelial loss can be minimal with such an approach.

Horizontal chop is the best approach in cases with an intumescent cataract with a freely spinning small nucleus. The surgeon must control the nucleus with the horizontal chopper and pin the opposite pole with the phaco needle in order to start chopping (Figure 2-19). These cataracts are usually brittle and chop very easily. There is plenty of room,

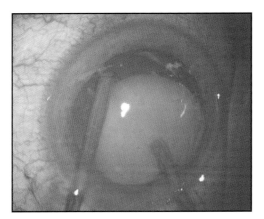

Figure 2-19. With a small, spinning intumescent cataract the nucleus is easily controlled and removed by horizontal chop.

so removing pieces is easy and visibility is not a problem. Horizontal chop is a very effective approach for such cases.

Proving that horizontal chopping is a safer approach is difficult because, in the hands of a good surgeon, all phaco-emulsification techniques have a very low capsular breakage rate. The author feels that his capsular breakage rate has decreased with phaco chop and he has documented, as have others, that appropriately used ultrasound energy can be dramatically reduced.[3] Furthermore, surgeons have been able to document that chopping approaches do significantly decrease the risk of wound burn.[4,5] It stands to reason, however, that if ultrasound and aspiration is never used near the capsule, iris, or the cornea, complications will be less likely.

Conclusion

Horizontal chop, as first described by Dr. Nagahara, is indeed an efficient, fast, and safe approach particularly suited to those patients who have a marginal cornea, weak zonules, hard cataract, or a small pupil. While there are distinct barriers that have resulted in resistance to this approach, the learning curve is really quite short if the beginning chop surgeon takes the proper steps, as outlined in this chapter.

References

1. Emery JM, Wilhelmus KA, Rosenberg S. Complications of phaco-emulsification. *Ophthalmology.* 1978;85:141-150.
2. Can I, Tamer T, Cakici F, Ozgul M. Comparison of Nagahara phaco-chop and stop-and-chop phacoemulsification nucleotomy techniques. *J Cataract Refract Surg.* 2004;30:663-668.
3. DeBry P, Olson RJ, Crandall AS. Phacochop and divide and conquer cataract extraction: a prospective comparison of phaco-emulsification energy. *J Cataract Refract Surg.* 1998;24:689-692.
4. Bradley MJ, Olson RJ. A survey about phacoemulsification incision thermal contraction incidence and causal relationships. *Am J Ophthalmol.* 2006;141:222-224.
5. Sorensen T, Chan CC, Bradley M, Braga-Mele R, Olson RJ. Ultrasound induced corneal incision contracture survey in the United States and Canada. *J Cataract Refract Surg.* 2012;38:227-233.

3

Vertical Chopping
Principles and Pearls

Louis D. "Skip" Nichamin, MD

Since the introduction of traditional phaco chop by Dr. Kunihiro Nagahara,[1] many authors have described technical variations and refinements that, when coupled with the latest generation of phaco technology, have led to an unprecedented level of efficiency in performing nuclear disassembly.

One seemingly subtle, yet important, modification would be a change in the direction in which one moves the chop instrument; specifically, from that of a horizontal to a vertical movement.[2]

This variation has come to be referred to as *Phaco Quick Chop*, a term coined by David M. Dillman, MD of Danville, Illinois. Interestingly, this technique was described nearly contemporaneously by several surgeons including Dr. Thomas Neuhann of Germany, Dr. Abhay Vasavada of India, and Dr. Vladimir Pfeifer of Slovenia. Dr. Fukasaku's snap and split variation, which is quite similar, may in fact represent the first iteration of this approach. As discussed in Chapter 1, all of these variations can be categorized as vertical chopping techniques, with Quick Chop being the classic example. In reality, this technique compliments rather than replaces traditional horizontal chopping. Many surgeons, myself included, utilize a combination of both approaches during a given case. Vertical chop is applicable

to a wide range of nuclear densities. Efficient disassembly is possible for all but the softest of lenses (which may be simply aspirated) or the rock hard cataract, which may be safely chopped after first debulking the central nucleus, thereby weakening its core. Dr. Dillman has termed this latter technique *Crater Quick Chop*.

Vertical chop appeals to many surgeons since it, to some degree, obviates the need to move the chop instrument out to the peripheral lens equator—a step that may be perceived as dangerous, particularly when visualization is not optimal. In reality, when performed with proper technique, the risk of inadvertent damage to the lens capsule is quite low (Figure 3-1).

As with traditional horizontal chop, the procedure begins by performing thorough hydrodissection with subsequent confirmation of rotational mobility to the lens. The chop instrument should be inserted through the sideport incision prior to engaging the nucleus with the phaco tip. If the nucleus is first impaled, its hold may be lost while manipulating the chopper into the eye. The longer distal tip of these manipulators may at first seem awkward when gaining entrance into the eye; the author finds it useful to invert the chopper 180 degrees prior to entering, and then rotate back into position once the instrument is within

Chang DF.
*Phaco Chop and Advanced Phaco Techniques: Strategies for
Complicated Cataracts, Second Edition* (pp 21-24).
© 2013 SLACK Incorporated.

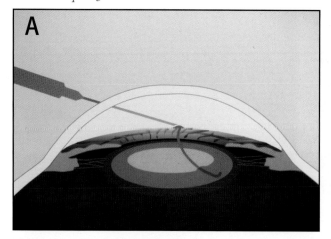

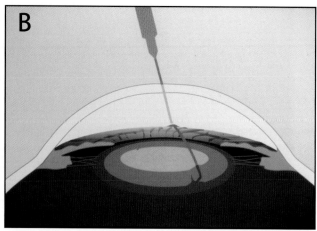

Figure 3-1. (A) By tilting the handle or proximal portion of the chop instrument toward the surgeon, the distal tip becomes parallel to the plane of the anterior lens capsule, making the excursion out to the periphery safer. (B) As the proximal portion of chopper is returned to an upright position, the distal tip slips around the lens equator and is now in good position to begin a horizontal chop.

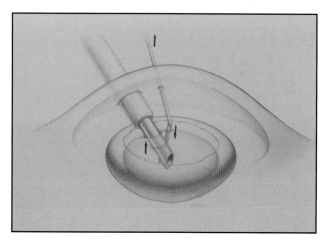

Figure 3-2. Vertical chop initiated post deeply impaling nucleus with phaco needle.

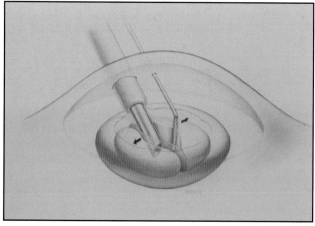

Figure 3-3. After vertical motion, instruments are separated laterally, propagating division.

the anterior chamber. The central nucleus is then deeply impaled using short bursts of pulsed phaco energy along with a steep angle of attack into the central lens substance. It is important to appreciate that at this time the phaco tip is intentionally occluded and, as such, thermal damage may occur at the wound site. In order to obtain a deep and secure hold on the nucleus, it is helpful to retract the silicone sleeve, exposing more of the metal needle, in order to maximize a deep purchase. The chop instrument is then placed just in front of or to the side of the buried phaco needle. Using the sideport incision as a fulcrum, the distal tip of the chop instrument is then pressed downward, assertively, into the nucleus as the phaco tip provides countertraction; a small degree of upward movement with the phaco tip helps to further initiate the nuclear division (Figure 3-2). As the cleavage plane is created, the chop instrument and phaco tip are then spread laterally apart, propagating the division entirely across the nucleus from one pole to the other, as well as down and through the posterior nuclear plate (Figure 3-3). It is extremely important to verify that each successive cleavage plane is completely

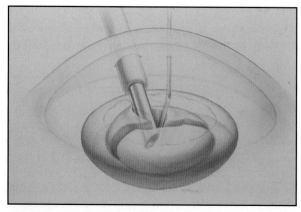

Figure 3-4. Process is repeated to create bite-sized nuclear segments for phacoaspiration.

through the lens by visualizing the red reflex of the fundus. One should not progress to the next chop unless this has been carefully verified.

The lens is then rotated, reimpaled, and the vertical down chop repeated (Figure 3-4). The more dense the

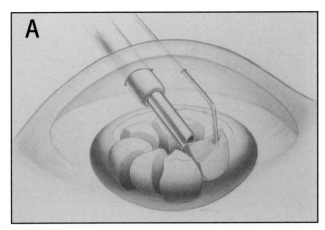
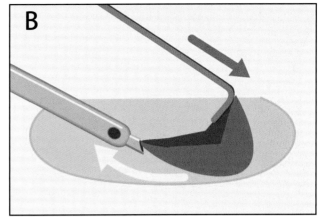

Figure 3-5. Purchase of chopped segments is facilitated by pushing peripherally with the chop instrument, thus sliding the posterior apical portion up to the phaco tip.

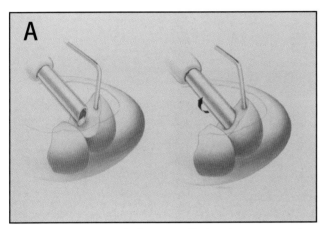
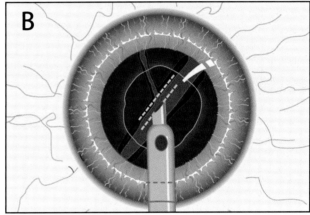

Figure 3-6. Rotation of phaco needle bevel to appose chopped segments. Parallel alignment of bevel to nuclear segments improves occlusion and purchase.

lens, the greater number of cleavage planes that are created. Once a section is chopped, the manipulator is used to push the chopped segment out toward the fornix of the capsular bag, causing the posterior apical portion of the chopped segment to present upward for easier purchase with the phaco tip (Figure 3-5). Adequate levels of vacuum and flow rate are used to evacuate these segments and are aided by short bursts of pulsed phaco energy to collapse the nuclear material into the phaco tip. The latest generation of phaco machines, along with proper crafting of both phaco and sideport incisions (to minimize leakage), allow for high fluidic levels, yet safe intracameral maneuvers. Purchase of chopped segments may also be facilitated by rotating the phaco instrument around its long axis to allow parallel alignment of the needle's bevel with the surface or facet of the nuclear segment, thus improving occlusion (Figure 3-6). As the purchased nuclear segment is drawn centrally from the capsular fornix, it may be further subdivided utilizing traditional (horizontal) maneuvers to create small bite-sized fragments, which are more easily aspirated.

Several additional points bear mention. As with any endocapsular technique, excellent hydrodissection is mandatory. Furthermore, hydrodelineation can create a concentric division plane between the hard inner endonucleus and the soft outer epinucleus; working within the cushioned confines of the epinucleus increases safety. Also, chopping the endonucleus creates smaller segments of nucleus, which makes subsequent purchase and removal easier. Evacuation of the epinucleus is performed by gradually debulking and trimming the epinuclear rim—mostly with aspiration and little, if any, phaco energy—until it spontaneously collapses in upon itself.

Choice of the chop instrument is also important. With traditional horizontal phaco chop, many surgeons prefer using a chopper that incorporates a blunt or bulbous distal tip to increase safety when passing the instrument out to the periphery. With vertical chopping techniques such as Quick Chop, a more pointed, beveled, or flattened tip will easily impregnate itself into the lens material. My current instruments of choice are the Nucleus Divider (Model #E 0726; Storz, St. Louis, MO) for soft to medium lenses and the Quick Chopper II (Model #8-14533; Rhein Medical, Tampa, FL) for dense cataracts.

CONCLUSION

The vertical phaco chop technique represents a simple but important refinement that may be used in place of, or more commonly in conjunction with, traditional horizontal chop in order to increase the overall ease, efficiency, and safety of the procedure.[3-9]

REFERENCES

1. Nagahara K. Phaco Chop film. Presented at International Congress on Cataract, IOL and Refractive Surgery. ASCRS, May 1993; Seattle, Washington.
2. Chang DF, ed. *Phaco Chop: Mastering Techniques, Optimizing Technology and Avoiding Complications.* Thorofare, NJ: SLACK Incorporated; 2004.
3. Koch PS, Katzen LE. Stop and chop phacoemulsification. *J Cataract Refract Surg.* 1994;20:566-570.
4. Chang DF. Converting to phaco chop: Why? Which technique? How? *Ophthalmic Practice.* 1999;17(4):202-210.
5. Fine IH, Packer M, Hoffman RS. Use of power modulation in phacoemulsification. Choo-choo chop and flip phacoemulsification. *J Cataract Refract Surg.* 2001;27:188-197.
6. Vasavada AR, Desai JP. Stop, chop, chop, and stuff. *J Cataract Refract Surg.* 1996;22:526-529.
7. Arshinoff SA. Phaco slice and separate. *J Cataract Refract Surg.* 1999;25:474-478.
8. Vasavada AR, Singh R. Step-by-step chop in situ and separation of very dense cataracts. *J Cataract Refract Surg.* 1998;24:156-159.
9. Vanathi M, Vajpayee RB, Tandon R, et al. Crater-and-chop technique for phacoemulsification of hard cataracts. *J Cataract Refract Surg.* 2001;27:659-661.

4

Comparing and Integrating Horizontal and Vertical Chopping

David F. Chang, MD

As previously discussed, both horizontal and vertical chop accomplish manual fragmentation of the nucleus. Although this is done in different ways, both methods offer the following important universal benefits:

- Reduced phaco power and time.
- Reduced stress on the zonules.
- Limitation of most ultrasound and vacuum to the supracapsular, central pupillary zone.
- Reduced reliance on the red reflex due to the more kinesthetic nature of the procedure.

This chapter will review the principles of each method and the relative advantages and disadvantages of these 2 contrasting strategies. Finally, the concept of combining the horizontal and vertical vectors into "diagonal" chopping will be discussed as a strategy for brunescent nuclei.

HORIZONTAL PHACO CHOP

Kunihiro Nagahara's original technique represents the classic horizontal chopping method. All subsequent variations of horizontal chop make use of the same principle whereby the chopper hooks the endonucleus inside the capsular bag and initially chops centrally toward the fixating phaco tip in the horizontal plane.

Stop and Chop

As discussed in Chapter 1, Dr. Paul S. Koch's "stop and chop" method is a hybrid of divide-and-conquer and horizontal chopping. His technique begins with sculpting a traditional deep, central groove in order to crack the nucleus in half (see Figures 1-5A and 1-5B). One then stops the divide-and-conquer method, and chops the heminuclei (see Figure 1-5C).[1] Although the Koch method utilizes some horizontal chopping, this author coined the term *nonstop chop* to differentiate and designate pure chopping techniques that eliminate all sculpting.[2]

The advantage of stop and chop is that it avoids the difficult first chop. As a result, one chops only across the radius, rather than the full diameter of the nucleus. Second, unlike with the initial nonstop chop, the phaco tip can be positioned within the trough up against the side of the heminucleus that is to be cleaved (see Figure 1-5C). Finally, the presence of the trough facilitates removal of the first fragment because it is not tightly wedged inside the capsular bag.

While chopping the heminuclei does partially reduce total ultrasound energy, the majority of sculpting during divide-and-conquer is used to create the first groove (see Figure 1-5A). Thus, stop and chop does not provide the full benefits of nonstop chopping listed previously. The

Chang DF.
Phaco Chop and Advanced Phaco Techniques: Strategies for Complicated Cataracts, Second Edition (pp 25-39).
© 2013 SLACK Incorporated.

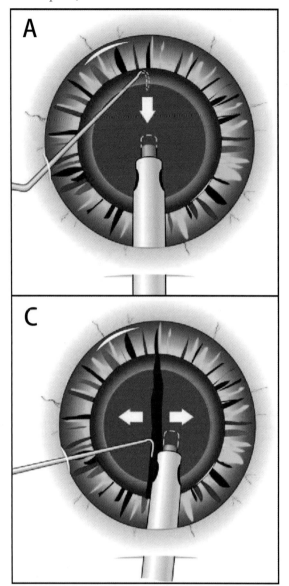
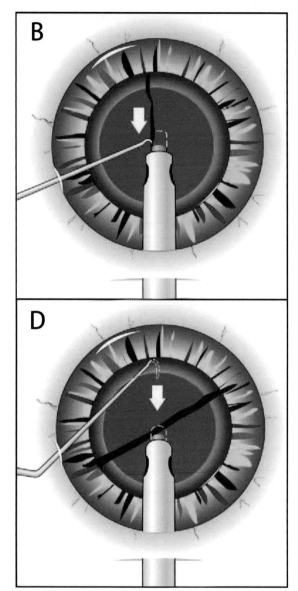

Figure 4-1. Schematic diagram of horizontal chop. (A) Horizontal chopper tip passes beneath the capsulorrhexis to hook the opposite nuclear equator within the epinuclear space. The phaco tip impales deeply. (B) The chopper tip passes directly toward the phaco tip. The initial compression force generates the fracture. (C) Sideways separation of the 2 tips extends the fracture through the rest of the nucleus, creating 2 separate heminuclei. (D) After slight rotation of the nucleus, the next chop is initiated by repeating this sequence of maneuvers.

remainder of this discussion will focus on pure, nonstop horizontal or vertical chop techniques.

Horizontal Chop Technique

The horizontal chop technique relies on compressive force to fracture the nucleus (Figure 4-1). This takes advantage of a natural fracture plane in the lens created by the lamellar orientation of the lens fibers. The key initial step is to use the chopper tip to hook the nuclear equator within the epinuclear space of the peripheral capsular bag prior to initiating the horizontally directed chop (see

Figure 4-1A).[2,3] Whether one first positions the chopper or the phaco tip is a matter of personal preference. Because chopper placement is the most difficult and intimidating step, many transitioning surgeons find it easier to position the chopper prior to impaling the nucleus with the phaco tip.

Initial Placement of the Chopper Tip

Following capsulorrhexis and hydrodissection, hydrodelineation should be performed in order to define and separate the epinuclear shell (see Figure 18-6). This is particularly important for horizontal chopping because

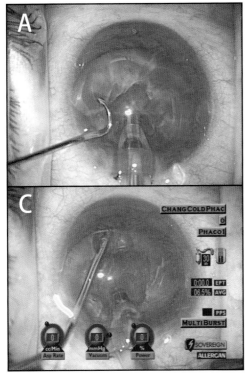

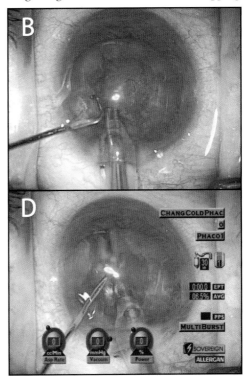

Figure 4-2. (A) Horizontal chop of a soft nucleus. (B) Aspirating the anterior epinucleus makes it easier to judge the capsulorrhexis position and the thickness of the nucleus. (C) After hooking the opposite equator with the horizontal chopper tip, the nucleus is deeply impaled as proximally as possible with the phaco tip. With a soft nucleus, simply pressing the phaco tip into the nucleus without ultrasound or vacuum is enough to embed it. (D) With a soft enough nucleus, the chop is completed without the need for ultrasound or vacuum.

it decreases the diameter of the endonucleus that must be peripherally hooked and divided by the chopper.[2] In addition, the separated soft epinucleus provides a working zone for the chopper. It is because of this epinuclear space that the horizontal chopper can be placed and manipulated peripheral to the endonuclear equator without overly distending and perforating the peripheral capsular bag. Later, after the endonucleus has been evacuated, the final step is to flip and aspirate the epinuclear shell (see Figure 9-9).

Prior to placing the chopper, the surgeon should first aspirate the central anterior epinucleus with the phaco tip in order to better visualize and estimate the size of the endonucleus and the amount of separation between the endonucleus and the surrounding capsular bag (Figures 4-2A and 4-2B). The chopper tip touches the central endonucleus and maintains contact as the surgeon passes it peripherally beneath the opposing capsulorrhexis edge (Figure 4-3A-C). This ensures that the tip stays inside the bag as it descends and hooks the endonucleus peripherally (Figure 4-3D). Although some surgeons tilt the chopper tip sideways to reduce its profile as it passes underneath the capsular edge, this is generally not necessary unless the capsulorrhexis diameter is small or the endonucleus is very large. The elongated horizontal chopper tip can be kept in an upright and vertical orientation because the

capsulorrhexis will stretch like an elastic waistband without tearing (see Figure 4-3C).

Once it reaches the epi/endonuclear junction, the chopper tip must be vertically oriented as it descends into the epinuclear space alongside the edge of the endonucleus (see Figure 4-3D). If it has not traveled peripherally enough, lowering the chopper will depress, not hook, the nucleus equator. The smaller the endonucleus, the larger the epinucleus, and the easier this step will be. Once in position, slightly nudging the nucleus with the chopper confirms that it is alongside the equator, and that it is within—rather than outside of—the bag (Figure 4-3E). Trypan blue capsular dye improves visualization of the anterior capsule for this step and is a useful teaching adjunct (see Figure 5-8).

Executing the First Chop

Next, the surgeon deeply impales the nucleus with the phaco tip. The phaco tip should be directed vertically downward and positioned as proximally as possible in order to maximize the amount of nucleus located in the path of the chopper (Figure 4-3F).[2] If the depth of the phaco tip is too shallow, sufficient compression of the central nucleus cannot occur. Once impaled, the phaco tip holds and stabilizes the nucleus with vacuum in foot pedal position 2. Although not as essential for horizontal chopping as with vertical chop, high vacuum improves the holding

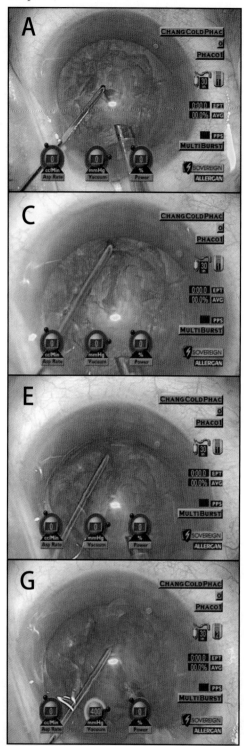
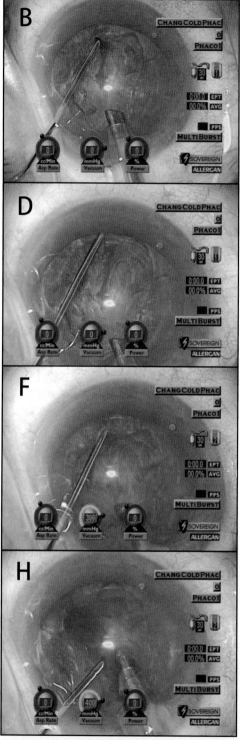

Figure 4-3. Horizontal chop of a firm 3+ nucleus. (A) Chopper tip is kept upright and touches the central endonucleus. (B) By maintaining contact with the endonuclear surface with slight downward pressure, the chopper tip will not pass outside the capsulorrhexis. (C) After reaching the capsulorrhexis margin, the upright chopper tip will slightly stretch and reflect the capsulotomy edge. (D) The upright chopper tip descends into the epinuclear space alongside the equator of the nucleus. The iris obscures the position of the chopper tip. (E) A slight nudge of the endonucleus confirms that the chopper tip is inside the capsular bag and alongside the equator. (F) With burst mode and high vacuum, the chopper tip is impaled as deeply and as proximally as possible. (G) The chop is executed by drawing the chopper tip directly toward the phaco tip until contact is made. High vacuum maintains the solid purchase so that the nucleus neither moves nor rotates. (H) Lateral separation of the instrument tips completes the fracture. High vacuum affords a strong grip of one hemisection.

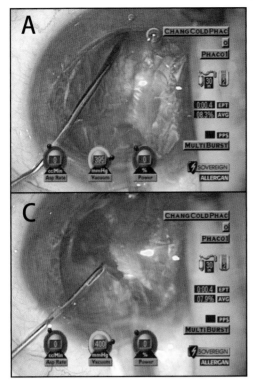
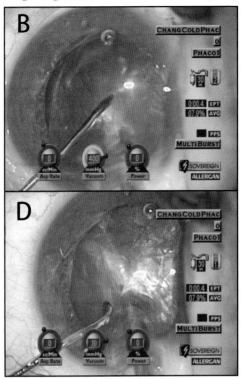

Figure 4-4. Horizontal chop of a brunescent 4+ nucleus. (A) A fracture is generated by the compressive force of the 2 instruments tips that must be positioned as deeply as possible. The linear track on the anterior nuclear surface was created by the chopper tip as it initially passed peripherally beneath the capsulorrhexis edge. (B) During the chop, the compressive forces are borne by the instruments, rather than the capsular bag. (C) Transecting the leathery posterior plate requires a long chopper tip and deep instrument placement. (D) Whitening of the tissue tract indicates the degree of compressive force exerted.

power and keeps the nucleus from wobbling or spinning during the chop (Figure 4-3G).

The surgeon pulls the chopper tip directly toward the phaco tip, and upon contact, moves the 2 tips directly apart from each other (Figure 4-3H). This separating motion occurs along an axis perpendicular to the chopping path and propagates the fracture across the remaining nucleus located behind the phaco tip (see Figures 4-1B and 4-1C). The denser and bulkier the endonucleus, the further the hemisections must be separated in order to cleave the remaining nuclear attachments. Thanks to the elasticity of the capsulorrhexis, even a wide momentary separation of large nuclear hemisections will not tear the capsular bag.

In order for the initial chop to succeed, a substantial amount of the central endonucleus must lie within the path of the chopper (see Figure 1-3A). It is easy to misjudge the depth of the 2 instrument tips, particularly if the anterior epinucleus has not been removed. If the phaco tip is too superficial or too central or if the chopper tip is not kept deep enough throughout the chop, the nucleus will not fracture.[2] Instead, the chopper will only score or scratch the anterior surface. The larger and denser the nucleus is, the more difficult proper positioning of the 2 instrument tips becomes. Fear of perforating the posterior capsule creates

a counterproductive but natural tendency to elevate the chopper tip during the chop.

The ergonomics and tactile "feel" of the horizontal chop will vary significantly as one advances along the nuclear density scale. A soft nucleus has the consistency of soft ice cream. Simply pressing the phaco tip into the nucleus can embed it deeply enough without the use of vacuum or ultrasound (see Figure 4-2C). In addition, no resistance is felt when the chopper is moved (see Figure 4-2D). With a medium density nucleus, the chopper encounters slight resistance as the chopping motion is initiated (see Figure 4-3G). This indicates that the desired compression is taking place.

This resistance becomes much greater when chopping denser 3 to 4+ nuclei. As the chopper presses toward the phaco tip, the surgeon recognizes that the nucleus is literally being squeezed between the 2 instrument tips (Figure 4-4A). This is followed by a sudden snap as the initial split occurs (Figure 4-4B). Like the forces leading up to an earthquake, the compressive force builds until the nucleus suddenly fractures along its natural cleavage plane, releasing the stored energy. With denser nuclei, the compressive force is evidenced by whitening of the nuclear tissue on either side of the chopper track (Figure 4-4C and

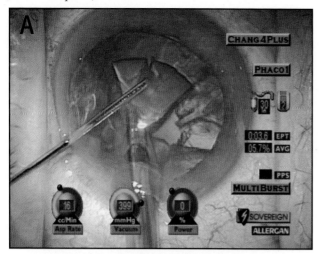
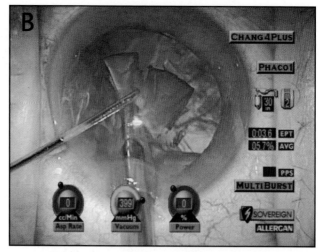

Figure 4-5. Horizontal chop to bisect mobile fragments. By compressing the piece between the 2 instrument tips, it cannot be dislodged.

4-4D). Correspondingly, more ultrasound power must be used in order for the phaco tip to be able to impale denser nuclei. Deeper penetration can be achieved by retracting the irrigation sleeve further to expose more of the metal tip.

Another key to developing sufficient compressive force is to move the chopper tip directly toward the phaco tip until they touch before commencing the sideways separating motion. As the instrument tips near each other, some surgeons tend to veer the chopper tip to the left so that the instruments never actually touch. While this may work for softer nuclei, this limits the compressive force and may impede fracturing a dense lens. This motion will also cause the nucleus to swivel and turn, which also undermines effective propagation of the fracture.

Removing the First Chopped Fragment

Upon completion of the initial chop, the nucleus should be completely fractured in half. If not, it can be rotated so that a second attempt can be made in a new area (see Figure 4-1D). The surgeon next uses the chopper tip to rotate the bisected nucleus 30 to 45 degrees in a clockwise direction and the opposite heminucleus is impaled with the phaco tip in a central location. If there is difficulty occluding the phaco tip, its bevel may need to be aligned parallel to and facing the surface it is about to impale (see Figures 7-10A and 7-10B). Repeating these same steps of hooking the equator and chopping toward the phaco tip will now create a small, pie-shaped fragment.

The strong holding force afforded by high vacuum will usually facilitate elevation of this first piece out of the bag. With firmer nuclei, this first piece can be difficult to remove because the pieces may interlock within the capsular bag like jigsaw puzzle pieces. In this case, one should attempt to make the first piece smaller than usual. Insufficient holding force may be the result of inadequate vacuum settings or failure to completely occlude the tip. With brunescent lenses, continuous phaco power tends to core out the tissue alongside the penetrating phaco needle,

which breaks the occlusion seal. As mentioned in Chapter 1, single burst mode can enhance the phaco tip's purchase of a firm nuclear piece by better preserving the initial seal around the opening (see Figure 4-4A).

Smaller and softer endonuclear pieces can also be difficult to extract because they adhere more to the epinucleus and tend to crumble. If portions of the fragment break off with attempted aspiration, the phaco tip will need to be advanced closer to the peripheral capsule in order to become reoccluded. In this case, it may be safer to manually tumble the piece out using the chopper. The same maneuver of hooking the endonuclear equator with the horizontal chopper tip is performed (see Figure 5-1E). However, instead of immobilizing the piece with the phaco tip, it is allowed to tumble forward into the center of the papillary plane (see Figure 5-1F). As the pie-shaped piece somersaults forward, it is pivoting upon its apex. This prevents even a sharp apical fragment tip from coming near the posterior capsule.

Each subsequent chop is a repetition of these same steps. Because of the need to hook the equator during every horizontal chop, it is advisable to remove each wedge-shaped piece as soon as it is created. Once half of the capsular bag is vacated, the phaco tip can impale and carry the remaining heminucleus toward the center of the pupil (see Figure 5-4C). This allows the horizontal chopper tip to be positioned alongside the outer edge under direct visualization, and without having to pass it beneath the anterior capsule (see Figures 5-4D and 5-4F). For obvious reasons, the initial chop is the most difficult to execute and the first fragment is the most difficult to remove. However, utilizing this technique means that if the nucleus is divided into 6 pieces, the chopper tip passes underneath the capsulorrhexis for only 3 of the chops.

One advantage of horizontal chopping, in particular, is that larger nuclear pieces can be repeatedly subdivided into smaller and smaller fragments (Figure 4-5). The size

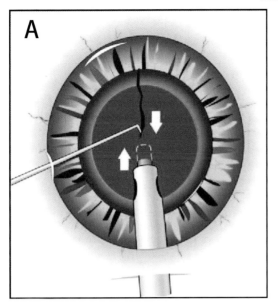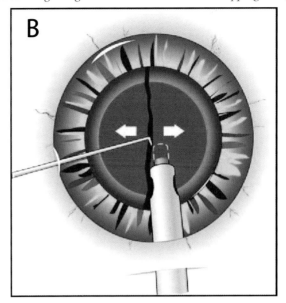

Figure 4-6. Schematic diagram of vertical chop. (A) Following deep impaling of the central nucleus, the sharp vertical chopper tip incises downward just in front of the phaco tip. A slight lifting motion of the phaco tip facilitates the shearing force. (B) Lateral separation of the hemisections completes the fracture.

of the pieces should be kept proportional to the size of the phaco tip opening. For example, just as one cuts a steak into smaller portions for a child's mouth, the nucleus should be chopped into smaller pieces if one is using a smaller diameter 20-gauge phaco tip. Poor followability and excessive chatter of firm fragments engaged by the phaco tip may indicate that the pieces are too large. Because of their greater overall dimensions, brunescent nuclei will need to be chopped many more times than soft nuclei.

VERTICAL PHACO CHOP

Hideharu Fukasaku, MD introduced his technique of "Phaco Snap and Split" at the 1995 American Society of Cataract and Refractive Surgery (ASCRS) meeting. Dr. Vladimir Pfeifer's "Phaco Crack" method of chopping is a similar technique that was introduced at the 1996 ASCRS meeting. This variation was renamed "Phaco Quick Chop" by David M. Dillman, MD. Abhay R. Vasavada, MD, FRCS published his "Stop, chop, chop, and stuff" technique in 1996,[4] and Steve A. Arshinoff, MD, FRCSC published his "Phaco slice and separate" method in 1999.[5] These are all examples of vertical chopping; when the chop is first initiated, the instruments move toward each other in the vertical plane (see Figure 1-4A).[2] Whereas the horizontal chopper moves inward from the periphery toward the phaco tip, the vertical chopper is used like a spike or blade from above to incise downward into the nucleus just anterior to the centrally impaled phaco tip (Figure 4-6).

The most important step in vertical chop is to bury the phaco tip as deeply into the center of the endonucleus as possible (Figure 4-7B). Depressing the sharp vertical chopper tip downward, while simultaneously lifting the nucleus slightly upward, imparts a shearing force that fractures the nucleus (Figure 4-8B and 4-8C). This is in contrast to the compressive force produced by horizontal chopping. After initiating a partial thickness split, the embedded instrument tips are then used to pry the 2 hemisections apart (Figure 4-7C and 4-7D). Just as with horizontal chopping, this sideways separation of the instrument tips extends the fracture deeper until the remainder of the nucleus is cleaved in half.

While the key to horizontal chop is adequate depth of the chopper tip, the most crucial factor in vertical chop is the depth of the phaco tip.[2] This is because the phaco tip must completely immobilize the nucleus against the incoming sharp chopper tip in order to generate enough shearing force to fracture it. This need for a strong purchase is also why high vacuum and single burst mode are more critical for vertical than for horizontal chop.

Slightly elevating the impaled phaco tip also prevents the descending chopper tip from pushing a firm nucleus against the posterior capsule. For a brunescent lens, the phaco tip must lollipop into the nucleus as deeply as possible in order to be able to lift it upward. Like spearing a potato with a fork, the phaco tip must aim for the center of the nucleus. Too superficial a tip location will provide insufficient support and leverage.

Much like a chisel would be used with a block of ice or granite, the vertical chopper tip can be used to cleave the nucleus into multiple pieces of variable size (Figure 4-7E-P). The vertically chopped edges may appear sharp, like pieces of broken glass, because the crushing

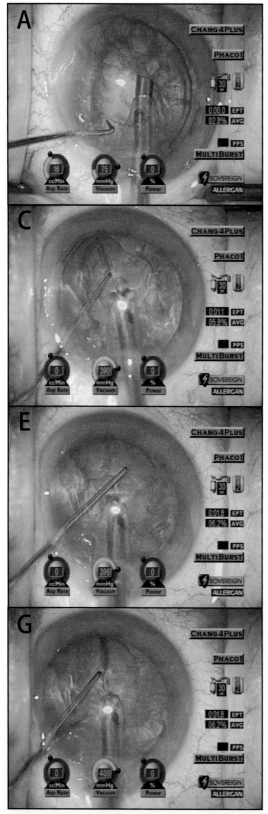
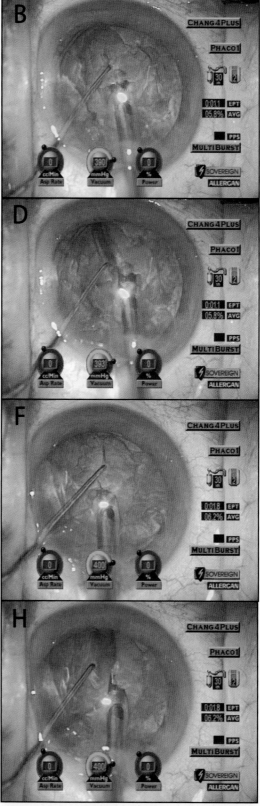

Figure 4-7. Detailed steps of vertical chop of a firm 3+ nucleus. (A) Anterior epinucleus is aspirated, affording improved visualization of the endonucleus. (B) Nucleus is deeply impaled centrally with burst mode and high vacuum. Retracting the irrigation sleeve exposes more of the tip. Sharp vertical chopper tip incises into the nucleus. (C) Initial fracture extends peripherally. (D) Sideways separation of the instrument tips completes the fracture. (E-G) After rotation, the second vertical chop is executed. The fracture is extending more peripherally with downward chop pressure. (H) Lateral separation completes the second vertical chop.

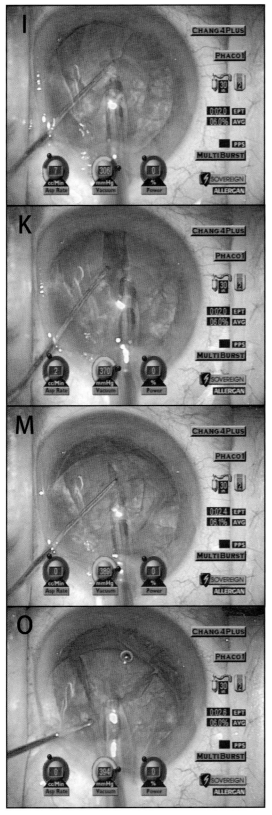
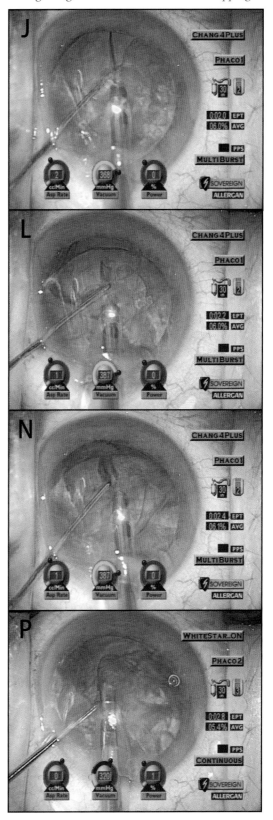

Figure 4-7 (continued). Detailed steps of vertical chop of a firm 3+ nucleus. (I, J) The subsequent chop is performed following rotation. (K) Note the sharp edges of the chopped pieces resemble cut glass. This indicates a shearing mechanism which differs from the compressive forces of horizontal chop (eg, Figure 4-4D). (L-N) Next chop is completed. By leaving the adjacent fragments in place, lateral stability is provided to the section being immobilized for chopping. (O) After completing all vertical chops, high vacuum is used to elevate the first piece out of the capsular bag. (P) All of the loose fragments are emulsified in the center of the pupil.

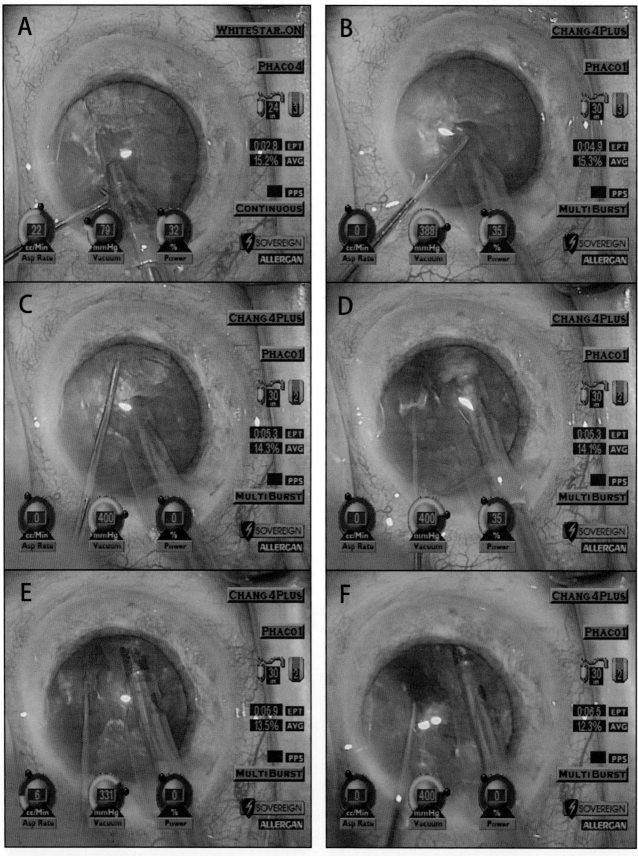

Figure 4-8. Vertical chop of a brunescent 4+ nucleus. (A) A small central pit is sculpted. (B) By impaling at the base of the pit, the phaco needle is able to penetrate to the deepest level. (C) Chop takes place more peripherally, where the nucleus is less thick. Capsular dye facilitates placement of chopper underneath the anterior capsule rim. (D-F) Following initial chop, repeated separating motions are necessary to extend the fracture through the posterior-most plate until the red reflex is seen.

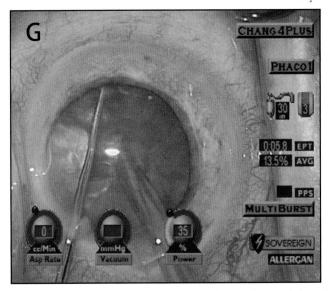
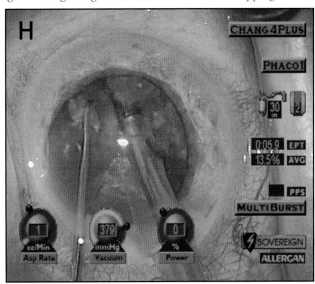

Figure 4-8 (continued). (G, H) For 4+ nucleus, a diagonal chopping vector is utilized.

force that characterizes horizontal chop is not involved (Figures 4-7H, 4-7K, 4-7N, and 4-7O). The sharp vertical chopper tip generally stays central to the capsulorrhexis and is always visualized, unlike in horizontal chopping, where the instrument passes underneath the anterior capsule or behind the iris.

When learning each of the 2 different chopping techniques, one should position the more important instrument first. For horizontal chop, this means hooking the nucleus with the chopper tip first. With vertical chop, the nucleus should first be impaled with the phaco tip. In horizontal chop, sequentially removing each newly created fragment provides the chopper with increased working space within the capsular bag. In contrast, one need not remove the vertically chopped pieces until the entire nucleus is fragmented (Figures 4-7O and 4-7P). This is because the presence of the adjacent interlocking pieces better stabilizes and immobilizes the section that is being chopped (see Figures 4-7E and 4-7N). In addition, since the vertical chopper is never placed peripheral to the nucleus equator, vacating space within the capsular bag early on provides no real advantage.

COMPARING HORIZONTAL AND VERTICAL CHOP

Although the author uses both techniques with equal frequency, they employ different mechanisms that have complimentary advantages and disadvantages. It is worth learning and utilizing both variations for this reason.

Vertical chopping requires a nucleus that is brittle enough to be snapped in half (see Figure 4-7D). The lack of firmness in soft nuclei explains the difficulty of performing vertical chop or divide-and-conquer techniques in these eyes. For example, in order to crack a grooved nucleus in half, there must be sufficient density to the nucleus remaining on either side of the trough. This is why one can snap a cracker in half, but not a piece of bread. The ability of the chopper tip to easily slice through a soft nucleus instead of fracturing it makes horizontal chopping an excellent method for these cases.

Horizontal chopping is also more advantageous for eyes with deeper than average anterior chambers, such as with high myopes or post vitrectomy cases. In such eyes, one must take measures to prevent or reverse lens-iris diaphragm retrodisplacement syndrome (LIDRS). The momentary pupillary block can be reversed or prevented by lifting the pupil edge off of the anterior capsule, so that irrigation fluid can flow into the posterior chamber. Nevertheless, the infusion force sometimes displaces the nucleus more posteriorly so that the phaco tip must approach it from a steeper angle. This can make sculpting a trough more difficult to perform and visualize. In addition, the vertical angle of the phaco tip makes it harder to lift and support the nucleus from behind during vertical chopping. In contrast, the maneuverable horizontal chopper is easily advanced back far enough to hook the lens equator. Even with a more vertical orientation, the phaco tip can still brace the nucleus against the incoming horizontal chopping motion. The difficulty of securing a strong purchase of the nucleus with the phaco tip because of the steeper angle of approach is less problematic for horizontal than for vertical chop.

Horizontal chop is this author's preference for weak zonule cases, such as traumatic cataracts (see Figure 14-9). Because of the inwardly directed and compressive instrument forces, horizontal chop produces the least amount of nucleus movement or tilt. This characteristic is invaluable when any nuclear tipping or displacement could tear the weakened zonules.

Finally, horizontal chop is more effective for subdividing smaller, mobile nuclear fragments, particularly if they are brunescent. Small mobile pieces are hard to fixate adequately for vertical chopping because there is insufficient mass for the phaco tip to impale. Attempting to vertically shear such fragments with a chopper will often dislodge the small piece instead. Trapping and then crushing the fragment between the horizontal chopper and the phaco tip will immobilize and divide it most effectively (see Figure 4-5).

The limitation of horizontal chopping is in its relative inability to transect thicker, brunescent nuclei. First, horizontal chopping should never be utilized in the absence of an epinuclear shell since there will be insufficient space in the peripheral bag to accommodate the chopper. In this situation, forcing the chopper tip into a tightly packed capsular bag risks tearing the capsulorrhexis. Second, the horizontally directed path of the chopper may not be deep enough to sever the leathery posterior plate of an ultra-brunescent nucleus. If this occurs, the pieces may seem freely separated at first, but are actually connected at their apex, like the petals of a flower. In such cases, it is best to try to inject a dispersive viscoelastic through one of the incomplete cracks in the posterior plate to distance it from the posterior capsule (see Figure 19-3). Since a dispersive viscoelastic resists aspiration, the surgeon can attempt to carefully phaco through the remaining connecting bridges that have been visco-elevated away from the posterior capsule.

Vertical and Diagonal Chop for Brunescent Nuclei

Because vertical chop is more consistently able to fracture the leathery posterior plate, it is this author's preference for denser nuclei (Figure 4-8A-H).[2] Returning to the log analogy from Chapter 1, the axe blade is driven into an upright log, but can only penetrate part way. Prying the 2 hemisections apart is necessary in order to extend the split through the remainder of the log. The same is true for the initial horizontal or vertical phaco chop, since it is impossible to position the phaco tip externally up against the posterior-most pole of the nucleus. Once the partial split is made by the chopper, it is the sideways separation of the instrument tips that extends the fracture along the natural lamellar cleavage plane through the remaining nucleus. In horizontal chop, this propagating fracture continues horizontally toward the surgeon, but it will not tend to advance further posteriorly. In contrast, with vertical chop, as the 2 halves are pried apart, the advancing fracture propagates downward in the vertical plane until it eventually transects the posterior-most layer.

With an ultra-brunescent lens, one can also slightly alter the angle of the vertical chop. Instead of incising straight down, like a karate chop striking a board, the vertical chopper should approach the embedded phaco tip more diagonally (Figure 4-8G). This provides more of a horizontal vector that pushes the nucleus against the phaco tip while the vertical vector initiates the downward fracture. This "diagonal" chop therefore combines the mechanical advantages of both strategies.

While it is possible to vertically chop a thick brunescent nucleus without doing so, it is generally easier to begin by sculpting a small, deep pit centrally (see Figure 4-8A).[6,7] By starting at the bottom of the pit, the phaco tip can be impaled more deeply than would have been possible without this preliminary debulking (see Figure 4-8B). Retracting the irrigation sleeve and using single burst mode further maximizes penetration of the phaco tip. Because of the steep angle of the phaco tip, maximal penetration advances the tip into the peripheral nucleus. Initiating the vertical chop in this thinner region better enables it to transect the posterior-most layer of an ultra-brunescent lens (see Figure 4-8C). However, this means that the chopper tip must pass peripherally beneath the capsulorrhexis before incising diagonally toward the phaco tip. Because of the poor red reflex, capsular dye helps in visualizing the anterior capsule for this purpose (see Figure 19-1E).

Once the diagonal chop commences, the hemisections are manually pried apart until the propagating fracture breaks through the leathery posterior plate in the periphery (see Figures 4-8D-F). Each time the separating motion is repeated, the chopper tip is repositioned more and more centrally. The posterior fissure will steadily unzip toward and across the central axis of the posterior plate (Figure 4-8F). One can then rotate the nucleus 180 degrees before repeating the same peripherally located diagonal chop. The nucleus will be completely bisected once the 2 oppositely initiated fractures connect in the center.

The large heminuclei are diagonally chopped into multiple fragments. As the loosened brunescent pieces are elevated out of the capsular bag, one often finds that they are still quite sizable. As mentioned earlier, horizontal chopping is more effective for subdividing mobile brunescent fragments (see Figure 4-5). This provides another reason to master both chopping variations. Not only does utilizing both methods allow surgeons to better handle the entire spectrum of nuclear density, but also both techniques can be employed for different stages of the same challenging case.

Comparative Risk of Complications

Improper technique can lead to complications with either chopping method. If a firm nucleus is not well supported by the phaco tip, downward force from a vertical chopper can push the nucleus against the posterior capsule. This can displace the bag enough to rupture the zonules. If one loses track of the anterior capsule location, one could perforate it with the vertical chopper. Finally, excessive

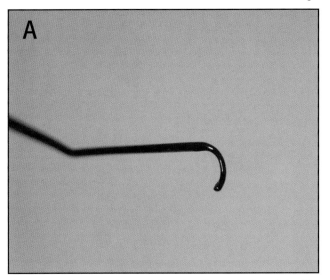

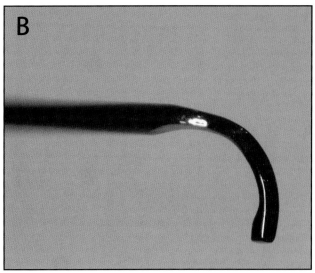

Figure 4-9. Close up views of the microfinger design of the Chang horizontal chopper tip (Katena Eye Instruments, Denville, NJ).

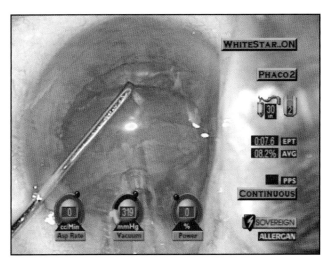

Figure 4-10. Curved microfinger tip conforms to and perfectly matches the shape of the nuclear equator. This minimizes distension of the capsular bag when the chopper is peripherally placed.

surge during removal of the final nuclear fragment or epinucleus could cause forward trampolining of the posterior capsule into the sharp vertical chopper tip.

Likewise, because the horizontal chopper tip is not visualized once it passes behind the iris, erroneous placement outside of the bag could occur. If the chop is initiated with the horizontal chopper placed outside of the capsular bag, a large zonular dialysis will result. Finally, as stated earlier, the absence of an epinucleus is a contraindication to placing a horizontal chopper tip in the peripheral capsular space.

Too small of a capsulorrhexis diameter increases the risk of tearing the continuous edge with the chopper tip or shaft, and the surgeon must be very cognizant of these risks. One should develop the habit of momentarily taking a mental "snapshot" of the capsulorrhexis shape and diameter once it

is completed. The capsulorrhexis contour will no longer be visible following hydrodissection and nuclear rotation, and the surgeon must therefore remember its location during sculpting or chopping. This is another reason why trypan blue capsular dye is helpful for transitioning surgeons.

Comparison of Horizontal and Vertical Choppers

The plethora of different chopper designs is particularly confusing for the transitioning surgeon. This area can be simplified by categorizing these many variants as either horizontal or vertical choppers. Since each works in dissimilar ways, their design principles are quite different.

Horizontal choppers usually feature an elongated but blunt-ended tip (Figure 4-9). A tip length of 1.5 to 2.0 mm is necessary in order to transect thicker nuclei, and the inner cutting surface of the tip may sometimes be sharpened for the purpose of incising denser lens material. The very end of the tip is always dull to diminish the risk of posterior capsule perforation. Many horizontal choppers have a simple right-angle tip design. However, this shape does not conform as well to the natural, curved contour of the lens equator and peripheral capsular bag. The author prefers the curved shape of an elongated microfinger because it can wrap snuggly around the lens equator without distending or stretching the peripheral fornices of the capsular bag (Figure 4-10).[2] The microfinger design also allows one to cup the nucleus equator so that it cannot slip away as compression begins.

Vertical choppers feature a shorter tip that has a sharpened point in order to penetrate denser nuclei (Figure 4-11). If the tip is too dull, it will tend to displace the nucleus off the phaco tip rather than incising into it. In contrast

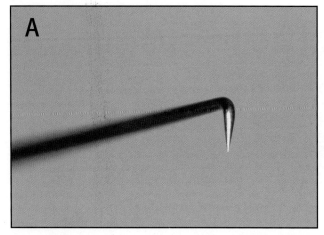
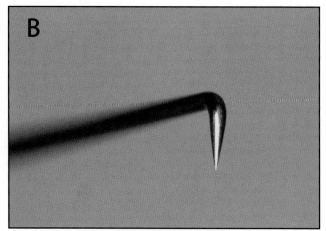

Figure 4-11. Close up views of sharp design of the Chang vertical chopper tip (Katena Eye Instruments).

to horizontal choppers, the length of the vertical chopper tip is shorter because it never encompasses one side of the nuclear segment.

The 3-dimensional (3D) motions required of the chopper are much simpler with vertical chop. Compared to horizontal chop, the chopper tip is not placed as peripherally and simply incises downward into the nuclear mass. The tip is always kept vertically oriented and is always visible until it descends into the nucleus. In contrast, the horizontal chopper tip is much longer, must execute a far more difficult set of motions, must pass underneath the capsulorrhexis, and must be blindly positioned behind the peripheral iris before initiating the chop.

Conceptually, the horizontal chopper's shape imitates the surgeon's left arm, hand, and finger. The long extended handle is the "upper arm." The first bend is the "elbow." The next shorter, straight extension is the "forearm." The next bend is the "wrist." Finally, in the case of the microfinger-shaped Chang horizontal chopper, the 1.75-mm long tip is curved like one's left index "finger" (see Figure 4-9A).

The sideport incision should always serve as the motionless fulcrum for the chopper shaft. In order to avoid displacing or distorting the sideport incision, somewhat counter-intuitive movements must be made with the horizontal chopper in particular. In the case of a right-handed surgeon operating temporally in a right eye, the chopper should be introduced through a paracentesis located 45 degrees to the left of the phaco tip, which is positioned at the 9 o'clock location for a right eye with a temporal corneal incision (see Figure 4-10). To move the chopper tip to the 3 o'clock nasal edge of the capsulorrhexis, both the chopper elbow and the surgeon's left elbow must be moved to the right. To drop the chopper tip down alongside the endonuclear equator, both the chopper elbow and the surgeon's elbow must be slightly elevated.

As the chopper is brought through the nucleus directly toward the impaled phaco tip, the chopper elbow should be gradually elevated and moved to the left. This causes the chopper tip's path to deepen slightly as it transects the center of the nucleus. Finally, the surgeon's fingers can be used to roll or rotate the handle to change the orientation of the tip. Although awkward at first, these 3D coordinated motions will become second nature with time. Until then, one should practice using the horizontal chopper for divide-and-conquer and perform practice chops in the anterior chamber, as will be described in the following chapter.

CONCLUSION

Horizontal and vertical chopping are variations that rely upon different mechanisms to provide complementary advantages and common benefits. The Chang double-ended combination choppers were designed to provide both a horizontal and a vertical chopper on a single instrument. This reflects the author's regular deployment of both techniques according to nuclear density, and together during the same case with the densest nuclei. The blunt-tipped Chang horizontal chopper is an elongated microfinger with a thinner tip profile to facilitate cutting. At the opposite end, the Chang vertical chopper is like a Sinskey hook with a sharp point to facilitate penetration into brunescent nuclear material. One can switch from using this sharp vertical chopper to the horizontal chopper as nuclear fragments are brought into the supracapsular space. This enables horizontal subchopping of large fragments and protects the posterior capsule from ever contacting the sharper vertical tip as the epinucleus is aspirated. The finger-shaped tip can also be used to engage and rotate the epinucleus counterclockwise with backhanded motions. The Seibel vertical chopper tip has the profile of a rounded blade (Figure 4-12). While the latter can vertically incise denser nuclear mass, there is no sharp point to come into contact

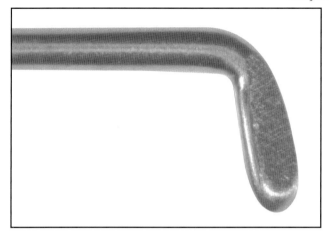

Figure 4-12. The Seibel Vertical Chopper is shaped like a blade, but with a rounded edge that would prevent capsule perforation upon incidental contact. (Reprinted with permission of Katena Eye Instruments.)

with the posterior capsule. For this reason, transitioning surgeons often prefer the Chang Horizontal/Seibel Vertical Chopper as their first combination chopper.

REFERENCES

1. Koch PS, Katzen LE. Stop and chop phacoemulsification. *J Cataract Refract Surg.* 1994;20:566-570.
2. Chang DF. Converting to Phaco Chop: Why? Which technique? How? *Ophthalmic Practice.* 1999;17(4):202-210.
3. Fine IH, Packer M, Hoffman RS. Use of power modulations in phacoemulsification. Choo-choo chop and flip phacoemulsification. *J Cataract Refract Surg.* 2001;27:188-197.
4. Vasavada AR, Desai, JP. Stop, chop, chop, and stuff. *J Cataract Refract Surg.* 1996;22:526-529.
5. Arshinoff SA. Phaco slice and separate. *J Cataract Refract Surg.* 1999;25:474-478.
6. Vasavada AR, Singh R. Step-by-step chop in situ and separation of very dense cataracts. *J Cataract Refract Surg.* 1998;24:156-159.
7. Vanathi M, Vajpayee RB, Tandon R, et al. Crater-and-chop technique for phacoemulsulsification of hard cataracts. *J Cataract Refract Surg.* 2001;27:659-661.

Please see companion narrated videos on the accompanying Web site at
www.Healio.com/phacochopvideos

5

Transitioning to Phaco Chop
Pearls and Pitfalls

David F. Chang, MD

To achieve a successful chop, the 5 interdependent objectives that must be accomplished and coordinated are as follows:

1. Proper initial placement of the chopper tip.

2. Proper placement of the phaco tip, utilizing vacuum to stabilize the nucleus.

3. Keeping the chopper tip adequately deep during the horizontal chop motion.

4. Optimizing chopper tip orientation and direction during the chop motion.

5. Manipulating the chopper shaft without deforming the sideport incision.

With both horizontal and vertical chop, the most challenging maneuvers are performed with the nondominant hand, which must display greater dexterity than is required for divide-and-conquer. For instance, inadvertently distorting the sideport incision with the chopper shaft will impede proper movement of the chopper tip and may compromise visibility and chamber stability. This bimanual skill set is the main reason why chopping is more difficult to master than divide-and-conquer, and why the learning curve is often much longer than surgeons expect.[1]

Phaco chop is an advanced phaco technique that should not be attempted until one has already mastered the divide-and-conquer method (Figure 5-1A-D).[2,3] Compared to chopping, the latter method is easier to learn because it is much less dependent upon bimanual instrument coordination. The phaco tip essentially performs a lamellar dissection of the nucleus as the central trough is sculpted. For this reason, experience with divide-and-conquer phaco teaches resident surgeons about the relative dimensions and densities of the entire spectrum of nuclei. Furthermore, if attempts at chopping the nucleus fail, divide-and-conquer becomes a reliable backup technique.

In divide-and-conquer, the second instrument is primarily used while in foot pedal position 1 (FP1). The surgeon alternates between using the phaco tip for sculpting and a second instrument for rotating. The only time they are used simultaneously is for the bimanual cracking maneuver, when neither ultrasound nor vacuum is engaged (see Figures 5-1A and 5-1B). Thus, in the divide-and-conquer method, the phaco tip is much more active than the spatula and there is far less reliance on bimanual dexterity and timing. In contrast, chopping requires synchronized bimanual instrument maneuvers that are simultaneously coordinated with FP2 and FP3.

Chang DF.
*Phaco Chop and Advanced Phaco Techniques: Strategies for
Complicated Cataracts, Second Edition* (pp 41-54).
© 2013 SLACK Incorporated.

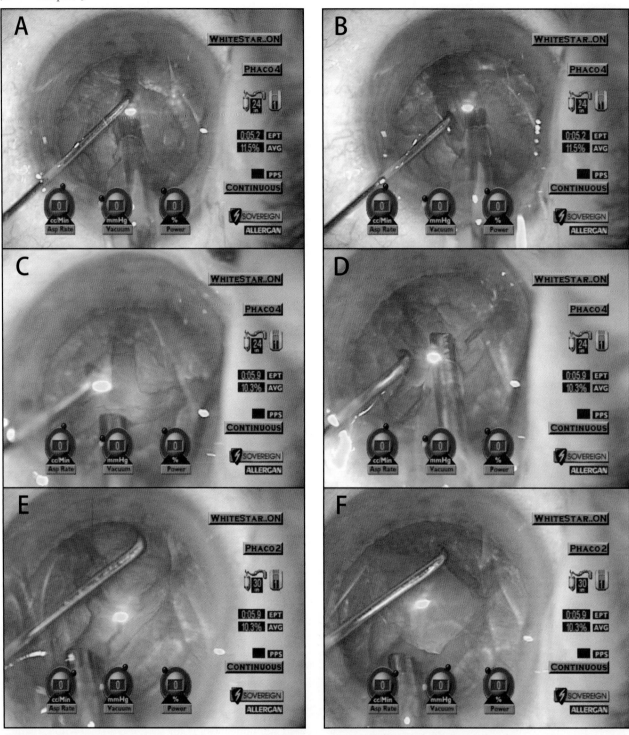

Figure 5-1. Initial steps of divide-and-conquer technique using horizontal chopper as a second instrument. (A) After sculpting a central trough, the long chopper tip is placed into the trench. (B) Sideways separation of the instrument tips cracks the nucleus in half. (C) A second groove is sculpted into one heminucleus. (D) The heminucleus is fractured into 2 quadrants. (E) As an alternative to aspirating the mobile quadrant, it is hooked with the horizontal chopper tip. (F) The quadrant is manually tumbled out of the bag. The sharp apex is the fulcrum about which the piece is tumbled out. It therefore cannot approach the posterior capsule.

WHICH METHOD TO LEARN FIRST?

While the authors advocate learning both horizontal and vertical chop for maximum versatility, there is no clear-cut consensus regarding which technique to learn first. For many surgeons, vertical chop is the easier technique to learn for 2 reasons. First, one is always able to visualize the vertical chopper tip because there is no need to place it blindly behind the iris. Second, less dexterity of the non-dominant hand is required for vertical chop. With horizontal chop, the chopper maneuvers are conceptually and mechanically more difficult to execute and are more likely to deform the sideport incision. However, vertical chop is more difficult to carry out on softer 2+ nuclei, and these otherwise forgiving lenses are not ideal for transitioning to vertical chop. Experience gained through our phaco chop instruction course suggests that transitioning surgeons are more likely to succeed by initially attempting to learn vertical prior to horizontal chop.

Horizontal chopping, in particular, involves repetition of the same fundamental maneuver.[1,2] Once the mechanics of this step are mastered, they can be readily applied to nuclei of all densities. In addition, horizontal chop more quickly teaches one to recognize the spectrum of nuclear size and density. This is because with horizontal chop, the surgeon must literally encompass one end of the nucleus with the chopper and will experience the tactile "feel" of fracturing progressively firmer nuclei. As with all phaco methods, the chop technique must be tailored according to the size and density of the nucleus. Therefore, one needs to be able to correlate how a nucleus appears at the slit lamp with how it will behave during surgery. This is true regardless of whether one is performing a phaco flip, phaco chop, or a divide-and-conquer procedure.

Because of the potential pitfalls encountered while learning either chopping technique, a successful transition requires both preparation and patience. Lacking these, many surgeons become intimidated or discouraged by the difficulties experienced. The purpose of this chapter is to provide a logical, stepwise game plan for transitioning to chopping and to describe the most common mistakes that must be avoided in order to be successful.

Case Selection for the Transitioning Surgeon

Most surgeons categorize nuclei according to their firmness—soft, medium, or dense. As viewed through the slit lamp exam, everyone understands that the color of the nucleus—as it progresses from yellow to gold to brown—correlates with increasing firmness and density. However, it is equally important to appreciate the size of the endonucleus—small, medium, or large. For example, compared to a medium-sized nucleus, soft lenses will have a smaller-diameter endonucleus that is not as thick. A proportionately thicker epinucleus surrounds the small endonucleus above, below, and on all sides. Chopping a small endonucleus is easier because of its reduced dimensions and the ample epinuclear space.

In contrast, the dimensions of brunescent endonuclei can range from small to medium to large. The size can also be determined at the slit lamp. High myopes with oil-droplet nuclear cataracts have only a tiny, central, opalescent endonucleus. Even as it starts to turn golden brown, it usually remains just as small, and most of the lens is therefore epinucleus. In other nuclear sclerotic cataracts, a golden or brunescent fetal nucleus is visible at the slit lamp, but the nucleus peripheral and anterior to it is pale yellow. This indicates an endonucleus of medium diameter and thickness surrounded by a relatively normal-sized epinucleus. Finally, there are nuclear sclerotic cataracts in which brunescence extends all the way forward to the anterior capsule when viewed at the slit lamp. This indicates a huge endonucleus with little to no epinucleus. It has both a larger diameter and a greater anterior-posterior thickness than the medium-sized endonucleus.

The key to differentiating these 3 endonuclear sizes at the slit lamp is to determine how far forward the brunescent color and opalescence extend from the fetal nucleus. Correctly anticipating the size of the endonucleus permits one to alter and adjust one's technique. For example, the sculpted trough must extend more peripherally and much deeper than usual in order to crack larger, denser nuclei when using divide-and-conquer. With chopping, the chopper and phaco tips must penetrate deeper than usual for a larger nucleus.[3] Otherwise, the chop will be too superficial and will fail to divide it.

Learning any new phaco technique is simplified and facilitated by optimal case selection. Soft to medium density endonuclei have a sizable epinucleus and are preferable for learning horizontal chop (Figure 5-2). However, vertical chop is more difficult to perform in soft nuclei. Because they provide little margin for error, large brunescent nuclei should not be attempted until one has mastered chopping less difficult cases. In the very beginning, surgeons new to chopping should avoid uncooperative patients and one-eyed patients. Finally, the transitioning surgeon might initially avoid eyes with problem characteristics such as pseudoexfoliation and loose zonules, excessively deep or shallow anterior chambers, deep-set eyes, small palpebral fissures, small pupils, intraoperative floppy iris syndrome, poor corneal clarity, or a poor red reflex.

TRANSITIONING TO HORIZONTAL CHOP

Preliminary Steps

Because it is the more difficult variation to master, this chapter will outline a stepwise approach for transitioning to horizontal chop. Like all phaco methods, chopping is easier to perform in the presence of a large pupil, a large capsulorrhexis, and a well hydrodissected and mobile nucleus. Hydrodelineation is particularly important in horizontal chopping because the chopper tip maneuvers within the epinuclear space. By demarcating the boundaries of the endonucleus, hydrodelineation also helps one to visualize proper placement of the chopper tip alongside the equator (see Figure 18-6). The technique of hydrodelineation should first be practiced and mastered with divide-and-conquer cases before attempting horizontal chopping.

The most difficult steps of horizontal chopping are the initial ones—the first chop across the entire unsculpted diameter of the nucleus and removal of the first segment. Each subsequent step becomes progressively easier as more and more space is vacated within the capsular bag. Logically, the safest strategy would allow surgeons to learn the steps in the reverse order—starting with the easiest maneuvers first.[1] In the proposed game plan, the component skills can be isolated, developed, and rehearsed while performing divide-and-conquer or stop and chop cases. These principles and the same stepwise learning progression are equally applicable to mastering vertical phaco chop.

Stepwise Game Plan for Horizontal Chop

Step 1. Practice using a chopper as the second instrument for divide-and-conquer (see Figure 5-1A-D). The larger profile of the chopper tip is both unfamiliar and intimidating for those accustomed to a spatula-like second instrument. In chopping, one must be able to manipulate the chopper shaft and tip without deforming the sideport incision. Excessive pressure or torsion can cause corneal striae, increased posterior pressure, and lateral displacement of the globe. In preparation for chopping, one can become comfortable and adept with the chopper by using it as the second instrument during divide-and-conquer. Indeed, its shape is well suited for reaching into the base of the sculpted trough to crack the nucleus in half. Two additional exercises can assist in developing the necessary horizontal chopper skills.

Step 2. When performing divide-and-conquer, use the microfinger-shaped chopper to tumble the quadrants out of the capsular bag (see Figure 5-1E and 5-1F). This provides practice hooking the equator of the endonucleus with the chopper. Because of the sculpted grooves, the quadrants are mobile instead of being tightly wedged within the capsular bag. One unnecessary concern raised by this maneuver is the possibility that the sharp apex of the fragment will perforate the posterior capsule. Because the apex serves as the fulcrum about which the fragment flips outward, it never gets close enough to puncture the capsule. This identical maneuver can later be used to tumble chopped fragments out of the bag if necessary. The second exercise is to explore

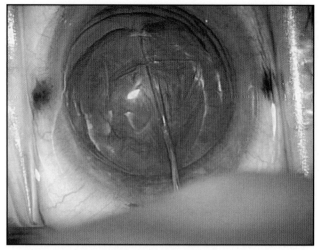

Figure 5-2. Hydrodelineation of a soft nucleus. The anatomic delineation between the endonucleus and the peripheral epinucleus is well visualized. It is at this line of demarcation that the horizontal chopper tip is positioned prior to the chop.

the capsular bag with the horizontal chopper when only the epinucleus is present (following removal of the endonucleus) (Figure 5-3A and 5-3B). The elongated tip can be placed in the peripheral capsular fornix to see that it does not distend it. It can also be used to palpate the central epinucleus. Surgeons are usually surprised at how deeply the chopper tip must be lowered in order to contact the central posterior capsule. This provides a mental picture of the margin of safety. Since fear of lacerating the posterior capsule with the chopper is something that every transitioning surgeon must overcome, visualizing and understanding this spatial relationship is invaluable.

Step 3. In divide-and-conquer, the first heminucleus is cracked into 2 quadrants that are elevated and emulsified in the pupillary plane.[4,5] Instead of immediately emulsifying them, use this opportunity to chop each quadrant into smaller pieces (Figure 5-4A and 5-4B). By holding the quadrant in the center of the pupil, one can visualize executing a horizontal chop in 3 dimensions without concern for the iris or the anterior or posterior capsule. One can readily envision how best to orient the horizontal chopper tip in order to trap the fragment against the phaco tip (Figure 5-5). A microfinger chopper should wrap around and cup the posterior slope of the equator. If the end of the tip instead rotates or shies away from the equator, sufficient compression cannot be generated. This subtle 3-dimensional (3D) concept of how to optimally orient the horizontal chopper tip is critical. Chopping these 2 mobile quadrants also allows the surgeon to experience the tactile feedback of the chopper as it cuts through nuclei of varying density. Developing this "feel" is helpful as one progresses toward chopping firmer and denser nuclei.

Step 4. After removing the first 2 quadrants, do not sculpt a groove into the remaining heminucleus. Instead,

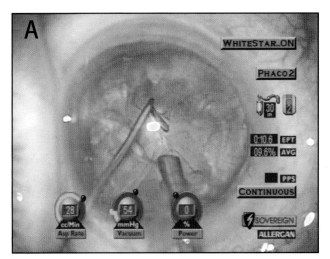
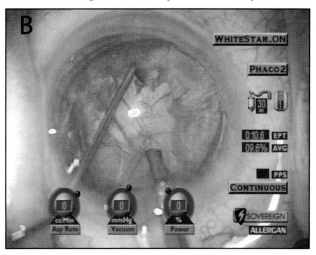

Figure 5-3. (A) After the nucleus is removed, the posterior epinucleus is touched with the horizontal chopper. (B) The chopper is likewise used to explore the peripheral bag. This demonstrates the surprising amount of space within the bag.

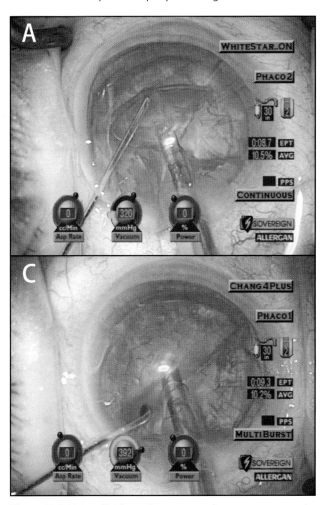
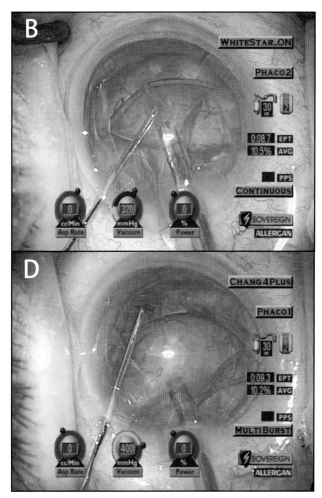

Figure 5-4. Using divide-and-conquer to learn component chopping skills in reverse order. (A, B) Chopping a quadrant allows one to practice the mechanics of horizontal chop without concern for the capsular bag or iris. (C) Instead of cutting a groove into the second heminucleus, it is carried to the center of the pupil. Note the separation from the epinucleus that has been hydrodelineated apart. (D) Chopping the second heminucleus can be done under complete visualization.

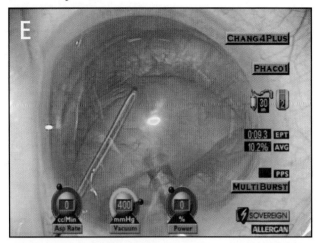
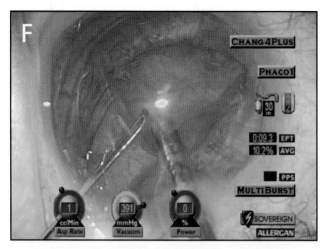

Figure 5-4 (continued). Using divide-and-conquer to learn component chopping skills in reverse order. (E, F) Chopping the second heminucleus can be done under complete visualization.

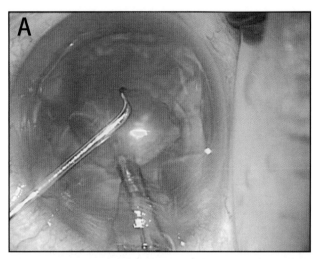

Figure 5-5. (A) Incorrect positioning of a horizontal chopper tip, which is flared outward. (B, C) Correct positioning of the chopper tip cups the equator and traps the nucleus so that it cannot avoid being transected.

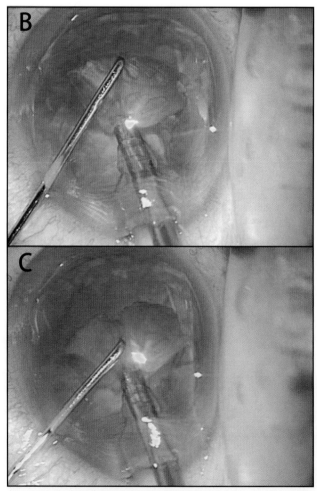

impale and carry the heminucleus to the center of the pupil (Figure 5-4C-F). A properly hydrodelineated endonucleus should easily separate from the epinucleus at this point. One can proceed to chop it into multiple pieces while directly visualizing the equator and without having to pass the chopper tip peripherally beneath the anterior capsule.

Step 5. The next step is to learn and master "stop and chop."[6] As with divide-and-conquer, first sculpt an adequately deep groove in order to crack the nucleus in half (see Figure 5-1A-D). After rotating the endonucleus slightly clockwise, start to chop the remaining halves. For the first time the transitioning surgeon must pass the chopper peripherally beneath the anterior capsule to hook the equator of the endonucleus. This is still considerably easier than chopping the entire unsculpted endonucleus for 3 reasons. First, one is chopping across a shorter distance (the radius instead of the diameter). Second, by placing the phaco tip into the trough and up against the side of the heminucleus,

proper position and depth of the phaco tip is assured. The nucleus will be sandwiched between the phaco tip on one side and the chopper tip on the other. Finally, the trough provides some vacant space which helps to mobilize the first chopped fragment.

Step 6. The next intermediate training step is what this author calls *half-trench* stop and chop (Figure 5-6).

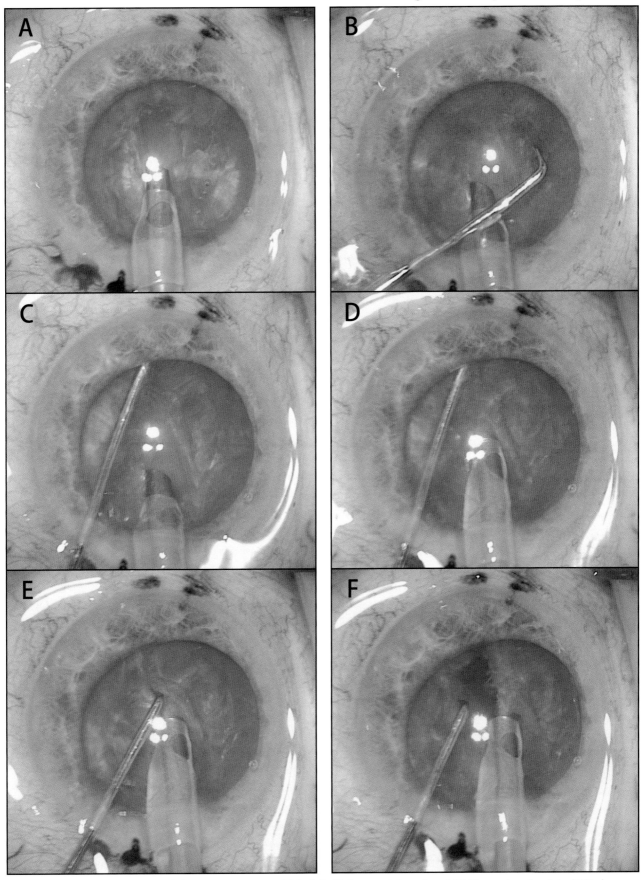

Figure 5-6. "Half-trench" stop and chop transition step. (A) Only half of a trench is sculpted. (B) The nucleus is rotated 180 degrees, but the remaining diameter is not sculpted. (C, D) The unsculpted half is chopped by first hooking the equator with the chopper and then impaling the phaco tip. (E) Horizontal chop is performed initially splitting the unsculpted half. (F) Separating the 2 chopped sections propagates the fracture along and through the proximal sculpted trench.

As originally described by Steven Dewey, one sculpts only half a groove[7] (see Figure 5-6A). The nucleus is spun for 180 degrees and the remaining unsculpted portion is chopped in the following manner (see Figure 5-6B). The phaco tip is first impaled into the remaining ledge of nucleus where the groove ended centrally (see Figure 5-6D). The partial groove assures that the phaco tip will be impaled at an appropriately deep level. One can draw the nucleus toward the phaco incision using a high vacuum purchase. This often exposes the distal equator of the endonucleus, which can be hooked with the horizontal chopper under direct visualization. Alternatively, the horizontal chopper can be placed before impaling the nucleus, as will be described later (see Figures 5-6C and 5-6D). The ensuing full thickness chop is easier, thanks to the partial groove (see Figures 5-6E and 5-6F). This is because after the unsculpted portion is chopped, the remaining proximal nucleus is thinner due to the sculpting. This minimizes resistance to fracturing of the remaining posterior plate. Unlike Dewey's original description for vertical chop, this half-trench technique for horizontal chop requires hooking the equator with the chopper. This skill is the key to the final remaining step.

Step 7. After mastering "classic" and "half-trench" stop and chop, one is now ready to progress to pure horizontal chopping, in which the entire nuclear diameter is cleaved in half without any sculpting.[1] For horizontal chop, softer and smaller endonuclei should be mastered before progressing to firmer and larger endonuclei (see Figure 5-2). Fortunately, if the initial chop fails, one can resort back to sculpting a trench for stop and chop. The remainder of this chapter will discuss pearls for mastering the pure, "non-stop" chopping maneuver.

Modifications for Vertical Chop

For vertical chopping, one should select 2 to 3+ density nuclei as initial cases because of the difficulty in using this technique with soft nuclei. In addition, it is difficult to vertically chop a loose quadrant or fragment without the stabilizing effect provided by the adjacent pieces of nucleus. One should therefore skip steps 2 and 3 from the previously described transitioning game plan. Finally, instead of using stop and chop as a transition technique, one can sculpt half trench or a central pit prior to attempting the first chop (see Figure 4-8A). This variation was discussed in Chapter 4 as a strategy for brunescent nuclei, but can be used with 3+ nuclei as well.[8,9] The centrally sculpted pit ensures deeper penetration of the phaco tip and makes it easier to transect the center of the posterior nuclear plate.

Pearls and Pitfalls in Learning Horizontal Chopping

As discussed in Chapter 4, horizontal chopping fractures the nucleus along a natural cleavage plane defined by the orientation of the lens lamellae. It requires that the bulk of the endonucleus be sandwiched and compressed between the chopper tip and the phaco tip. If positioned properly, the resulting compression force generated by one instrument moving toward the other initiates the fracture. The denser the nucleus, the greater the compression force required. Accomplishing a successful horizontal chop requires coordinating multiple instrument maneuvers and foot pedal positions.

To achieve a successful chop, the 5 interdependent objectives that must be accomplished and coordinated are as follows:

1. Proper initial placement of the chopper tip.
2. Proper placement of the phaco tip, utilizing vacuum to stabilize the nucleus.
3. Keeping the chopper tip adequately deep during the horizontal chop motion.
4. Optimizing chopper tip orientation and direction during the chop motion.
5. Manipulating the chopper shaft without deforming the sideport incision.

A failed chop is the result of mistakes with 1 or more of these objectives.[1]

Objective 1: Proper Initial Placement of the Chopper Tip

The first and most crucial step is to properly hook the equator of the endonucleus with the chopper. The chopper should pass below the capsulorrhexis edge and into the epinuclear space where it descends alongside the nuclear equator. If the chopper tip passes above the capsulorrhexis edge as it moves peripherally, it will cause a large zonular dialysis during the ensuing chop. This pitfall can be avoided by adhering to the following sequential steps.

The first step is to aspirate the anterior epinucleus. This improves visualization of the capsulorrhexis/anterior capsule location, the underlying endonucleus, and the amount of separation between the 2 (Figure 5-7A). Some surgeons prefer to keep the horizontal chopper tip in the same upright, vertical orientation throughout this maneuver. Pressing the dull chopper tip slightly downward as it moves peripherally maintains contact with the anterior endonuclear surface and prevents the tip from passing outside of the capsular bag (Figure 5-7B and 5-7C). As it reaches the edge of the anterior capsule, the upright tip will slightly stretch the capsulorrhexis before it descends into the epinucleus/endonucleus junction (Figure 5-7C and 5-7D). Hydrodelineation helps to define this junction. Trypan blue capsular dye also helps the novice to visually confirm that the chopper is passing beneath rather than over the capsulorrhexis edge (Figure 5-8).

First impaling the nucleus with the phaco tip prior to placing the horizontal chopper is another option. However, this tends to push the nucleus toward the distal capsular

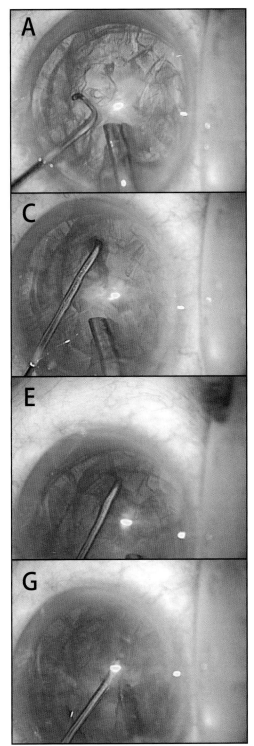
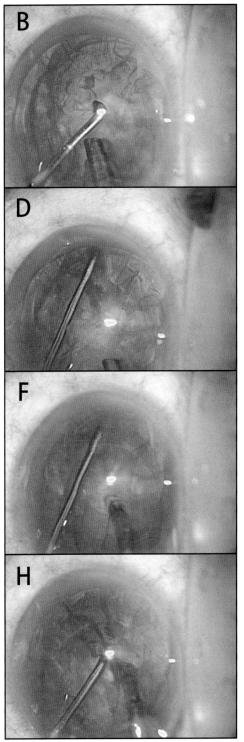

Figure 5-7. Avoiding pitfalls of the initial horizontal chop. Wide pupil allows good visualization of these details. (A) Aspirate the epinucleus to improve visibility of the first step. (B) Touch the central endonucleus with the tip in an upright position. (C) Contact with the endonuclear surface as the chopper moves peripherally to avoid placement outside of the capsulorrhexis. (D) The upright chopper tip descends alongside the equator at the epinuclear junction. The chopper rests within the epinuclear space. (E) Nudging the nucleus demonstrates that the equator is hooked and that the chopper tip is within the capsular bag. (F) The phaco tip must be impaled deeply. (G) During the chop, the chopper tip must stay deep and not elevate. It must aim directly toward, and contact, the phaco tip. (H) Sideways separation of the tips completes the full thickness fracture.

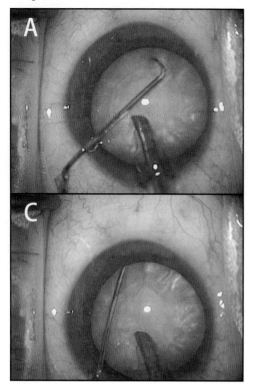
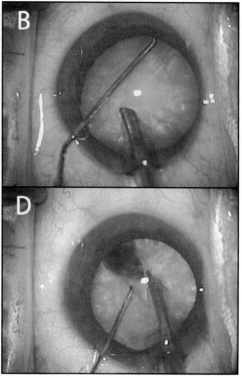

Figure 5-8. Trypan blue dye staining facilitates visualization of the anterior capsule as (A) the chopper passes beneath its edge and (B) then rotates to abut the equator. (C) Prior to initiating the chop, the dye staining allows confirmation that the chopper tip is inside the capsular bag. Note that the shaft of the chopper slightly stretches the smaller capsulorrhexis in this position. (D) As the heminuclei are pried apart, the dye staining permits visualization of the stretching of the capsulorrhexis that occurs with this maneuver.

fornix, thereby compressing the epinuclear space. Because horizontal chopper placement is the most intimidating step, positioning it first optimizes visualization of this maneuver. In addition, prior to impaling with the phaco tip, one can test the location of the chopper tip by slightly nudging the nucleus (Figure 5-7E). The anterior capsule should not move if the chopper tip is inside rather than outside of the capsular bag. A clear peripheral red reflex would result if the chopper was sitting in the zonular space. If the equator of the nucleus is hooked properly, it should move slightly with this "test" nudge. If it does not, the chopper is not peripheral or not deep enough and it will simply deflect over the anterior nucleus rather than compress and penetrate into it.

Objective 2: Proper Positioning of the Phaco Tip

Because it serves as the chopping block, the phaco tip must impale deeply enough into the nucleus to immobilize it against the incoming chopping motion. With a soft nucleus, the phaco tip can be advanced with manual pressure and vacuum alone. However, with a brunescent nucleus, maximum power and burst mode may be necessary to embed the tip deeply enough. The nucleus is fixated with high vacuum in FP2 to prevent it from wobbling or rotating during the chop.

The initial goal in horizontal chop is to position both instrument tips so as to maximize the amount of nucleus in the path of the chopper. The latter must slice through the center point of the nucleus in order to split it entirely. Sculpting habits create an undesirable tendency to advance the phaco tip centrally and superficially while in FP3. Instead, one must concentrate on starting the phaco tip just inside the proximal capsulorrhexis edge and aiming it posteriorly toward the optic nerve (Figure 5-7F). The larger and denser the nucleus, the greater the nuclear mass that is initially sandwiched between the chopper and phaco tips must be.

Objective 3: Maintaining Sufficient Tip Depth During the Chopping Motion

Fear of puncturing the posterior capsule creates a tendency to elevate the chopper tip as it moves toward the phaco tip. This is understandable because horizontal chop is a forceful, blind maneuver during which the surgeon cannot see the chopper tip or the posterior capsule. However, the result is that the central core of the endonucleus may not be compressed and divided during the chop motion. The chopper tip will instead scratch the anterior surface of the nucleus, rather than driving through the middle.

One must commit to keeping the chopper tip deep within the nucleus throughout the full course of the horizontal

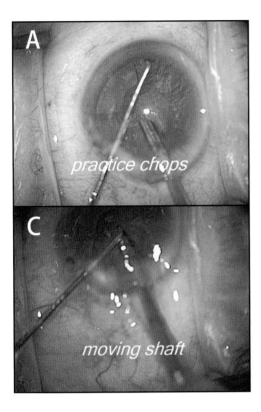

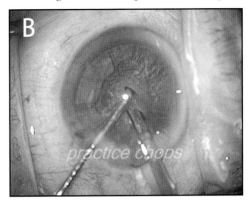

Figure 5-9. Practice chops performed in anterior chamber. (A, B) Like a practice golf swing, a practice chop imitates the proper instrument orientation during horizontal chopping under direct visualization. (C) A common error of displacing the globe by moving the chopper shaft, instead of just the tip, becomes evident during a practice chop.

chop. The confidence to execute a deep chop requires an understanding of the thickness of the nucleus, and of just how much posterior capsule clearance there truly is. Because of its convexity, the clearance is greatest centrally. In the crystalline lens, the central distance between the anterior and posterior capsules is approximately 4.0 to 4.5 mm. Even following removal of the anterior epinucleus, it is extremely difficult for a 1.5-mm to 2.0 mm-long chopper tip to reach the central posterior capsule with the nucleus present. As suggested earlier, exploring an empty capsular bag by gently touching the chopper tip to the posterior capsule after removing the nucleus will demonstrate this (see Figure 5-3A and 5-3B).

Objective 4: Optimizing Chopper Tip Orientation and Direction During the Chop

As the chop is executed, fear of contact with the posterior capsule causes transitioning surgeons to not only elevate the chopper tip, but to also change the angulation of the tip as well. Maximal cutting depth is achieved by having this tip vertically oriented from initiation to completion of the chopping motion. However, inexperienced surgeons may rotate the tip slightly toward or away from the phaco tip (see Figure 5-5A). While this provides better visualization of where the tip is, it reduces the depth of the chopping path through the tissue. This has the same counterproductive effect as elevating the tip during the chop.

As discussed in Chapter 4, one should move the chopper directly toward the phaco tip so that compression of

the encompassed nuclear material is sustained for as long as possible (see Figure 5-7F-H). During the initial chop, many surgeons tend to veer the chopper tip to the left of the phaco tip at the last moment. This is undesirable because it may create a counterclockwise torsion and rotation of the nucleus. In addition, the posterior-most part of the endonucleus may not fracture if the instrument tips never appose each other. This tendency may result from fear of damaging either the chopper or phaco tip. This should not happen because ultrasound is never utilized during the chopping motion and the 2 tips merely touch each other lightly.

To better understand this concept, imagine trying to bisect a thin pretzel stick with your thumb and index finger. If the 2 digits press directly against each other, the middle of the pretzel will be trapped, crushed, and then divided. However, if one were to instead snap their fingers at the last minute, the pretzel stick might spin and slip away without being divided. For denser nuclei, maximizing the compressive force of the initial chop is especially critical because this is the one situation where the phaco tip is not positioned against one side of the nuclear mass.

Objective 5: Avoiding Incisional Deformation by the Chopper Shaft

As stated earlier, the chopper should be maneuvered like a rowboat oar with the sideport incision serving as the stationary fulcrum. A common error is for the chopper shaft to push the globe away from the surgeon as he or she attempts to hook the opposite equator (Figure 5-9C). Displacing the globe to the edge of the microscope field compromises visibility. In addition, tilting the horizontal plane of the iris and endonuclear surface away from the surgeon impedes proper positioning of the phaco tip.

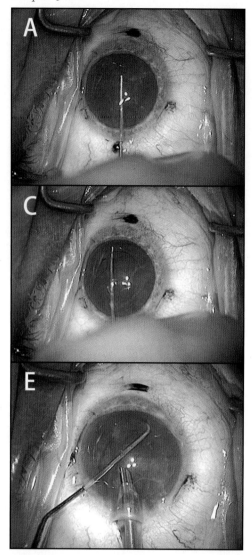
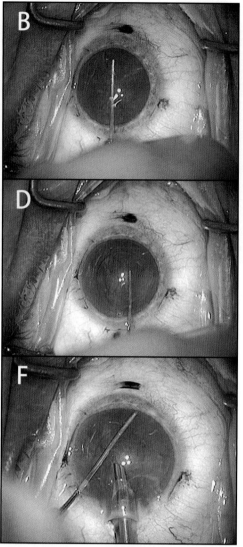

Figure 5-10. Partial viscodissection. (A-C) Dispersive ophthalmic viscosurgical device (OVD) (eg, sodium chondroitin sulfate [Viscoat]) is injected beneath the anterior capsule nasally. (D) This improves visualization by displacing the cortex and epinucleus. (E, F) Horizontal chopper placement is facilitated by further expanding the space between the endonucleus and the anterior and equatorial capsule.

ADDITIONAL PEARLS FOR THE SURGEON TRANSITIONING TO HORIZONTAL CHOP

Since horizontal chopping requires significant bimanual dexterity, another helpful exercise is to perform some "practice" chops in the anterior chamber above the nucleus prior to initiating the first chop (Figure 5-9). Much like a golfer's practice swings, this allows the surgeon to verify proper orientation of the chopper tip and shaft as he or she practices the full sequence of motions. This also allows the surgeon to develop some muscle memory and rhythm for the upcoming maneuver. For example, the surgeon should try to keep the elongated horizontal chopper tip vertically oriented throughout the entire chopping motion. If the surgeon finds that he or she is distorting, compressing, or displacing the incision, or that his or her hand position is awkward or uncomfortable, it is better to correct the problem at this point rather than after the chopper is inside the capsular bag (see Figure 5-9C).

As mentioned earlier, trypan blue dye permits visualization of the capsulorrhexis during horizontal chopper tip placement and movement (see Figure 5-8). This not only provides visual confirmation that the tip is inside the capsular bag, but also enables the surgeon to see if the chopper shaft is overly stretching the left side of the capsulorrhexis, which is often where the anterior capsule will be torn during horizontal chopping (see Figure 5-8C).

Finally, a variation of Dr. Dick Mackool's viscodissection concept can be used to facilitate horizontal chopper placement for the critical initial chop (Figures 5-10 and

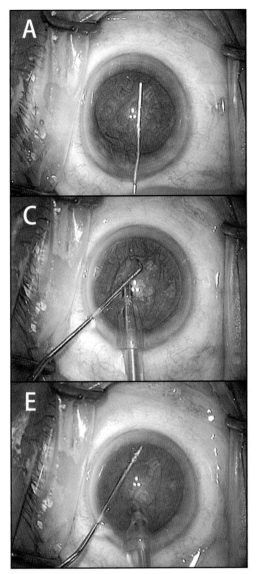
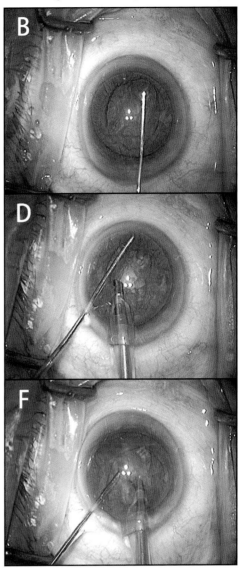

Figure 5-11. Initial placement and visualization of horizontal chopper tip is facilitated by partial equatorial viscodissection with a dispersive OVD.

5-11).[10] Rather than cohesive agents, one should use a dispersive OVD, such as Viscoat because it spreads evenly and resists aspiration. After the traditional hydro steps, the anterior epinucleus is aspirated. At this point, the dispersive OVD is injected just beneath the nasal capsulorrhexis edge until it reaches the equatorial fornix of the bag (see Figures 5-10A-C). This partial viscodissection maneuver widens and maintains the anatomic clearance between the endonucleus and anterior capsule and the nuclear equator and peripheral capsule. It also dramatically improves visualization by displacing any loosened cortical material that was stirred up by the hydro steps (see Figure 5-10D). The improved visualization and separation of the endonucleus from the capsular bag virtually insures proper intracapsular placement of the horizontal chopper tip (see Figures 5-10E and 5-10F). After execution of the first chop

and nuclear rotation, there is often enough remaining dispersive OVD to facilitate chopper tip placement for the second chop. Even the most experienced surgeons can resort to this maneuver whenever they encounter difficulty hooking the nuclear equator in a complicated case.

CONCLUSION

While one should not be overly aggressive with chopping techniques, neither can one afford to be timid and hesitant. There is a certain pace and rhythm used when performing these maneuvers that can be learned by observing experienced surgeons. Once a surgeon finally accomplishes his or her first successful chop, he or she will forever remember and recognize how it should look and feel. This is similar to the learning breakthrough that occurs after one successfully cracks a grooved nucleus for the first time. After one has mastered the basic horizontal or vertical chopping maneuver, the same step is simply repeated over and over again in order to fragment the remainder of the lens. In addition, whether one has mastered horizontal or vertical phaco chop first, learning the second variation becomes infinitely easier because the surgeon now possesses greater bimanual dexterity and a better understanding of the mechanics of chopping.

REFERENCES

1. Chang DF. Converting to phaco chop: why and how. *Ophthalmic Practice*. 1999;17(4):202-210.
2. Fine IH, Packer M, Hoffman RS. Use of power modulations in phacoemulsification. Choo-choo chop and flip phacoemulsification. *J Cataract Refract Surg*. 2001;27:188-197.
3. Vasavada AR, Desai, JP. Stop, chop, chop, and stuff. *J Cataract Refract Surg*. 1996;22:526-529.
4. Shepherd JR. In situ fracture. *J Cataract Refract Surg*. 1990;16:436-440.
5. Gimbel HV. Divide and conquer nucleofractis phacoemulsification: development and variations. *J Cataract Refract Surg*. 1991;17:281-291.
6. Koch PS, Katzen LE. Stop and chop phacoemulsification. *J Cataract Refract Surg*. 1994;20:566-570.
7. Dewey S. Transition to chop: a non-impaling technique. Video, American Academy of Ophthalmology Annual Meeting, 2003.
8. Vasavada AR, Singh R. Step-by-step chop in situ and separation of very dense cataracts. *J Cataract Refract Surg*. 1998;24:156-159.
9. Vanathi M, Vajpayee RB, Tandon R, et al. Crater-and-chop technique for phacoemsulsification of hard cataracts. *J Cataract Refract Surg*. 2001; 27:659-661.
10. Mackool RJ, Nicolich S, Mackool R Jr. Effect of viscodissection on posterior capsule rupture during phacoemulsification. *J Cataract Refract Surg*. 2007;33:553.

Please see companion narrated videos on the accompanying Web site at
www.Healio.com/phacochopvideos

6

Phaco Prechop

Takayuki Akahoshi, MD

PRINCIPLE AND HISTORY OF PRECHOP

Phaco prechop is a technique of mechanical nucleo-fracture performed under viscoelastic material prior to phacoemulsification. Without using any ultrasound or femtosecond laser energy, the nucleus is manually divided into fragments. Once the nucleus is divided, subsequent phacoemulsification can be performed quite easily and safely in a short time. Compared with the conventional grooving or divide-and-conquer technique, total ultrasound energy will be drastically reduced. As a result, there will be no thermal damage even through a sub-2-mm micro coaxial incision. The aspiration time and amount of balanced salt solution (BSS) irrigation will also be reduced significantly. This minimizes the risk of damage to the corneal endothelium and of elevated intraocular pressure (IOP) stressing the optic nerve. Because the total surgical time is remarkably reduced, the author believes that prechopping the nucleus before phacoemulsification is the most efficient and least invasive method of cataract surgery.

The author first developed this phaco prechop technique in 1992 at Mitsui Memorial Hospital in Tokyo and it received the American Society of Cataract and Refractive Surgery (ASCRS) Film Festival award in 1994. Since then all the author's cataract surgeries have been performed using this technique. The author currently performs nearly 60 cases per day and 8000 cases a year using prechop through a sub-2-mm incision as his routine procedure. The author first designed and commercialized special instrumentation for this technique in 1995. This Akahoshi Phaco Prechopper received an ASCRS Film Festival award in 1997. Because the author did not patent this instrument, there are dozens of different prechoppers and modified prechop techniques in use worldwide. However, the author continues to use only 2 prechoppers and 2 methods: the Karate Prechop with the Akahoshi Combo II prechopper for soft cataracts and the Counter Prechop with the Akahoshi Universal II prechopper for dense cataracts. These 2 instruments and techniques are suitable for the entire spectrum of cataracts.

Chang DF.
Phaco Chop and Advanced Phaco Techniques: Strategies for Complicated Cataracts, Second Edition (pp 55-76).
© 2013 SLACK Incorporated.

KARATE PRECHOP

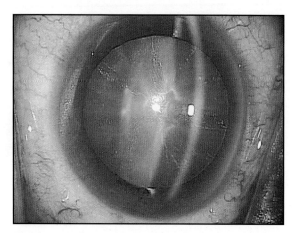

Figure 6-1. The Karate Prechop technique is used for Grade 1 and 2 soft cataracts with intact ciliary zonules.

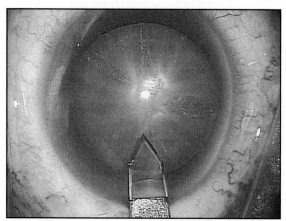

Figure 6-2. Under topical anesthesia, a temporal clear corneal incision is made with a trapezoid diamond keratome. According to the extent of the blade insertion, the incision size can be varied from 1.7 to 2.0 mm with a Nano Diamond Keratome (AE-8192; Asico, Westmont, IL) and from 2.0 to 2.3 mm with an Ultra Diamond Keratome (AE-8190). The appropriate blade should be selected considering the type of phaco tips and sleeves. For a soft cataract, a single plane keratome incision is made. A scleral tunnel that is too long may constrict the irrigation sleeve, and so the corneal tunnel length should be restricted to less than 1.0 mm long. A 2-step incision will be made for dense nuclei or eyes at risk for iris prolapse because of shallow anterior chambers or floppy iris syndrome.

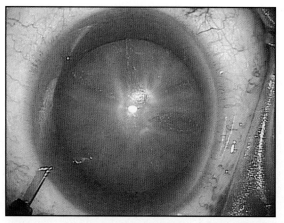

Figure 6-3. Using a diamond sideport keratome (AE-8131), a 0.6-mm sideport is made. To prevent ophthalmic viscosurgical device (OVD) leakage during IOL implantation, a small sideport is preferable.

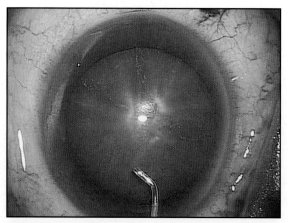

Figure 6-4. A 0.5% preservative-free lidocaine is injected into the anterior chamber. Although this step is not mandatory, the discomfort or pain caused by phacoemulsification in a myopic patient can be reduced.

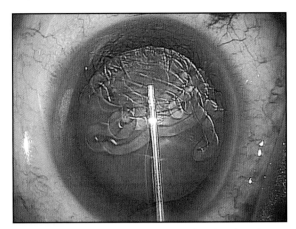

Figure 6-5. The anterior chamber is filled with a dispersive OVD such as sodium chondroitin sulfate (Viscoat). The technique of phaco prechop will not damage the corneal endothelium. However, protecting the endothelium with Viscoat is important because prechopped nuclear fragments will still circulate within the anterior chamber.

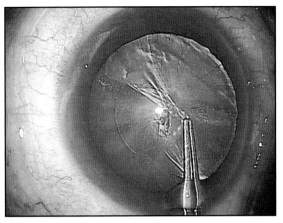

Figure 6-6. A continuous curvilinear capsulorrhexis (CCC) is made using Utrata capsulorrhexis forceps (AE-4344 or cross action AE-4345) that have thinner blades for easier manipulation through a small microcoaxial incision. The size of the CCC should be a bit smaller than the IOL optic diameter. For a 6.0-mm optic IOL, a 5.0-mm CCC is ideal. The CCC edge should always overlap the optic at the end of the surgery. This manner of IOL fixation is extremely important for achieving consistent refractive results and preventing posterior capsule opacification (PCO). For better visibility of the nucleus, carefully perform the capsulorrhexis without disturbing the underlying cortex.

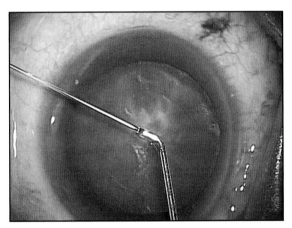

Figure 6-7. Hydrodissection is performed with a special 27-gauge hydrodissection cannula (reusable AE-7636 or disposable AS-7636) which is attached to a small 2.5-cc syringe. A pearl for successful hydrodissection is to use a small syringe to inject BSS most effectively. Because the tip of this cannula is bent and tapered, it is easy to introduce under the capsulorrhexis edge; this configuration also facilitates stromal incision hydration at the conclusion of surgery.

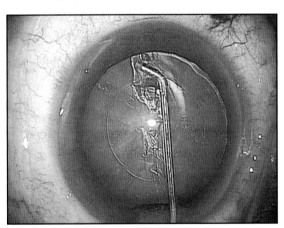

Figure 6-8. The cannula tip is introduced horizontally under the capsulorrhexis edge. The anterior capsule is slightly lifted so that the cannula tip is inserted just beneath the anterior capsule.

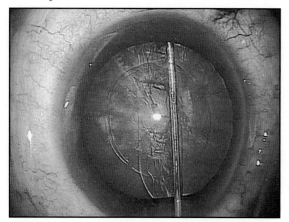

Figure 6-9. After rotating the cannula 90 degrees so that its tip is directed inferiorly, a small amount of BSS is quickly injected. When the fluid wave spreads toward the proximal end, the nucleus will start to subluxate into the anterior chamber. Push the nucleus downward so that the BSS in the space between the capsule and nucleus may spread uniformly within the capsular bag. Ascertain that the nucleus can be rotated freely in the capsular bag. Free rotation of the nucleus is mandatory at this point, because the nucleus will be more difficult to rotate after it has been prechopped into smaller pieces. With a posterior polar cataract, cortical cleaving hydrodissection should not be performed.

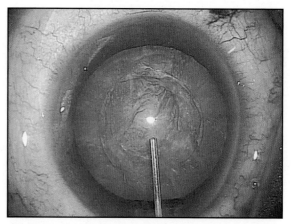

Figure 6-10. Fill up the chamber with Viscoat again. At this point, clear the cortex from the anterior nuclear surface for better visibility of the nuclear characteristics. For those who are not familiar with prechop, it is advisable to perform this under direct visualization of nucleus. If there is too much cortex blocking visibility of the nucleus, the anterior cortex may be preaspirated with an irrigation/aspiration (I/A) tip. However, once the surgeon has become more experienced with the technique, it will be possible to perform the prechop maneuver based more on "feel" and with less dependence on direct visualization.

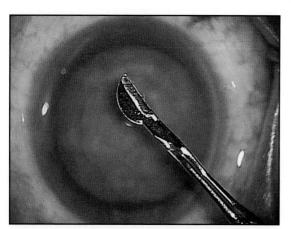

Figure 6-11. For the Karate Prechop technique, a Combo II Prechopper (AE-4190) will be used. The Combo Prechopper blade has 2 different edges—one that is sharp and angled and another that is blunt and rounded. The angular side is designed for incising into the nucleus. The rounded side can be used to safely separate the nuclear sections enough to confirm complete division.

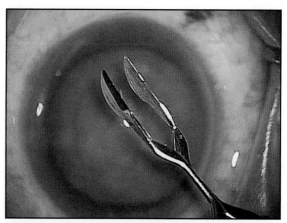

Figure 6-12. Compared to the conventional Combo Prechopper (AE-4284), the blades of the Combo II Prechopper can be widely opened through a much smaller incision, making it suitable for microcoaxial surgery. The Combo II can be used to prechop the nucleus through a corneal incision as small as 1.8 mm. Combo II is also suitable for use through a larger incision as well, and is the author's overall preference over the first generation Combo Prechopper.

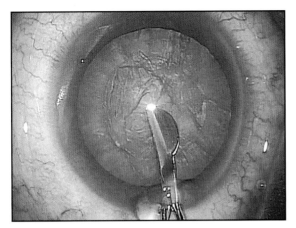

Figure 6-13. Introduce the prechopper horizontally. Because the blade height is 1.5 mm, it can easily fit through a 1.8 mm-incision.

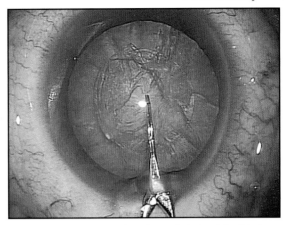

Figure 6-14. Place the sharply angled tip of the blade at the very center of the nucleus. By impaling the blade at this location, the stress on the zonules is equalized and minimized. From this center position, the blade is then incised downward.

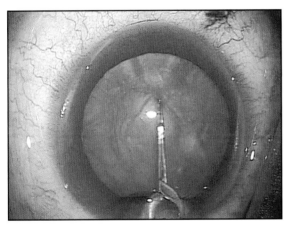

Figure 6-15. Impale the closed prechopper blades directly down into the nucleus. Insert the entire blade width into the nucleus. Because the height of the Combo Prechopper blade is 1.5 mm, the entire blade can be buried into the nucleus. If the nucleus is so dense that there is too much resistance, then the Karate technique will not work. Instead, for dense nuclei, the Counter Prechop technique should be used, in which counterfixation to the impaling prechopper is supplied by a second instrument.

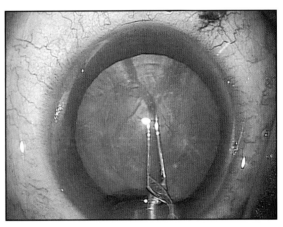

Figure 6-16. Open the blades gradually while pushing the nucleus slightly downward. An effective chop will not result if the blades are separated too quickly.

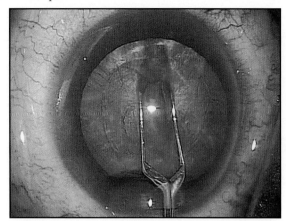

Figure 6-17. After the nucleus is completely prechopped, the posterior capsule can be observed between the 2 prechopped heminuclei. Merely making a crack in the nucleus is not enough. It is important to attain a complete division from the anterior to the posterior surface.

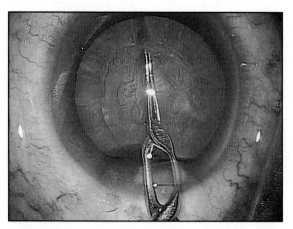

Figure 6-18. Insert the blades until they reach toward the distal end of the nucleus.

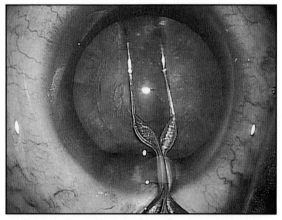

Figure 6-19. Open the blades to separate the distal part of the equator.

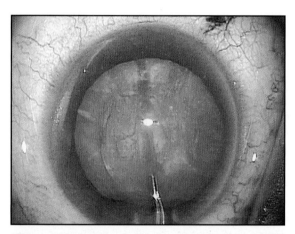

Figure 6-20. Position the blades closer to the proximal part of the nucleus.

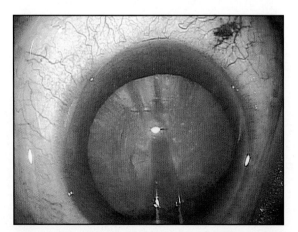

Figure 6-21. Open the blades to fracture the nucleus. The fracture propagates in 2 directions—from the proximal toward the distal equator and from the anterior surface through the posterior plate. The nucleus should now be completely bisected into 2 heminuclei.

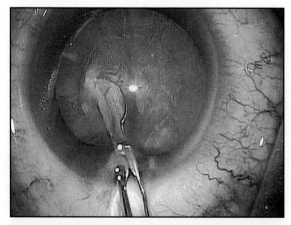

Figure 6-22. Reposition each prechopped nuclear fragment into its original location before rotation. Once the nucleus is bisected, nuclear rotation will be more difficult because of the increased nuclear volume within the capsular bag.

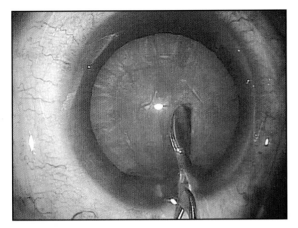

Figure 6-23. Using the angular side of the blade, rotate the nucleus 90 degrees. Slightly depressing the periphery of the nucleus facilitates nuclear rotation. If the hydrodissection is ineffective, then the nucleus may not rotate. Therefore, properly performing hydrodissection prior to prechopping is mandatory. Nuclear rotation will also be difficult if the OVD is burped out of the incision during the initial prechop maneuver. In this situation, the anterior chamber should be refilled with additional OVD or a second instrument can assist the rotational maneuver through the sideport incision.

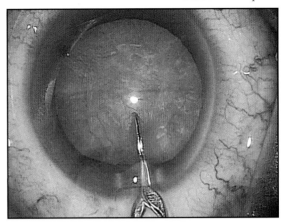

Figure 6-24. Place the angular side of the prechopper blade at the midpoint between the center of the nucleus and the edge of the anterior capsulorrhexis.

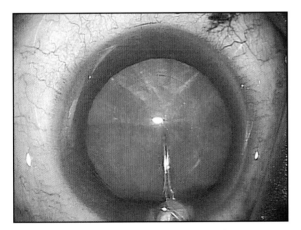

Figure 6-25. Impale the blades into the nucleus. Because the insertion point is slightly off center and the path of insertion is toward the posterior pole, the blades will be directed slightly obliquely as they are inserted. The distal half of the prechopped nuclear fragment will support the insertion of the blades into the proximal heminucleus. In the same way as the initial prechop, the surgeon should try to bury the entire blade into the mass of the nucleus.

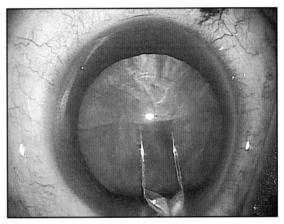

Figure 6-26. While pushing the nucleus obliquely down toward the posterior pole, open the blades slowly. Repeat this slow, opening action until the nucleus is completely prechopped from top to bottom.

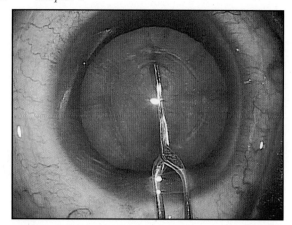

Figure 6-27. Insert the angular side of the closed prechopper blades into the distal heminucleus of the bisected lens. The point of prechopper insertion is at the center of the nucleus and the direction of insertion is downward.

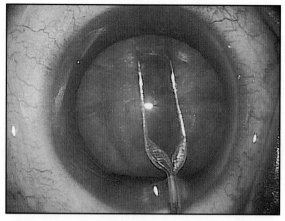

Figure 6-28. While pushing the nucleus downward, open the blades slowly. Confirm complete nuclear division from top to bottom and from the periphery to the center of the nucleus.

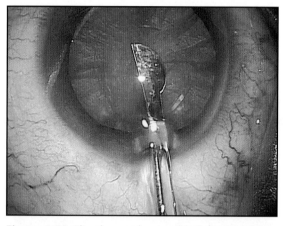

Figure 6-29. Flip the prechopper blade upside down. Using the rounded blunt side of the blade, one can safely nudge the fragments in order to confirm complete nuclear division.

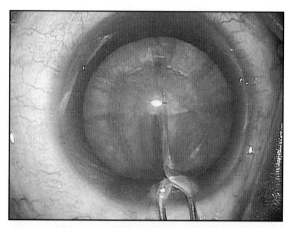

Figure 6-30. Insert the rounded side of the prechopper blades between the prechopped nuclear fragments and position them within the lower half of the nucleus. The rounded side of the blade is so blunt that it will not tear the posterior capsule on contact.

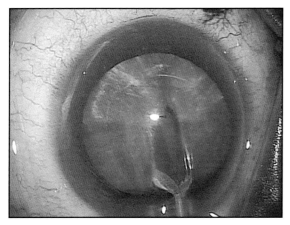

Figure 6-31. Open the blades within the lower half of the nucleus so that the posterior plate of the nucleus is completely separated. If the blades are positioned too superficially, then the posterior plate may not be transected even if the blades are widely opened. All of these dividing maneuvers are performed under a dispersive OVD and can be repeated as necessary until complete fragmentation has been achieved.

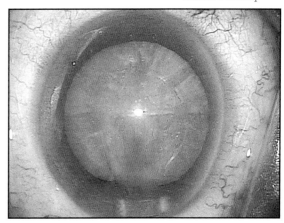

Figure 6-32. The nucleus has now been manually divided into 4 pieces without using any ultrasound energy. The creation of 4 prechopped quadrants is usually adequate to facilitate phacoemulsification. However, it may be desirable to create smaller fragments in order to reduce phaco time in complicated eyes, such as those with small pupils, intraoperative floppy iris, or Fuchs' corneal dystrophy. For example, following the initial transection into 2 heminuclei, one can rotate the nucleus 60 degrees instead of 90 degrees and sequentially perform 2 additional prechop maneuvers on the same heminucleus.

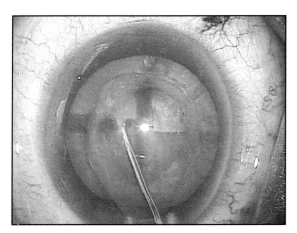

Figure 6-33. To more easily confirm complete separation of the nuclear fragments and to facilitate phacoemulsification, viscodissection may be performed. A cohesive OVD such as 1% sodium hyaluronate (Provisc) is injected between the chopped nuclear fragments and also into the potential space between the posterior capsule and nucleus. For this purpose, a cohesive OVD is more suitable than a dispersive one.

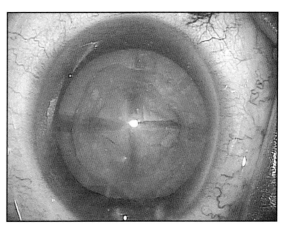

Figure 6-34. The nucleus is now completely prechopped and ready for phacoemulsification. It is important to note that even femtosecond laser nuclear fragmentation cuts cannot achieve complete nuclear division as can be done with manual prechopping. This is because femtosecond laser prechop cuts are restricted by the pupil size and the proximity of the posterior nuclear plate to the posterior capsule. In addition, it may not be possible to dock the laser to small or deep set eyes. Manual prechop techniques can achieve superior nuclear division with minimal cost and surgical time.

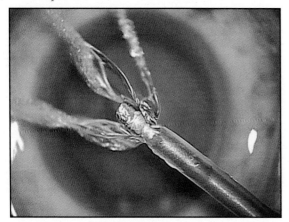

Figure 6-35. Because prechopping the nucleus drastically reduces ultrasound energy, phacoemulsification can be safely performed though a sub-2-mm incision using a Nano sleeve (Alcon Laboratories, Fort Worth, TX). Although any phaco tip can be used, this author prefers the reverse-Kelman style tip for the prechopped nucleus. The Kelman tip is bent away from the bevel to facilitate sculpting, while the reverse-Kelman tip is bent toward the bevel, which allows the bent tip to be positioned bevel down in order to facilitate occlusion.

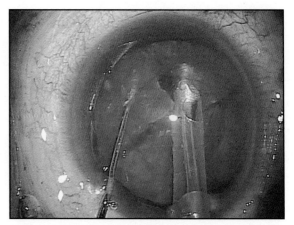

Figure 6-36. The author prefers bevel down positioning of the phaco tip for emulsification of the prechopped nucleus. With bevel down phaco, all of the ultrasound energy is effectively used to emulsify the nucleus as soon as the tip opening is completely occluded by it. Using the reverse-Kelman tip with a 30-degree bevel, it is very easy to occlude the phaco tip opening while its shaft is parallel to the incision. This lessens the risk of thermal damage or sleeve obstruction due to mechanical wound deformation. In terms of optimizing tip occlusion, the reverse-Kelman 30-degree beveled tip is more suitable than the 0 or 45 degree bevels.

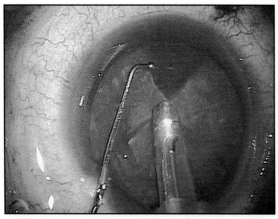

Figure 6-37. To minimize ultrasound energy, multiburst mode is recommended (see Figure 6-38). With this power modulation, the duration of phaco "ON" time (ON-T) is fixed, while the interval of the ultrasound emission is controlled linearly with the foot pedal. As the pedal is further depressed, ultrasound is emitted more frequently. However, it will never become continuous, even if the foot pedal is fully depressed. If the "OFF" time (OFF-T) is linearly decreased to 250 m/sec, there will still be 250 m/sec of corresponding OFF-T with maximum foot pedal depression. Remove the distal-most quadrant of the nucleus first in order to create vacant space into which to position the next nuclear fragment for phacoemulsification.

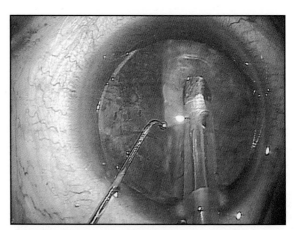

Figure 6-38. The bevel down phaco tip is first completely occluded with nucleus and the surgeon stays in foot pedal position two (FP2). Positioning the tip closer to the periphery of the nucleus (where more cortex is present) leads to a stronger occlusion. Once the higher-pitched sound from the phaco machine indicates that a maximum vacuum level has been reached, elevate the prechopped nuclear fragment from the capsular bag and emulsify it using FP3. Employing ultrasound energy without tip occlusion and higher vacuum levels is inefficient and ineffective for emulsifying the nuclear fragments.

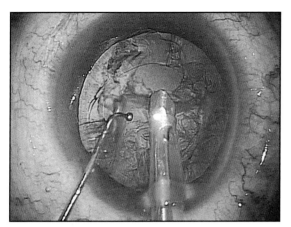

Figure 6-39. The Akahoshi Nucleus Sustainer (AE-2530; Asico) is a second instrument that is used to manipulate the nuclear fragments and to protect the posterior capsule. Since the sustainer has a tiny blunt ball at its tip, it can safely maneuver the nucleus. To avoid inadvertent contact of nuclear fragments with the endothelium, it is best to systematically elevate one fragment at a time out of the capsular bag. However, because the nucleus has been prechopped, the other loose fragments may tumble prematurely into the anterior chamber. Using the Nucleus Sustainer or other second-hand instrument can prevent this from happening.

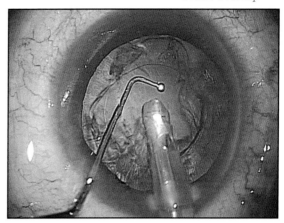

Figure 6-40. Although irrigation flowing through the inferior port of a 3-port infusion sleeve can help to keep the posterior capsule away from the phaco tip, placing the Nucleus Sustainer between the phaco tip and the posterior capsule as the last piece of the nucleus is emulsified will also block the posterior capsule from being snagged.

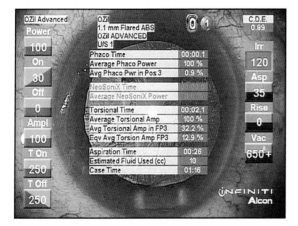

Figure 6-41. After the nucleus has been prechopped into smaller pieces, phacoemulsification can be performed using higher vacuum and aspiration flow rates. In this case the aspiration time was 26 seconds, total BSS consumption was 10 cc, and the total ultrasound energy was only 0.89%-seconds. The power setting will vary according to nuclear density, and the aspiration flow rate may be changed depending on anterior chamber depth and in consideration of any abnormalities of the corneal endothelium, iris, or zonules.

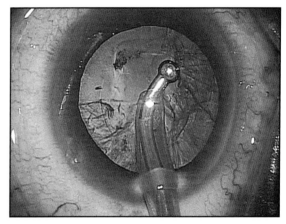

Figure 6-42. The cortex is removed with a curved ball I/A tip (AE7-3062). For sub-2-mm micro coaxial surgery, it is necessary to use an I/A tip with a smaller outer diameter. The outer diameter of this I/A tip shaft is 0.7 mm, which—when combined with the Nano infusion sleeve—can provide nearly 3 times more irrigation flow compared to using conventional I/A tips with a 1.0 mm shaft diameter.

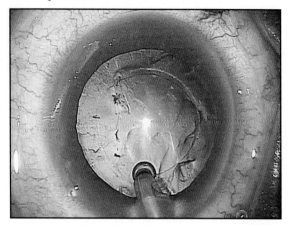

Figure 6-43. Because the tip is ergonomically curved, the subincisional cortex is easily removed without resorting to bimanual I/A.

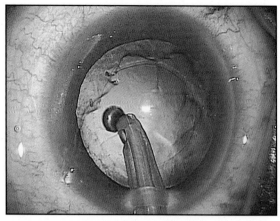

Figure 6-44. Because the I/A tip head has a spherical shape and the aspiration port is drilled at a 45-degree angle to the main shaft, the posterior capsule can be safely cleaned and polished using a lower vacuum setting.

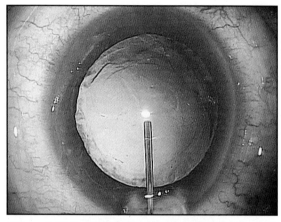

Figure 6-45. For IOL implantation, a cohesive OVD such as Provisc is preferable because it is easier to remove. It is important to refill the anterior chamber and capsular bag with sufficient OVD. This can be accomplished by continuing to inject OVD until it oozes out of the incision. Maintaining high intraocular pressure greatly facilitates IOL injection through a small incision.

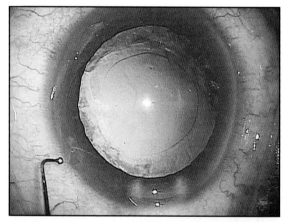

Figure 6-46. This author prefers using single-piece AcrySof IOLs such as the IQ (SN60WF), Toric (SN6ATx), ReSTOR (SN6AD1), and ReSTOR Toric (SND1Tx). The Acrysof platform can be implanted through a sub-2 mm incision using the Counter Traction Implant technique with a Monarch D-cartridge and Royale unihand injector (AE-9045LSP). Placing a second instrument through the sideport provides adequate counterforce to the cartridge as it is inserted.

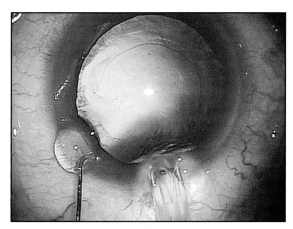

Figure 6-47. Even the smallest Monarch D-cartridge tip cannot be completely inserted into the anterior chamber though a 1.8-mm corneal incision. Only the protruding anterior lip of the cartridge tip can be inserted into the corneal tunnel. This makes countertraction with a second-hand instrument important for IOL injection.

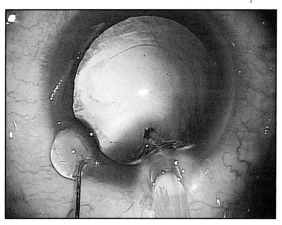

Figure 6-48. The IOL should be situated within the cartridge so that both haptics override the optic and so that the lens is curling downward as it exits the cartridge tip. In this way, the conoid elbow of the haptic will pass through the cartridge tip first, and stretch the incision in the process.

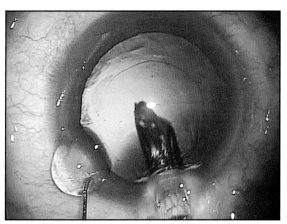

Figure 6-49. While injecting the IOL, push the plunger continuously until the lens is completely released into the capsular bag. Continue to provide the counter traction with the second instrument and make sure not to stop halfway. If this happens, the IOL could become stuck in the incision like a napkin inside a napkin ring, which can be a significant problem. If this occurs, the lens can either be pulled back out through the incision or pushed into the anterior chamber with forceps. If neither maneuver is successful, amputate that part of the IOL external to the incision and push the remainder of the IOL into the anterior chamber where it can be cut it into smaller pieces for removal.

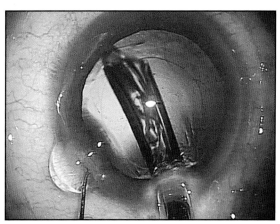

Figure 6-50. Proper placement of the AcrySof IOL into the cartridge is important. If the lens curls upward during placement, the plunger will pass underneath the lens optic and override it, rather than pushing against its edge. This in turn may result in overly abrupt exit of the IOL, which can traumatize the iris or tear the posterior capsule. Prior to docking the cartridge tip within the incision, it is important to confirm that the IOL moves smoothly as the plunger is advanced.

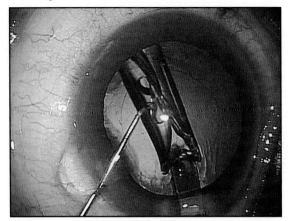

Figure 6-51. It is also important to maintain sufficient intraocular pressure during IOL implantation through a small incision. If the sideport incision is too large, OVD might leak out during insertion of the cartridge tip. This will soften the eye and proper tip insertion will fail. To minimize such OVD leakage through the sideport incision, a special 0.6-mm keratome (AE-8131) can be used. Because the Royale injector (Asico) has a long plunger, the lens position within the capsular bag can be manipulated with the extended plunger tip and the second hand instrument.

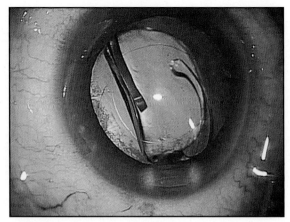

Figure 6-52. The AcrySof IOL opens slowly within the capsular bag. To prevent adhesion between the haptics and optic, the cartridge should be filled with sufficient OVD prior to inserting the IOL.

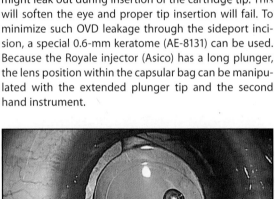
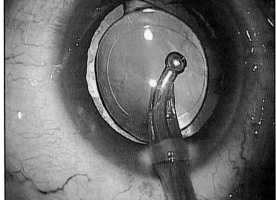

Figure 6-53. Remove the Provisc with the I/A tip. By tilting the IOL optic, any OVD behind the lens can be thoroughly removed.

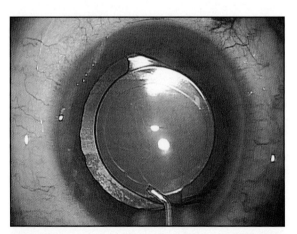

Figure 6-54. Using the hydrodissection cannula to irrigate the anterior chamber with BSS should wash out the Viscoat adherent to the endothelium. It is important to check for any small nuclear fragments which may be hidden within the residual Viscoat layer.

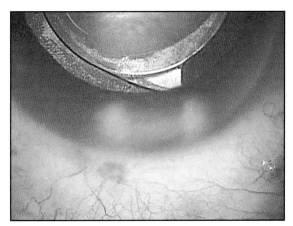

Figure 6-55. Prechopping the nucleus permits the cataract to be removed with minimal ultrasound energy. Because there is no thermal or mechanical damage, the incision is self-sealing without requiring stromal hydration.

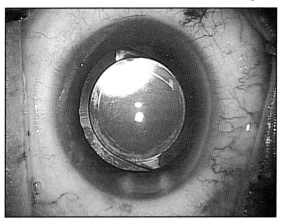

Figure 6-56. The eye is left unpatched at the conclusion of the surgery.

COUNTER PRECHOP

The aforementioned Karate Prechop technique is contraindicated for brunescent nuclei harder than Grade 3, and for eyes with weak zonules (eg, pseudoexfoliation, Marfans, trauma, prior acute angle closure glaucoma, prior vitreoretinal surgery), or a torn capsulorrhexis. In these challenging cases, prechop should only be performed when the nucleus is supported by a second instrument. This technique of bimanual prechopping utilizing nuclear counter support is called Counter Prechop. Both the Karate and Counter Prechop methods can be used for routine cases. However, Counter Prechop must be used for the complicated cases where standard Karate Prechop is contraindicated.

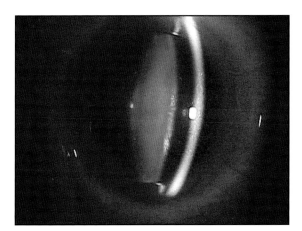

Figure 6-57. In transitioning to Counter Prechop, it may helpful to stain the anterior capsule with dye to highlight the capsulorrhexis edge.

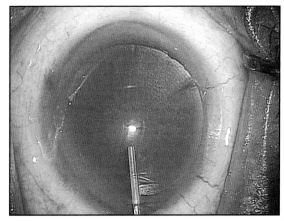

Figure 6-58. After fashioning a 2-step temporal clear corneal incision with a trapezoid diamond keratome, 0.5% preservative-free lidocaine is injected intracamerally. A small 0.6-mm sideport incision is made and the anterior chamber is filled with Provisc. It is important to use a cohesive OVD such as Provisc rather than a dispersive OVD when capsular staining is planned.

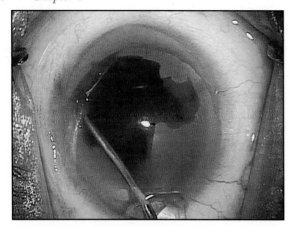

Figure 6-59. An off label Visco-ICG solution dissolved in Provisc is painted on the lens capsule using a Visco-ICG cannula (AE-7272). A small amount of Visco-ICG solution can be applied effectively on the capsule, as it has a hole on the inferior side of the curved cannula. The corneal endothelium is protected by the partition of Provisc. Because the ICG is dissolved in Provisc, it persists longer within the anterior chamber and minimizes any chance for the dye to leak into the vitreous cavity. To create the Visco-ICG solution, 25 mg of sterile ICG powder is completely dissolved in 1.0 cc of distilled water by shaking the vial for 3 minutes. The solution is aspirated into a 2.5-cc syringe. One vial (0.7 mL) of Provisc is added into the syringe and shaken vertically for another 3 minutes.

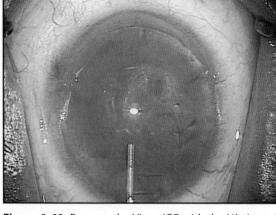

Figure 6-60. Remove the Visco-ICG with the I/A tip and refill the anterior chamber with Viscoat. It is important to thoroughly remove any Visco-ICG behind the iris.

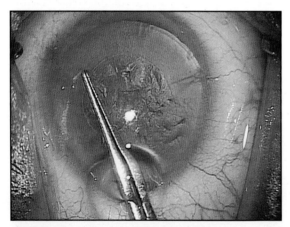

Figure 6-61. Make a 5.0-mm capsulorrhexis.

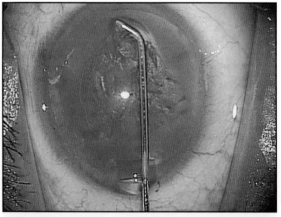

Figure 6-62. Perform cortical cleaving hydrodissection with a 27-gauge cannula (eg, reusable AE-7636 or disposable AS-7636) attached to a small syringe. It is important to confirm that the nucleus rotates freely within the capsular bag before continuing.

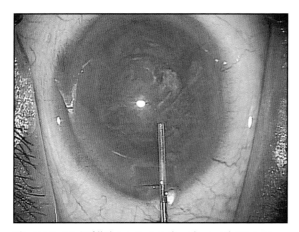

Figure 6-63. Refill the anterior chamber with Viscoat.

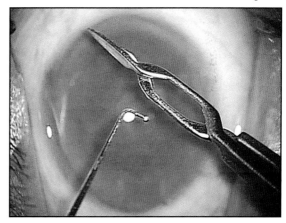

Figure 6-64. The Universal II Prechopper (AE-4192) and the Nucleus Sustainer (AE-2530) are used for the bimanual Counter Prechop technique. This prechopper has thinner and sharper blades that are able to open wider through a small incision compared to the conventional Universal Prechopper (AE-4282). There are many different types of prechoppers available in the market; however, 2 prechoppers, the Combo II (AE-4190) and the Universal II can manage virtually any type of cataract. The Nucleus Sustainer is used to support the nucleus and provide counterfixation against the impaling force of the prechopper. Because the sustainer has a tiny dull ball at its tip, it can safely support the nuclear equator without risk of puncturing the posterior capsule.

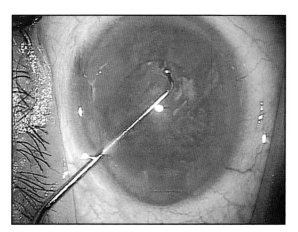

Figure 6-65. Carefully introduce the sustainer under the distal capsulorrhexis edge until it drops into the epinuclear space to brace the equator of the nucleus. Accidentally placing this instrument outside the bag will result in a zonular dehiscence. Therefore, visualization of the capsulorrhexis edge is important and capsule staining may be necessary in some cases.

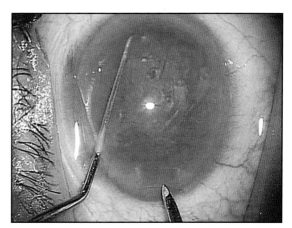

Figure 6-66. Pass the Universal II Prechopper through the incision with the blades oriented horizontally.

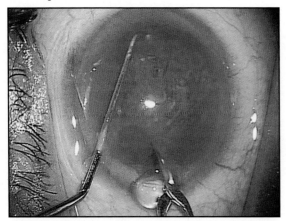

Figure 6-67. Insert the prechopper directly into the nucleus. To provide enough counterforce, the entire equator of the nucleus should be supported. This means that the tips of the second instrument and the prechopper must be positioned deeply enough to surround the hardest central core of the nucleus. A nuclear sustainer with a longer tip (AE-2530L) can be employed for highly myopic eyes with a deep anterior chamber, or in cases with a large-sized nucleus.

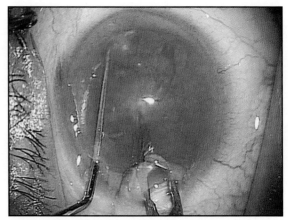

Figure 6-68. Advance the 2 instrument tips toward each other. The tip of the closed prechopper blade and the tip of the sustainer should surround and bracket the central part of the nucleus. If the nucleus was supported too superficially, the sustainer cannot provide proper counterforce to the prechopper. Such misalignment of the instrument tips may stress the zonules. Inserting the prechopper deeply into the core of the nucleus without adequate nuclear counter support may excessively displace the nucleus to the point of tearing the proximal zonules.

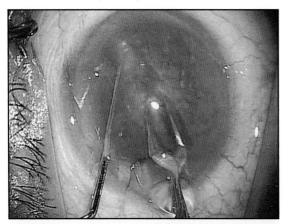

Figure 6-69. Open the prechopper blades once they have reached the center of the nucleus. If the nucleus is not bisected by this initial maneuver, reposition the prechopper at the bottom of the nuclear valley created by the 2 incompletely separated fragments. The goal is to open the prechopper blades within the bottom half of the nucleus; separating the blades while they are positioned too superficially within the anterior half of the nucleus will not achieve complete division. Slowly open the blades several times until complete separation of the posterior plate is achieved. The posterior capsule should become momentarily visible once complete nuclear division has been attained.

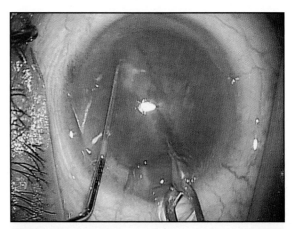

Figure 6-70. Reposition the closed prechopper blades within the proximal part of the nucleus.

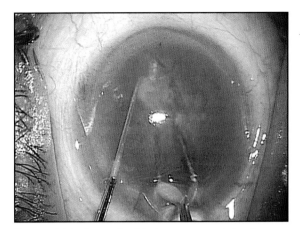

Figure 6-71. Open the blades to extend the fracture plane entirely through the proximal half of the nucleus until the equator is reached. Repeat the same maneuver for the distal half of the nucleus. Confirm that the nucleus has been completely bisected from top to bottom and from one equatorial pole to the other.

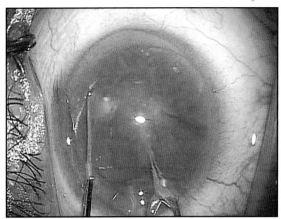

Figure 6-72. Use the 2 instruments to rotate the nucleus 90 degrees. Maintain adequate chamber depth by reinjecting OVD as necessary.

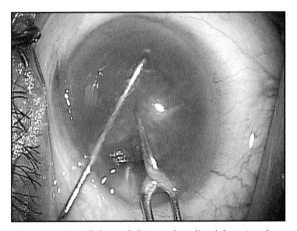

Figure 6-73. While stabilizing the distal heminucleus with the closed prechopper blades, carefully position the sustainer beneath the anterior capsular rim and alongside the distal equator of the nucleus.

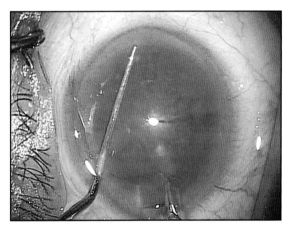

Figure 6-74. Impale the closed blades of the prechopper into the nucleus adjacent to the proximal edge of the capsulorrhexis. Again, the tips of the sustainer and of the prechopper should be aligned along the same depth and axis of the central nuclear core.

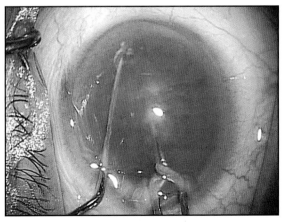

Figure 6-75. Once the prechopper blade tips have penetrated into the central nucleus, open the blades in order to bisect the proximal heminucleus.

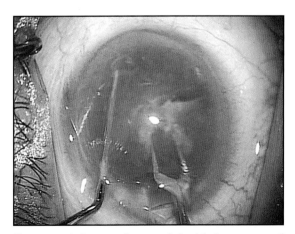

Figure 6-76. Repeatedly spread the blades apart until the proximal heminucleus is completely bisected.

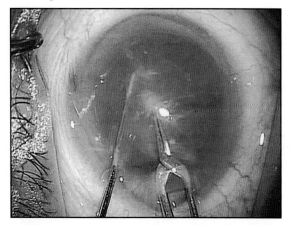

Figure 6-77. Insert the closed prechopper blades into the central core of the distal heminucleus. The sustainer should abut the nuclear equator to provide counterfixation to the impaling force of the prechopper blades. Advance the 2 instrument tips toward each other. Sometimes the sustainer may act as the active phaco chopper while the closed prechopper blades function like a stationary phaco tip to hold and brace the nucleus.

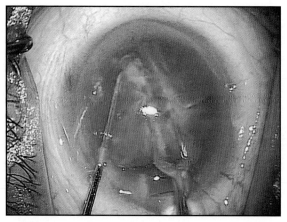

Figure 6-78. Open the blades in order to bisect the distal heminucleus. Repeat the opening action until complete division is confirmed.

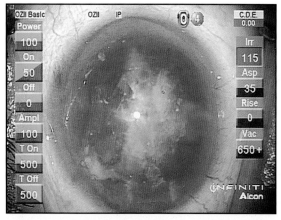

Figure 6-79. In cases with a dense nucleus, each nuclear fragment may be further bisected into smaller pieces to facilitate nuclear emulsification. By continually reinjecting more dispersive OVD and repeating the preceding steps, the nucleus can be further prechopped into 8 fragments before initiating phaco.

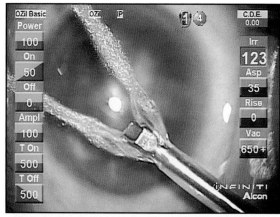

Figure 6-80. Both longitudinal and torsional ultrasound ON-T will be set for longer periods in the case of dense cataracts. The duration of OFF-T between bursts is also lengthened in order to increase the cooling time for the tip.

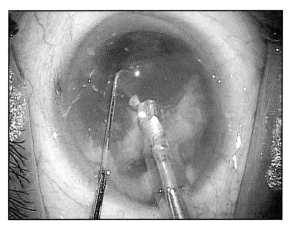

Figure 6-81. The basic principle of phacoemulsification for the dense cataract is the same as for the soft one. Always achieve complete tip occlusion by engaging the nucleus with the bevel down. Ultrasound energy should be utilized only after the tip is occluded and the vacuum level has risen. The Square Wobble tip, which has a decentered shaft, creates a wobbling phaco tip motion with the OZil handpiece. Because the square edges of the tip head can emulsify the nucleus more efficiently than the conventional round tip, use of this tip modification is recommended for dense cataracts. During phacoemulsification, if one discovers that the nucleus is not completely bisected, the prechopping maneuver may be repeated after refilling the chamber with dispersive OVD.

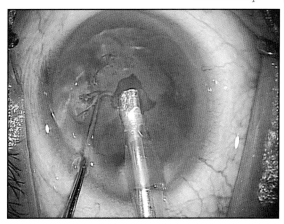

Figure 6-82. As the last nuclear fragments are removed, the sustainer tip is used to block the phaco tip in order to prevent the posterior capsule from being aspirated because of momentary postocclusion surge.

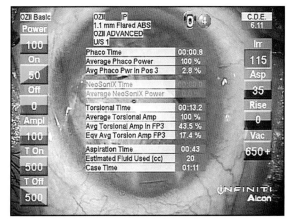

Figure 6-83. By prechopping this very dense nucleus into smaller pieces, the aspiration time in this particular case was only 43 seconds. BSS consumption was 20 cc with a cumulative dissipated energy of 6.11.

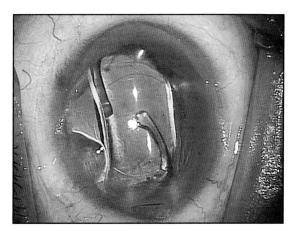

Figure 6-84. A 6.0-mm optic single-piece AcrySof is implanted using the Counter Traction implantation technique described previously.

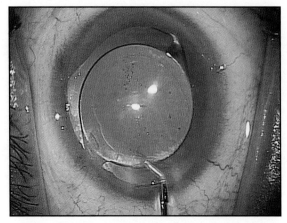

Figure 6-85. The anterior chamber is lavaged with BSS and reformed with the hydrodissection cannula.

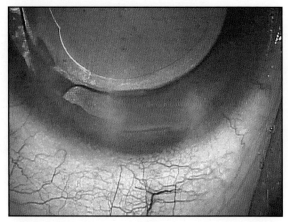

Figure 6-86. Even if the nucleus is very dense, prechopping it into smaller pieces will minimize ultrasound energy while avoiding any thermal or mechanical damage to the incision. Because of this, the wound is self-sealing without any need for stromal hydration.

The author wishes to acknowledge Dr. David F. Chang for his extensive assistance in editing this chapter.

SUGGESTED READINGS

Akahoshi T. Farewell to Bimanual. Developing a Sub-2 mm Coaxial Phaco and IOL Insertion Technique. *Cataract Refract Surg Today.* 2005(6 suppl):1-4.

Akahoshi T. Phaco prechop: manual nucleofracture prior to phaco-emulsification. *Op Tech Cataract Ref Surg.* 1998;1:69–91.

Akahoshi T. *Phaco Prechop: Mechanical Nucleofracture Prior to Phacoemulsification. The Frontier of Ophthalmology in the 21st Century.* Tianjin, China: Tianjin Science and Technology Press; 2001:288-322.

Akahoshi T. The Countertraction Technique: implanting a 6mm AcrySof lens through a sub-2mm Incision. *Cataract Refract Surg Today.* 2006(4):1-3.

Albert DM, Lucarelli MJ. *Clinical Atlas of Procedures in Ophthalmic Surgery.* 2nd ed. New York, NY: Oxford University Press; 2011:27-42.

Buratto L, Werner L, Zanini M, Apple DJ, eds. *Phacoemulsification: Principles and Techniques, Second Edition.* Thorofare, NJ: SLACK Incorporated; 2002.

7

Biaxial Microincision Chopping

Mark Packer, MD, FACS, CPI

HISTORY OF BIAXIAL MICRO-INCISION CATARACT SURGERY

The historical development of biaxial microincision cataract surgery (B-MICS) began in the 1970s when Louis J. Girard, MD attempted to separate infusion from ultrasound and aspiration but abandoned the procedure because of thermal injury to the tissue.[1,2] Shearing and colleagues successfully performed ultrasound phaco through 2 1.0-mm incisions using a modified anterior chamber maintainer and a phaco tip without the irrigation sleeve.[3] They reported a series of 53 cases and found that phaco time, overall surgical time, total fluid use, and endothelial cell loss were comparable to those measured with standard phaco techniques. Crozafon described the use of Teflon-coated phaco tips for bimanual high-frequency pulsed phaco and suggested that these tips would reduce friction and therefore allow surgery with a sleeveless needle.[4] Tsuneoka et al determined the feasibility of using a 1.4-mm (19-gauge) incision and a 20-gauge sleeveless ultrasound tip to perform phaco.[5] They found that outflow around the tip through the incision provided adequate cooling and performed this procedure in 637 cases with no incidence of wound burn.[6]

Additionally, less surgically induced astigmatism developed in the eyes operated with the bimanual technique. Agarwal and colleagues developed a bimanual technique called *phakonit* using an irrigating chopper and a bare phaco needle passed through a 0.9-mm clear corneal incision.[7] They achieved adequate temperature control through continuous infusion and use of a cooled balanced salt solution poured over the phaco needle.

Soscia et al have shown in cadaver eye studies that phacoemulsification with the Sovereign WhiteStar system (Abbott Medical Optics [AMO], Santa Ana, CA), using a bare 19-gauge aspiration needle, does not produce a wound burn at the highest energy settings unless all infusion and aspiration is occluded.[8,9] WhiteStar represents a power modulation of ultrasonic phacoemulsification that reduces the production of thermal energy by limiting the duration of energy pulses to the millisecond range.

ADVANTAGES OF BIAXIAL MICRO-INCISION CATARACT SURGERY

The advantages of B-MICS include enhanced chamber stability due to a more nearly perfectly closed system, better

Chang DF.
Phaco Chop and Advanced Phaco Techniques: Strategies for Complicated Cataracts, Second Edition (pp 77-83).
© 2013 SLACK Incorporated.

followability due to separation of infusion and aspiration, access to 360 degrees of the anterior segment with either infusion or aspiration by switching instruments from one hand to the other, the ability to use the flow of irrigation fluid as a tool to move material within the capsular bag or anterior chamber (particularly from an open-ended irrigating chopper of manipulator), prevention of iris billowing and prolapse in cases of intraoperative floppy iris syndrome, and significantly decreased chance of vitreous prolapse in the case of a posterior capsular tear, zonular dialysis, or subluxed cataracts, due to maintenance of a pressurized stream of irrigation from above.

The many advantages of B-MICS are easily accessible to the skilled cataract surgeon. Regardless of the final incision size required for intraocular lens (IOL) insertion, B-MICS stands on its own as a superior technique.

Separation of irrigation from the aspirating phaco needle allows for improved followability by avoiding competing currents at the tip of the needle. In some instances, the irrigation flow from the second handpiece can be used as an adjunctive surgical device, flushing nuclear pieces from the angle or loosening epinuclear or cortical material from the capsular bag. In refractive lens exchange (RLE), the lens material may be washed completely out of the bag and extracted with aspiration and vacuum only, so that no ultrasound is used and no instrument enters the endocapsular space, increasing the safety profile of this demanding procedure.[10] The flow of fluid from the open end of an irrigator represents a very gentle instrument that can mobilize material without trauma to delicate intraocular structures.

Another benefit of a separate infusion stream comes to bear in scrubbing troublesome plaques from the posterior capsule (Figure 7-1). Focusing the flow of fluid on the posterior capsule and putting the tissue on stretch facilitates capsule polishing with either a roughened or silicone-covered aspiration tip. The taut posterior capsule shows less inclination to become entrapped in the aspiration port, and the subcapsular plaque material is more easily stripped away.

Perhaps the greatest advantage of the biaxial technique lies in its ability to remove subincisional cortex without difficulty. As originally described by Brauweiler, by switching infusion and aspiration handpieces between 2 microincisions, 360 degrees of the capsular fornices are easily reached and cortical clean-up can be performed quickly and safely.[11] The ability to switch hands also represents a significant advantage to instructors of phacoemulsification, who may find that they must take over a case from a resident with opposite manual dominance.

Utilization of B-MICS as we have described for RLE and routine cataract surgery offers an enormous advantage of maintaining a more stable intraocular environment during lens removal. This may be especially important in patients with a high degree of myopia who are at a greater risk for retinal detachment following lens extraction. By

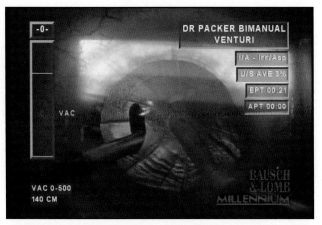

Figure 7-1. Utilizing xenon slit beam illumination (OPMI VISU 160; Carl Zeiss, Dublin, CA) highlights this posterior subcapsular plaque. The stream of irrigation fluid from the irrigating chopper is directed posteriorly to put the capsule on stretch while the silicone-sleeved aspiration tip is used to scrub away the material.

maintaining a formed and pressurized anterior chamber throughout the procedure, there should be fewer tendencies for anterior movement of the vitreous body with a theoretical lower incidence of posterior vitreous detachment occurring from intraoperative manipulations. Future studies will need to be performed in order to document a significant reduction in posterior segment morbidity utilizing this method of lens removal.

B-MICS is advantageous when intraoperative floppy iris syndrome (IFIS) occurs. Keeping the irrigator high in the anterior chamber tamponades the iris and keeps it from becoming floppy. As long as we irrigate above the iris, it will not billow. Alternatively, we can hydroexpress the cataract out of the capsular bag and carousel the endonucleus in the plane of the capsulorrhexis. Therefore, the epinucleus holds the iris back. In those IFIS cases where we cannot hydroexpress the lens, we dilate the pupil widely with sodium hyaluronate 2.3% (Healon 5), do our hydro steps, and then perform one endolenticular chop. Next, we bring the nuclear material up to the irrigating chopper, which is kept above the iris, for disassembly and mobilization. Very frequently, by restricting ourselves to foot pedal position 3 (FP3) in occlusion or FP1 with a clearance of occlusion, the Healon 5 can remain in the eye, keeping the pupil dilated. After epinucleus removal, the pupil tends to constrict; however, we redilate it with Healon 5. By keeping the aspiration tip in occlusion, we go circumferentially around the capsulorrhexis, mobilizing cortex from the capsular fornices without bringing it out of the eye. Maintaining occlusion of the tip immobilizes Healon 5, thus allowing the pupil to remain dilated. After the cortex has been removed from the fornix, we then remove it from the eye.

Though the advantages described previously relate principally to separation of irrigation from aspiration, some

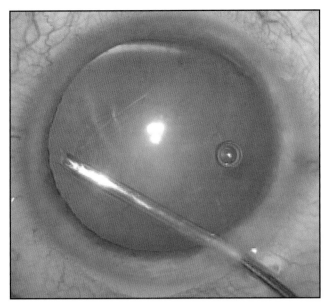

Figure 7-2. The capsulorrhexis is nearly complete in this eye with a history of trauma and 90 degrees of zonular dialysis visible temporally. The wrinkling of the capsule is a clear sign of absent tension. Nevertheless, because of the increased control allowed by the microincisions, which do not allow prolapse of viscoelastic, the capsulorrhexis will be centered, round, and smaller in diameter than the IOL.

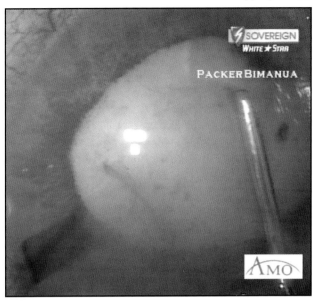

Figure 7-3. Capsular dye and microincisions help to control the capsulorrhexis in this eye with a hypermature cataract.

BIAXIAL MICROINCISION CATARACT SURGERY TECHNIQUES

of the other major advantages we have seen from B-MICS do relate to incision size. For example, there has been an improvement in control of most of the steps involved in endocapsular surgery due to increased chamber stability. Because viscoelastics do not leave the eye easily through these small incisions, the anterior chamber is more stable during capsulorrhexis construction and there is much less likelihood for an errant rhexis to develop. This added margin of safety is particularly noticeable in cases of zonular compromise such as pseudoexfoliation, traumatic zonular dialysis, and status post glaucoma filtering surgery, as well as in cases of intumescent cataract and nanophthalmos with a very shallow anterior chamber (Figures 7-2 and 7-3). The added chamber stability can also make a difference in control of the capsulorrhexis in high myopia with an extremely deep anterior chamber and floppy capsule. The adoption of microincision techniques has also served as a catalyst for instrument manufacturers, who have developed delicate, exquisite forceps for the construction of the capsulorrhexis. The result has been unparalleled surgical control. Hydrodelineation and hydrodissection can also be performed more efficiently by virtue of a higher level of pressure building in the anterior chamber prior to eventual prolapse of viscoelastic through the microincisions.

In order to reap the benefit of these advantages, strict attention to detail is required. The first technique to master is construction of the incision. There is variability in incision size among surgeons who employ 20-, 19-, and even 18-gauge instrumentation. The author prefers 20-gauge because it offers greater control. Because the outer diameter of the 20-gauge tip is 0.9 mm, the circumference of the tip is 2.8 mm and the incision must measure 1.4 mm. An incision smaller than 1.4 mm stretches and tears, causing loss of self-sealability. These microincisions are converted from a line to a circle upon introduction of the tip, and we want them to resume the configuration of a line when the tip is withdrawn. Compromise of the corneal collagen by stretching or tearing will reduce the likelihood that the incision will resume its virgin architecture at the end of the case. This can be minimized by using only trapezoidal-shaped incisions. Diamond and metal knives specially designed for construction of 20- or 19-gauge incisions are now available from a variety of manufacturers. It behooves the surgeon to purchase and learn to use this instrumentation, whether constructed of steel, diamond, or other material.

Capsulorrhexis construction represents the initial hurdle in the biaxial learning curve. However, microincision capsulorrhexis forceps permit a greater degree of precision and control, so much so that we advocate their use with any size of incision. The pinch-type initiation of the capsulorrhexis is particularly valuable in cases of zonular compromise because the forces acting on the capsule remain balanced. Even with a severely wrinkling capsule due to traumatic zonular dialysis, these extraordinarily delicate forceps permit moment-by-moment control of the capsulorrhexis. With new technology IOLs, such as the Crystalens (Bausch + Lomb, San Dimas, CA) and the Synchrony (Visiogen, Irvine, CA), we have found capsulorrhexis size to be an important determinant of final lens position and therefore postoperative refractive status. Using microincisions enhances the precision of capsulorrhexis construction not only because of the improvements in instrumentation but also because there is not a tendency for the chamber to shallow, as often occurs with a 2.5-mm incision due to burping of viscoelastic.

As stated previously, the goal of cortical cleaving hydrodissection is to lyse the equatorial capsular–cortical connections, which will generally allow aspiration of the cortex, along with the mobilization of the epinucleus. Hydrodelineation is performed to allow free mobility of the endonucleus within the epinuclear shell, allowing endocapsular nuclear disassembly within the safety cushion of the epinucleus. Hydrodissection and hydrodelineation may be performed just as described previously for standard small-incision surgery; the microincisions do allow egress of viscoelastic during this step so that there is not an increased risk of blowing out the posterior capsule due to overpressurization. Of note, we found that the intraocular pressure during hydrodissection, as measured in the vitreous cavity of a cadaver eye, varies around means of 78 to 223 mm Hg, regardless of whether a standard small incision or microincision is employed.[12] These were among the highest pressures we recorded during the entire phacoemulsification and IOL implantation procedure. Clearly, if viscoelastic is prevented from exiting the eye, there is adequate pressure to rupture the capsule. This represents a special concern to users of high zero-shear viscosity ophthalmic viscosurgical devices (OVDs), who should insure that a path for egress is prepared with a track of balanced salt solution from the cannula tip to the incision.

CHOPPING IN BIAXIAL MICROINCISION CATARACT SURGERY

A variety of irrigating choppers are now available for microincision surgery. How to place the blade or paddle of the chopper through the incision is not always immediately apparent. With the canoe paddle-shaped Tsuneoka Chopper (Du-02317, MicroSurgical Technologies [MST], Redmond, WA), for example, the paddle must be placed parallel to the incision, inserted into the chamber, and then rotated to allow full entry. Surgical videos are generally available from industry for instructional purposes. Placing the phaco tip through the incision may also be harder than it first appears. A 30-degree tip may be inserted into the incision bevel down and then rocked gently from side to side to permit passage into the chamber.

The surprising fact about horizontal and vertical chopping techniques with biaxial phaco is how little they differ in terms of hand movement from standard small-incision coaxial phaco. Seeing the bulkier irrigating chopper in the eye and getting used to the heavier feel in one's hand represent the major differences; the actual chopping techniques are the same. The stream of irrigation fluid from the chopper or manipulator can function as an efficient tool within the eye and is one of the most significant advantages of biaxial phaco, a key reason we do not want to go back to coaxial. In particular, washing subincisional endonuclear or epinuclear material into range of the phaco tip permits enhanced safety and control. A great example is RLE with an accommodative IOL in high myopia, probably the situation in which we are most concerned about maintaining the integrity of the capsule. Not only would compromising the capsule increase the risk of posterior segment complications but it may also result in an inability to implant the IOL of choice for the procedure. With biaxial RLE, no instrument other than a cannula and a stream of fluid ever need enter the endolenticular, or endocapsular space; we can hydroexpress the soft lens material into the anterior chamber with the stream of irrigation fluid and carousel it safely from the eye with fluidics alone. With cortical cleaving hydrodissection we can achieve a clean capsule without ever placing an aspiration tip below the level of the capsulorrhexis. The absence of ultrasound energy allows for the safest minimally invasive procedure possible. The margin of safety is further enhanced by this approach.

If there is a breach of the posterior capsule, residual lens material can generally be removed while maintaining irrigation in the anterior chamber and disallowing vitreous prolapse. With biaxial phaco we have the option of switching from a phaco tip to an aspirator to a vitrector if necessary without ever compromising chamber stability. The approach, once a tear is recognized, consists of continuous irrigation in the anterior chamber while lens material is removed from the bag. Once the bag is clean, a dispersive viscoelastic is injected at the level of the posterior capsule while irrigation is still maintained; only once the viscoelastic has fully tamponaded the break and filled the chamber is the irrigator removed. The IOL can then be inserted into the ciliary sulcus or the capsule through a standard temporal clear corneal incision. In the case of sulcus placement, the optic is pushed posteriorly through the capsulorrhexis prior to final clean-up. Once viscoelastic is removed, the triamcinolone staining technique described by Burk et al is utilized to insure a completely vitreous-free environment in the anterior segment.[13]

Table 7-1.

SAMPLE PHACO PARAMETERS FOR BIAXIAL MICROINCISION CATARACT SURGERY

MEMORY	VARIABLE WhiteStar Phaco mem 1 (use for hard cataracts)	CHOP Phaco mem 2	TRIM Phaco mem 3	FLIP Phaco mem 4	IRRIGATION AND ASPIRA-TION, SILICONE CURVED TIP	VISCOAT REMOVAL, SILICONE CURVED TIP
Power	40	40	20	20	n/a	n/a
Flow	30 Panel	30 Panel	22/16 Panel	24/16 Panel	22 Panel	40 Linear
Vacuum	500/380 Case B Panel	500/380 Case B Panel	200/50 Linear	200/80 Linear	500 Linear	500 Panel
Ramp	30%	30%	30%	30%	85%	85%
Mode (unoccluded or occluded)	Variable WhiteStar CN/CL/CF/CD 18%/20%/ 33%/43%	Linear WhiteStar CL	Linear WhiteStar CL	Linear WhiteStar CL	n/a	n/a
Other	ICE with 7% power kick	ICE with 7% power kick	Continue irrigation	Continue irrigation	Continue irrigation	Continue irrigation
Bottle height	30 inches	30 inches	30 inches	30 inches	30 inches	30 inches

ICE = increased control efficiency

We have found this technique to be simple, efficacious, and safe because most of the lens extraction is occurring in the plane of the iris, away from the posterior capsule and the corneal endothelium. Whether surgeons employ 18- or 21-gauge incisions, the principle advantages of B-MICS phaco arise from the separation of infusion and aspiration. No matter how small the incision, these advantages cannot be achieved with coaxial techniques.

CASE STUDY: BIAXIAL MICROINCISION CATARACT SURGERY VERTICAL CHOP

Examining each step in a model case enhances understanding. Following hydrodissection and hydrodelineation, the phaco needle is first embedded proximally with high vacuum and 40% power (Table 7-1). In the left hand is a vertical chopper that will be used to split the nucleus in 2. As vacuum builds to occlusion, a rapid rise time enables the phaco needle to quickly grasp the endonucleus. At the point occlusion is reached, the aspiration flow rate drops to 0. We

then move into FP2 so that high vacuum is maintained and the power goes to 0 (Figure 7-4). The blade of the irrigating vertical chopper is brought down just distal to the phaco tip as we lift up slightly with the phaco needle. As a full-thickness cleavage plane develops, dividing the nucleus in 2 pieces, we separate our hands to insure a complete chop (Figure 7-5). In this case, the heminucleus to the left is larger and is therefore addressed first.

The lens can then be rotated with the irrigating chopper so that the first heminucleus can be chopped and consumed. If there is a disparity in size, the larger half is moved distally. The phaco needle is now embedded to the right using high vacuum and low levels of power. A quadrant-sized piece is chopped off and consumed (Figure 7-6). The remaining quadrant of the first heminucleus is then impaled with the phaco tip and aspirated (Figure 7-7). Total effective phaco time (EPT) to this point is less than half a second. EPT is a useful parameter for surgeons to follow. It cannot be compared across different machines made by different manufacturers; however, when using one machine it can be compared from case to case as a sign of surgical efficiency. EPT is the amount of time that ultrasound would have been turned on had it been running on 100% continuous power. That means that we used about half a second

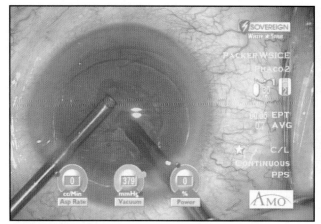

Figure 7-4. The 20-gauge phaco needle is embedded in the endonucleus as the irrigating chopper is prepared to incise and split the lens.

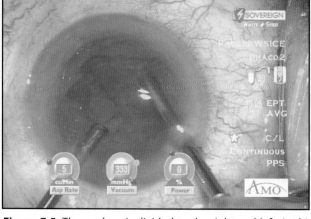

Figure 7-5. The nucleus is divided to the right and left. In this case, a posterior shelf has developed; it is particularly important to separate the instruments fully to insure a complete chop in this situation.

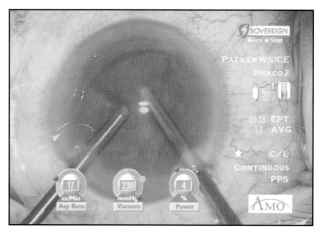

Figure 7-6. After a second chop has divided one of the heminuclei, the first quadrant is mobilized.

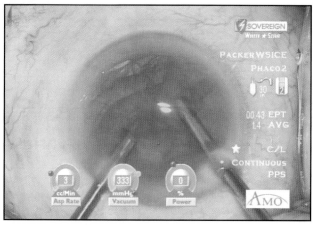

Figure 7-7. The irrigating chopper is used to hold the epinucleus back as another quadrant is aspirated.

of the maximum ultrasound power that the machine can produce to remove half the nucleus. Continuous power can produce thermal energy, but using WhiteStar Technology, or micropulsed phaco, there is no risk of wound burn. Despite the tightness of the incisions, minimal incisional outflow is present and has a cooling effect around the phaco needle.

To address the second half of the nucleus, it is first rotated with the irrigating chopper so that it is in the distal capsule. The phaco needle is embedded in the smaller heminucleus and it is subdivided with the irrigating chopper, again using high vacuum and low levels of power (Figure 7-8). As the final quadrant is grasped and pulled centrally for aspiration, the sharp blade of the irrigating chopper is turned sideways as a safety precaution (Figure 7-9).

When addressing the epinucleus, we reduce our settings, turn down the vacuum and flow rate, and trim the rim of the epinucleus, disallowing the epinucleus from flipping into the phaco needle with the stream of irrigation fluid or the irrigating chopper itself. The advantage of the trimming procedure lies in the aspiration of cortical material from behind the epinuclear shell. In most cases this step eliminates the need for irrigation and aspiration (I/A) prior to IOL insertion. Once 3 quadrants of the epinuclear shell have been rotated and trimmed, the final quadrant is used to flip the epinuclear bowl into the phaco needle (Figure 7-10). Following aspiration of the epinucleus, the capsule is entirely clean of cortex (Figure 7-11). The asteroid hyalosis in the vitreous cavity is obvious.

B-MICS with a vertical chop technique allows efficient lens extraction with rapid visual rehabilitation. This procedure demonstrates some of the tangible benefits of separating inflow from outflow, use of irrigation fluid as an instrument to mobilize material, and reduced EPT.

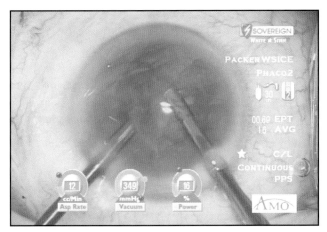

Figure 7-8. A segment of the second heminucleus is aspirated.

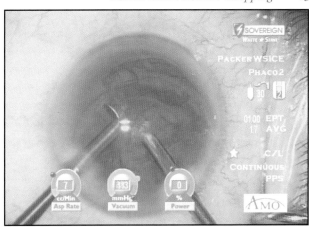

Figure 7-9. As the final quadrant is aspirated, the chopper is turned sideways and the flow of irrigation fluid is directed posteriorly to keep the posterior capsule at safe distance.

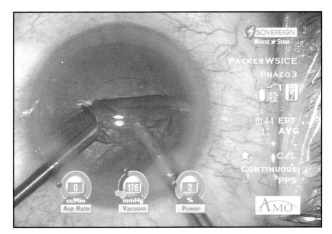

Figure 7-10. The epinucleus is grasped with the phaco needle at reduced power, flow, and vacuum and then flipped.

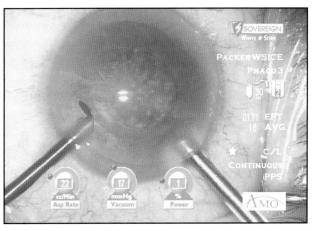

Figure 7-11. The capsule is clean; asteroid hyalosis is visible in the vitreous cavity.

REFERENCES

1. Girard LJ. Ultrasonic fragmentation for cataract extraction and cataract complications. *Adv Ophthalmol.* 1978;37:127-135.
2. Girard LJ. Pars plana lensectomy by ultrasonic fragmentation 1984, part II: operative and postoperative complications, avoidance or management. *Ophthalmic Surg.* 1984;15(3):217-220.
3. Shearing SP, Relyea RL, Loaiza A, Shearing RL. Routine phacoemulsification through a one-millimeter non-sutured incision. *Cataract.* 1985;2:6.
4. Crozafon P. The use of minimal stress and the Teflon-coated tip for bimanual high frequency pulsed phacoemulsification. Paper presented at: 14th Meeting of the Japanese Society of Cataract and Refractive Surgery; July 1999; Kyoto, Japan.
5. Tsuneoka H, Shiba T, Takahashi Y. Feasibility of ultrasound cataract surgery with a 1.4 mm incision. *J Cataract Refract Surg.* 2001;27(6):934-940.
6. Tsuneoka H, Shiba T, Takahashi Y. Ultrasonic phacoemulsification using a 1.4 mm incision: clinical results. *J Cataract Refract Surg.* 2002;28(1):81-86.
7. Agarwal A, Agarwal A, Agarwal S, Narang P, Narang S. Phakonit: phacoemulsification through a 0.9 mm corneal incision. *J Cataract Refract Surg.* 2001;27(10):1548-1552.
8. Soscia W, Howard JG, Olson RJ. Bimanual phacoemulsification through 2 stab incision. A wound-temperature study. *J Cataract Refract Surg.* 2002;28(6):1039-1043.
9. Soscia W, Howard JG, Olson RJ. Microphacoemulsification with WhiteStar. A wound-temperature study. *J Cataract Refract Surg.* 2002;28(6):1044-1046.
10. Fine IH, Hoffman RS, Packer M. Optimizing refractive lens exchange with bimanual microincision phacoemulsification. *J Cataract Refract Surg.* 2004;30(3):550–554.
11. Brauweiler P. Bimanual irrigation/aspiration. *J Cataract Refract Surg.* 1996;22(8):1013–1016.
12. Khng C, Packer M, Fine IH, Hoffman RS, Moreira FB. Intraocular pressure during phacoemulsification. *J Cataract Refract Surg.* 2006;32(2):301–308.
13. Burk SE, Da Mata AP, Snyder ME, Schneider S, Osher RH, Cionni RJ. Visualizing vitreous using Kenalog suspension. *J Cataract Refract Surg.* 2003;29(4):645–651.

SECTION II

Phacodynamics of Chopping

8

Understanding the Phacodynamics of Chopping

Barry S. Seibel, MD

Chopping has numerous advantages as described throughout this book, particularly with regard to decreasing the amount of ultrasound energy required for cataract removal. However, despite the technique's longevity of over 2 decades as well as the intense interest in the topic evidenced by the high attendance at this faculty's phaco chop courses, chopping continues to be practiced routinely by a minority of surgeons. Many other surgeons may have abandoned the technique in frustration without having the benefit of the meticulous description of key components of the technique as described in this book. In particular, their phaco machines were likely not optimized for chopping, and they may even have been set in such a way as to compromise effective chopping. The study of the fundamental principles underlying not only the machine technology but also the individual microsurgical maneuvers is called phacodynamics, and it provides a logical context of reasoning to guide the setting of machine parameters. Phacodynamics further allows the surgeon to readily adapt to anatomical and procedural variations as they present by logical reasoning as opposed to rote memorization of a set of steps or settings.

Phacodynamic goals in chopping may be roughly grouped into 3 categories. First, the surgeon must achieve an adequate grip of the nucleus in order to facilitate impaling and splitting by the chopping instrument. This goal is achieved by correlating applied vacuum to the nuclear density as assessed intraoperatively and by optimizing the vacuum seal on the phaco tip's aspiration port. The second goal is to control postocclusion surge when using high vacuum by proper use of machine parameters as well as such hardware options as fluidic resistors and dual linear pedal control. The third goal is the maximization of mechanical advantage for all surgical maneuvers by utilizing proper instrument placement as well as movement.

In understanding the machines that we will be using, we need to first ascertain whether we are using a flow pump or a vacuum pump; all current and likely future machines may be clinically classified into one of these 2 categories. Furthermore, the clinical roles of flow and vacuum must be defined. Flow, or aspiration outflow, is the volume of fluid per unit time that exits the anterior chamber through the phaco tip's aspiration port. It is measured in cubic centimeters or milliliters per minute and is compensated for by an adequate bottle height to ensure chamber stability. The clinical role of flow is to attract lens material to the aspiration port and to remove it from the eye if that material can deform sufficiently to fit through the phaco needle. For material that cannot readily deform sufficiently to be removed from the eye by aspiration outflow, vacuum

Chang DF.
Phaco Chop and Advanced Phaco Techniques: Strategies for Complicated Cataracts, Second Edition (pp 87-97).
© 2013 SLACK Incorporated.

provides the necessary deformational force, augmented as necessary by ultrasound energy. Vacuum, measured in millimeters of mercury (mm Hg), provides the grip for lens material that is occluding the aspiration port. This grip allows ultrasound energy to more efficiently emulsify the material, and it also allows manipulation and fixation of the lens fragment so that chopping instruments can efficiently subdivide it.

With a flow pump, such as a peristaltic system, a surgeon commands a flow rate in cubic centimeters or milliliters per minute and also sets a vacuum limit in millimeters of mercury. The vacuum limit does not command the machine to automatically produce that level of vacuum but rather limits vacuum build-up past that amount with occlusion of the phaco tip's aspiration port. Therefore, flow pumps attempt to maintain the commanded flow rate while the vacuum varies with the degree of tip occlusion up to the vacuum limit. When setting flow rate in a flow pump, the surgeon is actually setting the rotational speed of the pump head as its rollers traverse the aspiration line tubing in order to propagate fluid. When the aspiration port is completely unoccluded, the actual aspiration outflow rate is proportional to this commanded flow rate or pump speed. By increasing pump speed with the machine's flow rate control, nuclear fragments are more strongly and rapidly attracted to the phaco tip. However, as the aspiration port becomes progressively occluded, the pump has increasing difficulty pulling the same amount of fluid through an effectively smaller opening until finally flow ceases completely with complete tip occlusion. Even with complete occlusion of the phaco tip, flow rate control is still a useful parameter because it proportionately varies the rise time (the time required for vacuum to build to the preset limit once the tip is completely occluded). For example, a longer rise time, produced by a slower commanded flow rate (pump speed), gives the surgeon more time to react in case he or she did not achieve the desired occlusion geometry or in case of inadvertently occluded material such as iris or capsule.

As opposed to a flow pump that directly controls flow as the vacuum varies up to the preset limit, a vacuum pump directly controls the vacuum level while the flow varies. Vacuum pumps represent the second main category of phaco pumps, with examples being the rotary vane pump, the diaphragm pump, and the venturi pump. These pumps may be differentiated from flow pumps in a number of ways. First, as already mentioned, a surgeon using a vacuum pump is unable to directly command a flow rate; in fact, vacuum pumps do not typically have a flow rate in cubic centimeters or milliliters per minute anywhere on their display panel. Second, as already mentioned, the surgeon directly commands the actual vacuum level (not just a vacuum limit) in millimeters of mercury on a vacuum pump as opposed to commanding flow (in cubic centimeters or milliliters per minute) on a flow pump. Third, vacuum pumps are usually indirectly linked to the fluid in the aspiration

line via their drainage cassette. In other words, air in the drainage cassette is between the pump and the aspiration line, as opposed to a flow pump's rollers being directly connected to the aspiration line, which is in direct contact with the aspiration fluid. Fourth, as opposed to the flexible drainage pouch employed with flow pumps, vacuum pumps must have a rigid drainage cassette or pouch that will not collapse with applied commanded vacuum from the pump.

The applied vacuum in a vacuum pump's drainage cassette proportionately produces flow when the aspiration port is unoccluded. When the tip is completely occluded, flow ceases and the vacuum is transferred from the cassette down the aspiration line to the occluded tip. In contrast to using a flow pump, a vacuum pump surgeon will command a given vacuum while the flow varies according to fluidic resistance at the aspiration port of the phaco tip (recall that a flow pump produces a commanded flow rate, whereas a vacuum varies according to fluidic resistance at the tip). For example, if a surgeon commands a vacuum level of 140 mm Hg, the pump will produce this level of vacuum in the machine. If the material entering the tip is viscous (dense nuclear emulsate and/or viscoelastic, both with high fluidic resistance), the subsequent flow will be relatively low. However, once this viscous material passes through, the same commanded vacuum level would result in a faster flow rate as less viscous balanced salt solution traverses the fluidic circuit. Therefore, for a given level of aspiration port occlusion or viscosity, a low commanded vacuum will produce a lower aspiration outflow rate, and a higher commanded vacuum will produce a higher aspiration outflow rate.

A phacodynamic analysis of the various parts of the procedure determines what parameters are effective and active at different stages. Suppose that the surgeon has chopped a fragment and wants to attract it to the tip; the most relevant parameter for this function is flow. In Figure 8-1, the green bar in the vacuum meter would represent the preset vacuum limit in a flow pump, and it would represent the actual commanded vacuum in the rigid drainage cassette in a vacuum pump. Red bars in this vacuum meter represent the actual vacuum present inside the phaco tip, but only one bar is present because there is very little actual vacuum inside of the tip due to the lack of significant fluidic resistance to the low-viscosity aqueous. If the clinical goal were to attract the fragment more strongly to the phaco tip, the surgeon would create a stronger anterior chamber current (purple arrows) by increasing the commanded flow rate with a peristaltic pump (ie, flow pump) or alternatively increasing the commanded vacuum level in a venturi pump (vacuum pump), which would in turn produce an increased outflow rate as described in the preceding paragraph. Although the function for vacuum is limited when attracting a fragment in this setting, it does require a minimum level, particularly in flow pumps, in order to clear the aspirated viscoelastic and

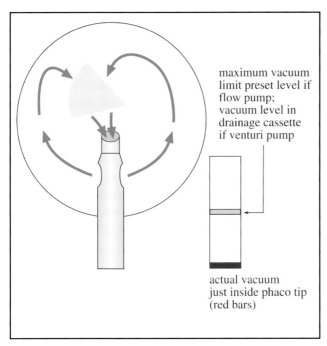

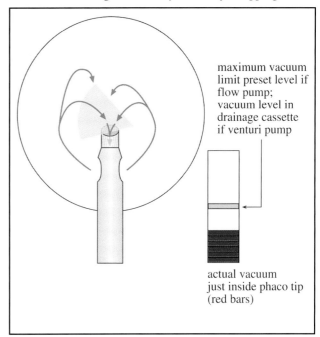

Figure 8-1. With low viscosity aqueous traversing the unoccluded aspiration port, there is little resistance flow and therefore only low actual vacuum just inside of the phaco tip.

Figure 8-2. With partial occlusion of the aspiration port by the nuclear fragment, flow resistance is increased. As a result, the actual vacuum just inside of the phaco tip is also increased.

any existing lens emulsate in the aspiration path between the aspiration port and the pump. Otherwise, the resistance from this material might produce enough vacuum to reach an inadequate preset limit, causing the pump to interrupt flow in order to avoid going past this vacuum level; the interrupted flow would, of course, interfere with the clinical goal of attracting the chopped fragment.

Figure 8-2 represents a chopped fragment that has been attracted to the phaco tip's aspiration port using flow as described previously. At this point, the surgeon may wish to phaco-aspirate the fragment, using the attractive fluidic forces of flow and vacuum to overcome the repulsive force of the axially vibrating ultrasonic needle, particularly with traditional longitudinal ultrasound. With denser nuclei, the surgeon may experience chattering of the fragment, indicating that flow and/or vacuum need to be increased or that ultrasound actually has to be decreased. Figure 8-2 may also represent a nuclear fragment that has been mobilized centrally to allow chopping into still smaller fragments; in this case, a strong vacuum grip is needed to immobilize the fragment during the chopping maneuver. If the attempted chop prematurely dislodges the fragment prior to completing the chop, the grip would have been insufficient, and the surgeon might mistakenly think that more vacuum is needed. However, note that although more vacuum is present (more red bars in the vacuum meter) than in Figure 8-1, it has still not reached the preset level represented by the green bar because of the incomplete occlusion at the aspiration port; part of the machine's vacuum is producing a flow through the smaller effective surface area at the partially

occluded aspiration port. Therefore, increasing the vacuum limit on a peristaltic pump or increasing the commanded vacuum on a venturi pump will only change the level of the green bar on the vacuum meter but will not change the actual vacuum inside of the tip and will therefore not affect the amount of clinical grip of the fragment.

In order to achieve a stronger grip than was present in Figure 8-2, the phaco needle must be more deeply impaled into the nuclear fragment in order to completely occlude the aspiration port, as shown in Figure 8-3. This is a critical example of the importance of optimizing surgical technique prior to dogmatic reliance on machine technology; this prioritization insures that the lowest, and therefore safest, effective parameter is used for each stage of surgery. Note that the red bars in the vacuum meter have risen to the point of the green bar, reflecting the absence of flow with complete tip occlusion and the transfer of all of the machine's vacuum and gripping force to the fragment occluding the aspiration port; many phaco machines give audible feedback to this event with an occlusion bell or tone. If the surgeon experiences insufficient grip at this point, it makes sense to increase the vacuum parameter further.

In addition to understanding fluidics as described previously, chopping surgeons are aided by a phacodynamic understanding of ultrasonic technology, in which the phaco needle vibrates at a frequency of thousands of times per second over a stroke length of a few thousandths of an inch in order to produce acoustic breakdown of lens material. Traditional ultrasound drives the needle longitudinally along the axis of the phaco handpiece, whereas more recent

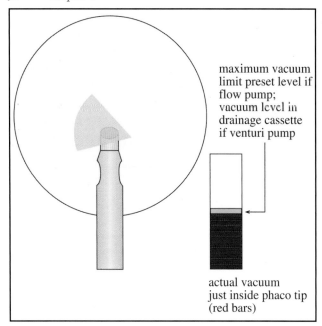

maximum vacuum
limit preset level if
flow pump;
vacuum level in
drainage cassette
if venturi pump

actual vacuum
just inside phaco tip
(red bars)

Figure 8-3. With full occlusion of the aspiration port, flow ceases completely, and vacuum just inside of the tip increases to the maximum preset level.

ultrasound variations translate the needle in a rotatory fashion (OZil, Alcon Laboratories, Fort Worth, TX) or in an ellipsoidal path (Signature, Abbott Medical Optics [AMO], Santa Ana, CA). Early phaco machines had a fixed amount of power available in pedal position 3; this power level was set on the machine panel. For over a decade, surgeons have been able to vary the power in a linear fashion by modulating pedal travel in position 3, thereby achieving a higher level of intraoperative finesse. Still newer adjustments for ultrasound involve the power modulations of pulse mode and burst mode. Burst mode allows the surgeon to vary the number of bursts of power per unit time with a constant amount of power set on the panel; the duration of the burst can vary widely (eg, from 5 to 1000 ms, with the latter being continuous power). Pulse mode allows the surgeon to vary the phaco power with linear control with a fixed number of pulses per second that is set on the panel. Pulse mode ranges from 1 to 20 pps with a 50% duty cycle and linear control of power. Remember to use pulse or burst modes only during full occlusion impaling or phaco-aspiration; these modes should not be used for sculpting, for which linear continuous power is appropriate. However, a more recent evolution of pulse mode, coined *hyperpulse* by David F. Chang, MD, uses duty cycles that are shorter than the 50% of regular pulse, along with higher potential pulses per second (up to 60 or more).[1] These modulations allow improved followability, better thermal protection, and applicability to all phases of cataract surgery including sculpting.

A discussion of potential incisional burns is particularly relevant to phaco chop methods. Such burns are associated with friction produced by the translation of the ultrasonic needle, particularly in the more confined space of the cataract incision, where the needle might rub directly against the irrigating sleeve, which is itself in direct contact with the cornea or sclera. Predisposing factors for an incisional burn are those that either increase potential friction or decrease tip cooling. Examples of the former would be high levels and/or continuous application of ultrasound power. Examples of increased friction would be an excessively tight incision or, alternatively, pulling the phaco handpiece/needle against a roof or side of the incision instead of centering it within the incision and oar-locking as needed. Finally, decreased tip cooling occurs when fluid flow is decreased or stopped, as with viscous emulsate beyond the capability of the given vacuum parameter or complete occlusion of the aspiration port. The former situation can be mitigated by judiciously limited use of highly retentive viscoelastics such as sodium hyaluronate 2.3% (Healon 5), as well as implementation of Dr. Steve Arshinoff's soft shell viscoelastic method, which utilizes an easily aspirated central core of cohesive viscoelastic such as Healon or 1% sodium hyaluronate (Provisc).[2] Moreover, such evacuation of viscoelastic would ideally take place just prior to initiation of phaco power using aspiration alone. Complete occlusion of the aspiration port, which is a relative risk factor for incisional burns, is an integral part of phaco chop, because it is used to achieve a vacuum seal when burying the tip to enable a strong grip on the cataract for chopping. Therefore, optimization of all other risk factors is particularly important, and relatively low levels of hyperpulsed power should be used for this purpose.

Another choice regarding ultrasonic equipment involves the style and size of phaco needle, with the most basic decision involving the angulation at the distal tip, illustrated in Figure 8-4. Traditional teaching informed us that a less angulated tip (eg, 0-degree tip) occluded more easily, whereas a more angulated tip (eg, 45 degrees) cut or sculpted more effectively. The latter might be true (no effective studies substantiate the claim), but the former is false for a number of reasons. In order to understand this statement, it is first necessary to define a good or effective occlusion: a complete impaling of the aspiration port into a given nuclear fragment such that the port is uniformly embedded across its entire surface area and such that an effective grip is achieved. In Figure 8-5, the upper 2 diagrams illustrate good occlusions as defined above with both a 0-degree tip as well as with a 45-degree tip. The lower 2 diagrams illustrate poor, difficult occlusions such that in order to achieve at least the same depth of occlusion in one area of the aspiration port as in the upper drawings, the opposite side of the port had to be buried much deeper, utilizing much greater ultrasound energy. These difficult occlusions are illustrated with a 0-degree tip as well as a 45-degree tip. Therefore, the differentiation is not the tip angulation but rather the relationship of that angulation or the aspiration port to the cataract surface to be occluded.

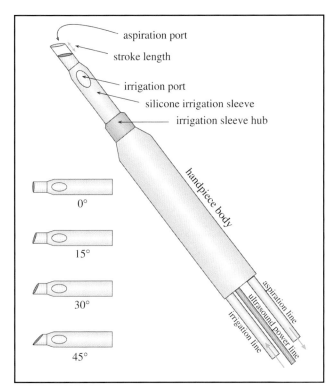

Figure 8-4. Phaco tip angulations routinely vary between 0 and 45 degrees. Tip angulation by itself is not a determinant of effectiveness of occludability.

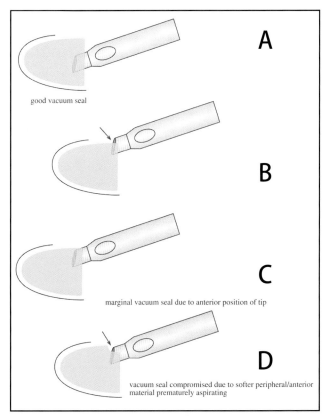

Figure 8-6. Various states of phaco tip occlusion.

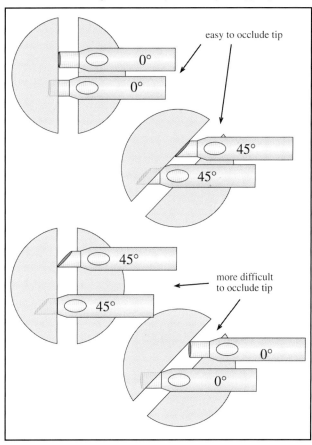

Figure 8-5. Effective occlusion of the phaco tip's aspiration port, regardless of tip angulation, is achieved by rotating the phaco tip and the surface to be engaged such that they are parallel, as seen in the upper 2 diagrams.

As long as these surfaces are made to be parallel by tip rotation and nuclear manipulation, an effective occlusion can be achieved regardless of tip angulation, as illustrated in the upper 2 diagrams in Figure 8-5.

Another key element in achieving an effective grip is attaining a solid vacuum seal. Figure 8-6A illustrates an excellent seal with the aspiration port parallel to the surface that was occluded and the needle buried 1 to 1.5 mm into the central nucleus, which is densest and therefore best allows higher vacuum for gripping. Figure 8-6B shows an improperly anterior placement of the tip that does not even allow complete occlusion of the aspiration port, thereby precluding efficient transfer of the phaco machine's vacuum and holding power. Figure 8-6C allows complete aspiration port occlusion but is still too anterior such that the softer peripheral (anterior) nucleus is preferentially aspirated under high vacuum load, leading to a break in the vacuum seal and a loss of effective grip as shown in Figure 8-6D.

Figure 8-7A-1 shows a good central placement of the phaco tip, but it has not been buried a sufficient amount into the nucleus; with minimal manipulation, the vacuum seal is broken and the effective grip is lost, as seen in

Figure 8-7A-2. Dr. I. Howard Fine has suggested the use of burst mode phaco to overcome timidity in achieving a sufficiently deep impaling.[3] An alternative is to simply use linear ultrasound control with pulse mode while visually titrating the depth of penetration. A useful gauge is recalling that the external diameter of a standard phaco needle is about 1 mm; prior to starting the case, simply retract the silicone irrigating sleeve around the needle such that the length of exposed needle from the closest point of an angulated aspiration port is the same or slightly longer than the needle diameter. Figure 8-7B shows an excellent vacuum seal that starts identically to that which was seen in Figure 8-6A; however, that seal has eroded and grip has been lost in transitioning to the step shown in Figure 8-7C. The problem could be traced to overuse of 2 machine parameters. If the applied vacuum is excessive for the engaged nuclear density, abrupt and uncontrolled aspiration just around the tip will occur as shown, illustrating the importance of titrating vacuum according to astute intraoperative observation of the tip. In addition, if ultrasound energy is applied in excessive amounts or for excessive time, the resultant overcavitation will also erode the vacuum seal as shown, leading to loss of grip. Similar vigilance is needed for tip observation with regard to titrating the correct amount of ultrasound energy. Furthermore, the surgeon must remember to cease ultrasound completely by returning to pedal position 2 once the desired seal has been obtained; good grip and control is very difficult to achieve with a vibrating phaco needle in position 3. To summarize, phaco needle angulation is somewhat arbitrary, and most variations can be used effectively with the foregoing principles.

In addition to distal tip angulation, the surgeon may choose the tip dimensions. For approximately the first 2 decades of phaco, almost all work was done with a 19-gauge straight needle. When newer options are now chosen, the surgeon must appreciate the clinical implications of the different designs. For example, the 20- or 21-gauge microneedles have some fluidic benefits because of the increased fluidic resistance, and therefore surge control, consequent to their smaller internal diameter. However, the smaller aspiration port surface area resulting from the smaller diameter means that the surgeon will have less grip on occluding nuclear material for a given vacuum setting relative to a standard 19-gauge needle. The most recent needles have compound dimensions in which the distal aspiration port diameter is larger than the main shaft internal diameter. The larger distal opening allows the machine to operate more efficiently because any given vacuum is applied over a larger surface area, thereby producing a stronger grip, whereas the small internal shaft diameter simultaneously results in fluidic benefits in terms of surge control. As surgeons try a new technology, they must be aware of how these new designs may affect their technique. For example, the preceding discussion illustrates why a surgeon who previously used a standard 19-gauge

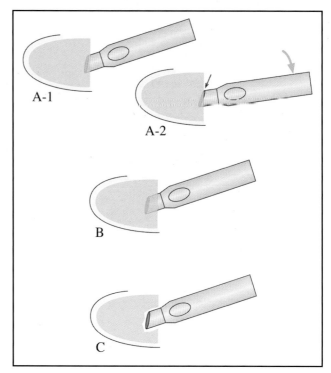

Figure 8-7. Various states of phaco tip occlusion.

needle should anticipate the need for higher vacuum settings (approximately 30%) when transitioning to a 21-gauge needle. Another example would be the aspiration bypass tip (Alcon Laboratories), which places a tiny hole in the needle within the anterior chamber so that some small flow is always maintained even with complete distal aspiration port occlusion, thereby enhancing surge control for a given vacuum setting. However, this bypass port effectively precludes a complete occlusion, thereby reducing the effective grip for a given vacuum setting; the surgeon must anticipate this differential and compensate accordingly with increased flow and vacuum settings.

In addition to adjusting machine parameters as described above, the chopping surgeon may need further machine refinement in response to observing postocclusion surge. This phenomenon occurs when vacuum builds to high levels between the machine pump and an occlusion at the aspiration port. The high vacuum levels partially collapse the aspiration line tubing, with the change in tubing volume divided by the change in applied vacuum being defined as compliance (Figure 8-8A). When the occlusion breaks down due to applied ultrasound, the potential energy of the re-expanding tubing adds additional outflow pull to the flow, which had been balanced to bottle height at a steady-state condition; therefore, the chamber may shallow, dimple, or even collapse if the additional outflow is excessive (Figure 8-8B). When observing surge, the surgeon should first respond by raising the bottle height to provide additional infusion pressure to better keep up with the observed excess outflow rate. If this adjustment is inadequate, then

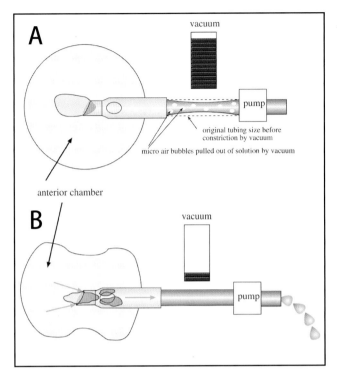

Figure 8-8. (A) High vacuum between the pump and full occlusion of the aspiration port. (B) Postocclusion surge with anterior chamber shallowing.

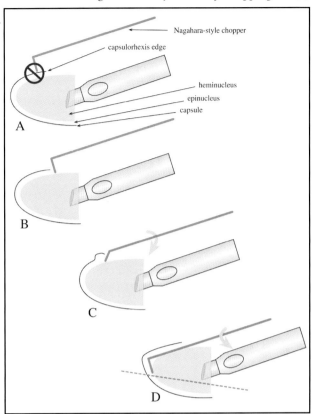

Figure 8-9. Cross-sectional analysis of steps in the Nagahara horizontal chop method.

the vacuum level must be lowered. Another option is to change to a more resistive phaco needle (eg, microflow or flare tip) or a more resistive tubing set (eg, Intrepid, Alcon); needless to say, these choices are ideally made prior to a case rather than in the middle of one.

Figure 8-9 is a schematic of a side view from a stop and chop maneuver in which the goal is to engage and chop a heminucleus. Note the correct placement of the phaco needle in the anterior–posterior center of the nucleus with its aspiration port parallel to the nuclear face and observe how it is buried an appropriate amount of about one needle diameter, or 1 mm. Note that the chopper tip is placed against the nucleus at a point central to the capsulorrhexis to avoid damage to the anterior capsule. David F. Chang, MD has suggested the use of capsule stain for transitioning chopping surgeons to aid in the identification of the capsulorrhexis edge.[1] As the chopper is moved peripherally, the tip is kept in contact with the anterior nuclear surface in order to push under the capsule rather than accidentally jumping on top of it; this constant contact will have the effect of creating a gentle scoring mark on the nuclear surface, and an interruption in this score mark should alert the surgeon to the possibility that the capsule may have slipped under the chopper. Another important point regarding this peripheral movement of the chopper is its temporary rotation such that the angle between the chopping tip and main instrument shaft is more parallel with the iris plane in order to better slip under it; as the nuclear periphery is

reached, the chopper tip is rotated back such that it points posteriorly in order to maximally engage the nucleus. Note how the dashed line connecting the bottom of the chopping tip with the bottom of the phaco needle encompasses the bulk of the nucleus anterior to the line (see Figure 8-9D). As the chopper tip is then drawn toward the phaco tip along this dashed line (in a horizontal direction for horizontal chopping), the nucleus is compressed between the 2 instruments, producing maximum efficiency in propagating the chop's fracture line. Beginning chopping surgeons may often make the mistake of having one or both instruments anterior to this dashed line or starting in the correct position but then drawing the chopper anterior to the dashed line rather than along it; either of these incorrect maneuvers will typically result in an incomplete chop due to lack of the compressive effect as described previously.

Although Figure 8-9 illustrates proper instrument placement for chopping, it also illustrates some of the reasons behind the slow adoption of this technique by the ophthalmic community. First, it is somewhat challenging to dissect the relatively large chopping tip under the capsulorrhexis and iris in order to reach the proper positional endpoint just prior to the chop. Furthermore, it can be seen that the chopping tip is somewhat uncomfortably close to the posterior capsule in this position, and even though the tip

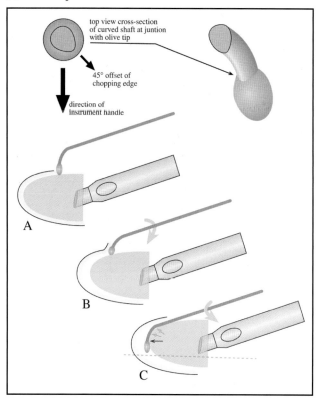

Figure 8-10. Dr. Paul Koch's stop and chop method utilized vacuum to centrally displace the heminucleus to facilitate easier placement of the chopping instrument at the nuclear periphery.

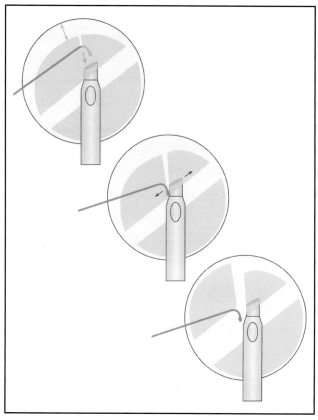

Figure 8-11. Anterior (surgical microscope) view of the stop and chop method.

is not sharp, most chopper tips have a small enough surface area to provide uncomfortably high pressure in case of inadvertent contact with the capsule. Both of these liabilities are addressed in Figure 8-10, which illustrates the use of vacuum to grip the heminucleus and pull it away from the periphery so that the chopper placement is more easily facilitated with less dissection and with better visualization of the peripheral endpoint; this maneuver was independently described by Paul Koch of the United States as the stop and chop technique and Ron Stasiuk of Australia as the mini-chop method.[4] Furthermore, a Seibel chopper (Rhein Medical, St. Petersburg, FL) is illustrated with its distal olive-shaped tip, providing a significant safety margin over a standard chopper in case of contact with the capsule due to the greater size and therefore tip surface area. Therefore, this tip also gives greater nuclear manipulating and pushing force when needed with less of a tendency to inadvertently penetrate the nucleus compared to the smaller distal tip of standard choppers. Note also the curved distal shaft, which contains the chopping edge (shown in Figure 8-10 offset for a right-handed surgeon). This curve not only engages and fits the nuclear periphery in a more anatomically correct manner relative to the abrupt right angle of a standard chopper but it also is much easier to insert and remove through the paracentesis incision.

Figure 8-11 illustrates the same stop and chop technique. Note the space between the peripheral capsule and the centrally displaced heminucleus. High vacuum is needed for a strong grip in order to move the heminucleus into this position, but once the chopper engages the periphery and is drawn horizontally toward the phaco tip, the heminucleus becomes mechanically fixated between the 2 instruments. The vacuum level at this point can conceivably be lowered to a safer and more appropriate level for carouseling phaco-aspiration of the chopped fragment with less likelihood for postocclusion surge compared to maintaining the now unnecessarily high vacuum level that was originally needed to mobilize the heminucleus centrally. A significant machine technology that allows this safe and appropriate moment-by-moment titration of vacuum (as well as other parameters) is the dual linear pedal control on the AMO Signature and the Bausch + Lomb Stellaris (Rochester, NY). A standard phaco pedal has fluidics and ultrasound located sequentially within a single plane of travel, up and down or pitch (Figure 8-12A). This configuration has 2 fundamental liabilities. First, each parameter of fluidics and ultrasound has a small range of pedal travel and therefore limited control sensitivity; pushing the pedal a small distance quickly traverses whatever range of linear control that might be present. Second, even if linear control of the vacuum is

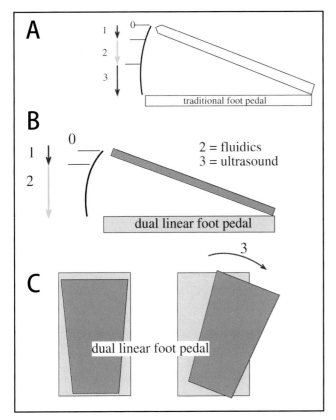

Figure 8-12. Dual linear pedal control expands the range of position 2 (fluidics) for more control sensitivity, and transposes position 3 (ultrasound) from a pitch to a yaw (sideways) motion, enabling independent control of fluidics and ultrasound.

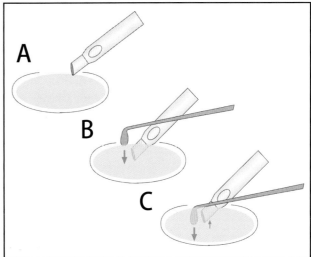

Figure 8-13. Vertical chop method, Stage 1. The phaco tip is embedded into the nuclear center with high vacuum, and the chopper vertically impales the nucleus.

present in position 2, only the maximum vacuum level is typically carried into and throughout position 3, thereby precluding a balanced moderate titration of both parameters. The dual linear pedal overcomes these liabilities by separating fluidics and ultrasound into 2 planes of pedal movement, pitch (up and down) and yaw (side to side), as seen in Figures 8-12B and 8-12C. This design offers enhanced control sensitivity because of the increased range of travel for both fluidics (either vacuum or flow) and ultrasound. Even more important, the parameters may be simultaneously and independently controlled in a linear fashion, so that the surgeon may choose high vacuum and high ultrasound for initially impaling the heminucleus, high vacuum and no ultrasound for centrally displacing the heminucleus, moderate vacuum and no ultrasound for the actual horizontal chop, and then moderate vacuum and moderate ultrasound for carouseling phaco-aspiration of the chopped fragment.

Vertical chopping, as described in detail in Chapters 3 and 4, has somewhat different phacodynamic requirements than horizontal chopping due to the different vector forces involved. As seen in Figure 8-13A, vertical chopping starts out in a similar manner to horizontal chopping in that the phaco tip is imbedded into the center of the nucleus.

However, rather than dissecting a horizontal chopper to the nuclear periphery, the vertical chopper is placed close to the center of the pupil just in front of the phaco tip. It is then pushed posteriorly to fully imbed it, as shown in Figure 8-13B, at which point continued downward force to the chopper and slight upward force to the phaco tip (both with only slight actual movement) work to begin the chop (Figure 8-13C). These chopping forces are augmented by the simultaneous horizontal movement and separation shown in Figure 8-14. By slightly rotating the nucleus 45 to 60 degrees, another chop can be quickly made to create the first fragment, and this process can be continued to divide the nucleus into 6 to 8 pieces prior to removing any one of them. The completely chopped nucleus is relatively unstable in the capsular bag, and the first piece is therefore relatively easy to remove by first impaling with the phaco tip and pulling with vacuum and then phaco-aspirating closer to the center of the chamber. This ease contrasts with the occasional difficulty of removing the first chopped fragment in a horizontal chop method that is held tightly in place by the residual ring of intact nucleus. Although the nucleus could conceivably also be first completely chopped into 6 or more fragments as described for vertical chopping, this is not as convenient because of the additional movement and dissection attendant to horizontal chopping.

The initial placement of the vertical chopper significantly affects the ease and efficiency of the procedure. Figure 8-15A shows 2 potential initial vertical chopper placements, one just distal to the phaco tip and one further from the phaco tip and closer to the capsulorrhexis edge. Note the short blue arrows superimposed on the chopper tips that represent the vector force required to penetrate this particular nuclear density. However, this force will also have the effect of inducing a torque on the nucleus around

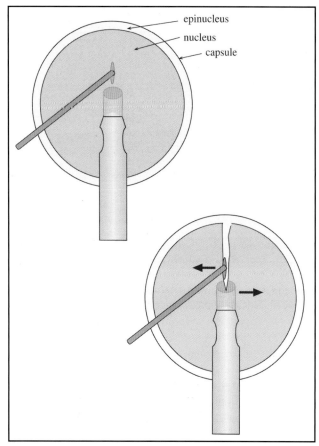

Figure 8-14. Vertical chop method, Stage 2. A slight horizontal separation of instruments completes the chop.

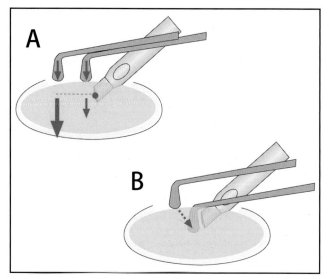

Figure 8-15. (A) Placing the vertical chopper closer to the phaco tip reduces torque that could break the vacuum seal and grip. (B) A variation of Dr. Steve Arshinoff's "slice and separate" method applied to vertical chop.

the pivot point created by the phaco tip (see blue dot). Furthermore, as dictated by Newtonian physics, torque is equal to the applied force times the lever arm, which is the distance from the applied force to the pivot point. Therefore, the more distally placed chopper will induce a greater torque (see larger blue vector arrow in nucleus) that will be more likely to break the vacuum seal at the phaco tip and preclude an efficient chop. The correct vertical chopper placement, therefore, is about 1 mm distal to the phaco tip, a position that minimizes induced torque but provides a slight buffer against the initial chopper placement, itself inducing a premature fracture plane that breaks the vacuum seal, a situation that could occur if the chopper were directly juxtaposed to the phaco tip. In Figure 8-15B, the vertical chopper is placed more distal to the phaco tip but is drawn toward the tip as it is impaled into the nucleus. This variation of Steve Arshinoff's slice and separate technique helps the chopper to "bite in" to the cataract as it progresses toward the same positional endpoint as Figure 8-15A.[5]

Even with ideal chopper placement, note the fundamentally different vector forces involved with vertical chopping as opposed to horizontal chopping in that the latter causes mechanical entrapment of the nucleus as the chopper and phaco tip are drawn horizontally together. This mechanical entrapment allows for a reduced vacuum level during the actual chop. Vertical chopping, however, utilizes opposed forces (up and down, apart) that never mechanically trap the nucleus and therefore requires a sustained high vacuum level to maintain a stabilizing grip of the nucleus until the chop is completed. Therefore, compared to horizontal chopping, the higher vacuum levels that are sustained longer until the completion of the chop can lead to more potential surge and chamber instability; recall the compensatory phacodynamic mechanisms previously discussed to deal with such postocclusion surge.

Most of the authors of this book use both horizontal and vertical methods, often within a single case, and this practice underscores the importance of correct instrument selection for each method in order to maximize efficiency and safety. Figure 8-16 illustrates both types of choppers as present on either end of the double-ended instrument manufactured for this author by Rhein Medical (#05-4065-R). In the side view, both tips are somewhat similar in that they are rounded distally. However, the top view illustrates the profound difference between them that is a direct corollary of their function in the 2 different procedures. The Seibel horizontal chopper has an olive-shaped tip that provides maximum safety in case of contact with the capsule; its large surface area minimizes the chance of inadvertent penetration because of reduced pressure at any given amount of force. This expanded surface area is also beneficial in nuclear manipulation such as rotation and cracking because the tip effectively pushes the nucleus with minimal tendency to inadvertently penetrate into it, as might the smaller tip of a standard chopper. The chopping edge on

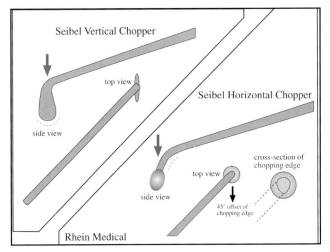

Seibel Vertical Chopper

top view

side view

Seibel Horizontal Chopper

top view

side view

cross-section of
chopping edge

45° offset of
chopping edge

Rhein Medical

Figure 8-16. The side views of the vertical and horizontal choppers are similar, but the top view reveals a dramatic difference reflective of their specialized applications within the 2 different methods.

the inner curvature effectively cleaves the nucleus when drawn in a horizontal fashion. This tip, however, would be a very poor choice for vertical chopping for the very reason that it is so effectively safe for horizontal chopping; its large surface area and subsequent high resistance to tissue penetration means that it would be very difficult to impale into the nucleus from above as is required for vertical chopping. For this purpose, vertical choppers have a relatively sharp posterior edge. However, most vertical choppers achieve this sharpness by a slim conical shape resembling an ice pick. Though this design is successful for vertical chopping, it nevertheless sacrifices the safety margin in case of inadvertent capsule contact. The Seibel vertical safety chopper addresses this issue by having a beveled edge on

the perimeter of a curved, flat distal surface. The flatness and beveled edge allow the design to work in all but the very densest, brunescent nuclei, but the rounded curve ensures that any capsule contact will be distributed over a larger surface area relative to a standard vertical chopper, thereby enhancing the safety margin and reducing the chance for inadvertent capsule penetration.

CONCLUSION

Phacodynamics offers a framework of logical reasoning with which to approach not only the various chopping techniques but all aspects of surgery. Once surgical goals are clearly defined for each step of the operation, machine parameters can be logically optimized to provide maximum safety and efficiency. Furthermore, surgical instruments can be logically chosen and applied to achieve the desired results while minimizing unnecessary movements that can prolong the case and frustrate the surgeon. These principles will ensure that the instruments and phaco machine will always be working for the surgeon in a proactive and predictable manner.

REFERENCES

1. Chang DF. *Phaco Chop: Mastering Techniques, Optimizing Technology, and Avoiding Complications.* 1st Edition. Thorofare, NJ: SLACK Incorporated; 2004.
2. Arshinoff S. ASCRS Film Festival Award Winner; 1996.
3. Fine IH. Choo-choo chop and flip phacoemulsification. In: *Phaco and Foldables.* Thorofare, NJ: SLACK Incorporated; 1997:1-3.
4. Koch P. ASCRS Film Festival Award Winner; 1993.
5. Arshinoff S. Slice and separate technique; *J Cataract Refract Surg.* 1999;25(4):474-478.

All figures in Chapter 8 have been reprinted with permission from Seibel BS. *Phacodynamics.* 4th ed. Thorofare, NJ: SLACK Incorporated; 2005.

9

Optimizing Machine Settings for Chopping Techniques

David F. Chang, MD

Machine settings—both ultrasound and aspiration—should be customized according to each surgeon's equipment, technique, and experience. The same surgeon may also adjust machine parameters according to the density of the nucleus. Simply copying someone else's settings without understanding the rationale may therefore be inappropriate. For example, the higher flow and vacuum settings of an experienced surgeon may be too aggressive for a novice. However, as phaco technology evolves, the expansive array of programming options can be intimidating. This chapter will review general concepts that should guide one making the transition to phaco chop using a peristaltic pump system.

PHACODYNAMICS: THE 4 OBJECTIVES

How much benefit is derived from modifying and customizing machine parameters? With the availability of high vacuum and advanced phaco power modulations, the advantages of such maneuver-specific specialization are significant. As with a point-and-shoot camera, the simplicity of using a fixed set of parameters for the entire case is appealing. However, just as professional photographers know how to optimize their equipment for special situations, so too can phaco surgeons. As the requirements change during the course of the case, one should dynamically modify the pump fluidics, the phaco power, and the ultrasound mode. Thanks to multiple, preprogrammed memory settings and even dual linear systems, surgeons can now use the foot pedal to seamlessly alter these parameters intraoperatively.

Every phaco technique combines multiple maneuvers with different phacodynamic requirements. As a conceptual framework for understanding fluidic and ultrasound strategies, one should consider the following 4 separate objectives that sequentially change in priority during any phaco case:

1. Sculpting efficiency
2. Impaling/holding power
3. Followability
4. Chamber stability

With the exception of sculpting, chopping and divide-and-conquer share these same objectives. If possible, one should assign a separate phaco memory setting for each objective. This allows one to preprogram a package of fluidic and ultrasound parameters that are optimized for each specific goal.

Chang DF.
Phaco Chop and Advanced Phaco Techniques: Strategies for Complicated Cataracts, Second Edition (pp 99-110).
© 2013 SLACK Incorporated.

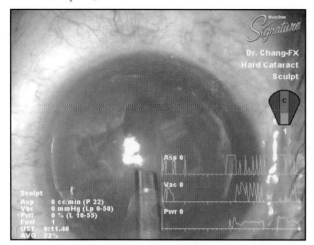

Figure 9-1. Video overlay demonstrating that during sculpting, aspiration, flow, and vacuum are kept low. The green graph shows the aspiration flow rate over time, with the left end of the timeline denoting the past and the far right end denoting the present. The blue graph shows the vacuum level over time. The yellow graph shows the ultrasound power over time. This screen captures a momentary pause during sculpting (zero power and the foot pedal is in position 1). The bottom left white numbers show the settings. In this mode, the aspiration flow rate is set at 22 cc/min, the maximum vacuum setting is 50 mm Hg, and continuous ultrasound is under linear control from 10 to 55%.

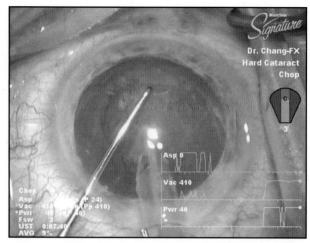

Figure 9-2. During chopping, burst mode and high vacuum (410 mm Hg) result in maximum purchase and holding power for a brunescent nucleus. At this moment (see far right of the time line) there is a single burst of 40% ultrasound (yellow graph) and the vacuum has reached 410 mm Hg (blue graph), while aspiration flow has dropped to zero (green graph).

OPTIMIZING FLUIDICS FOR CHOPPING

The first major area for parameter adjustment is pump fluidics. Of the peristaltic pump's 2 aspiration variables, flow rate (measured in cc/min) governs the pump speed and therefore the speed of the procedure. Higher flow rates better attract particles to an unoccluded phaco tip and cause vacuum to build more rapidly after the tip is occluded. However, if things are happening too quickly, one should decrease the flow rate.

Vacuum (measured in mm Hg) builds within the aspiration line in between the occluded phaco tip and the pump, and will not exceed a maximum programmed level called the vacuum limit. With a peristaltic pump, the vacuum level cannot rise to the maximum level until the tip is occluded with tissue. Clinically, vacuum determines the strength with which the phaco tip grips nuclear material. The vacuum could be increased if the pieces keep falling off.

Objective 1: Sculpting Efficiency— Fluidics

This objective applies to divide-and-conquer and stop and chop, but not to pure chopping techniques. During the sculpting stroke, the tip does not occlude as long as it keeps moving and does not become embedded within the nucleus

(Figure 9-1). This prevents the vacuum level from rising. Aspiration flow helps to keep the tip path clear of debris, which improves visibility. Eventually, the tip slows down and must submerge into the peripheral lens as it passes beneath the capsulorrhexis edge. At this point, particularly with soft lenses, a sudden rise in vacuum can cause the peripheral nucleus and equatorial capsular bag to rush into the tip. For this reason, one should operate on a low vacuum setting for sculpting. Since holding power is superfluous during sculpting, high vacuum adds unnecessary risk to this step.

Phaco Chop Objectives

With both horizontal and vertical phaco chop, there are 3 sequential steps used to remove the endonucleus. The first step is chopping the nucleus into progressively smaller fragments. Second, the phaco tip elevates and carries these fragments out of the capsular bag and into the pupillary plane. Finally, these mobilized pieces are removed by "phaco-assisted" aspiration in the supracapsular location at a safe distance from the posterior capsule. For the first 2 maneuvers, the key fluidic attribute is holding power. For the last maneuver, followability and chamber stability are the primary objectives. As stated earlier, these 3 objectives assume different priorities during the course of the case.

Objective 2: Holding Power—Fluidics

During a chop, the phaco tip performs 2 distinct maneuvers that are facilitated by high vacuum. First, the tip impales the nucleus to immobilize it against the incoming chop (Figure 9-2). A strong purchase will prevent the chopper from dislodging or torquing the nucleus. This is

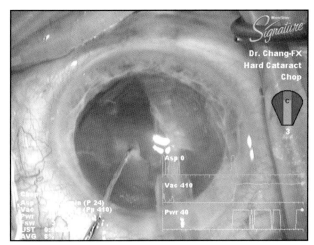

Figure 9-3. High vacuum maximizes gripping ability for moving fragments, such as during the separating maneuver following a vertical chop. At this moment (see far right of the timeline) there is a single burst of 40% ultrasound (yellow graph) and the vacuum has reached 410 mm Hg (blue graph), while aspiration flow has dropped to zero (green graph).

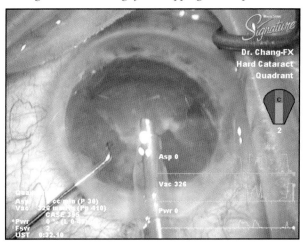

Figure 9-4. High vacuum in Quadrant setting (410 mm Hg maximum vacuum setting) provides excellent holding power for elevating fragments from the bag. At this moment (see far right of the timeline), with the foot pedal in position 2, there is partial occlusion with the vacuum level reaching 326 mm Hg.

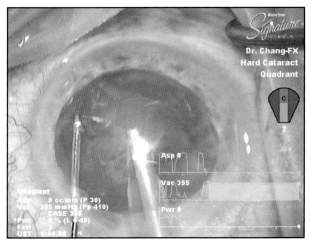

Figure 9-5. Setting for emulsifying mobile fragments utilizes transversal nonlongitudinal mode (Ellips with the Signature [Abbott Medical Optics {AMO}, Santa Ana, CA]). The CASE antisurge algorithm (see Chapter 11) reduces the vacuum level to 355 mm Hg prior to occlusion break to reduce the likelihood of postocclusion surge.

Objective 3: Followability—Fluidics

The third and final maneuver is scavenging and emulsifying the mobile chopped fragments (Figure 9-5). By increasing the force by which material is pulled through the tip, higher vacuum levels decrease the requirement for phaco energy during this stage. However, because the tip is frequently unoccluded or partially occluded, flow rate is more important here. A higher flow rate helps attract loose fragments to the phaco tip and allows the tip to re-engage a piece that momentarily deflects away. Ideally, pieces should gravitate toward a stationary and centrally held phaco tip. If there is continuing difficulty engaging mobilized fragments or if it seems as though the phaco tip must repeatedly chase pieces into the periphery, the flow rate might be too low and may need to be increased.

Objective 4: Chamber Stability—Fluidics

As progressively more of the nucleus is removed, the posterior capsule becomes increasingly exposed to the phaco tip. As the final fragments are removed, any forward trampolining of the posterior capsule is dangerous, and chamber stability becomes crucial. This is especially true if the epinucleus is thin or absent, or if the zonules are lax. Since holding power is unnecessary at this stage, high vacuum becomes a liability and should be lowered to eliminate any chance of surge (Figure 9-6). This lower vacuum setting will also be appropriate for the epinucleus and for soft nuclei, where holding power is less important.

particularly important for vertical chopping where a shearing motion is generated. Second, the tip must grip and separate one hemisection from the other (Figure 9-3). While flow rate is less important for these steps, high vacuum increases surgeon control of the chopping and separating motions. Next, the chopped fragments are elevated out of the capsular bag, with the first interlocked pieces being the most difficult to extract. As it does for elevating quadrants in the divide-and-conquer technique, high vacuum maximizes holding power for this step (Figure 9-4).

Postocclusion Surge

As stated earlier, high vacuum provides 2 sets of advantages that benefit all techniques. First, it increases the strength with which a nuclear piece is held at the tip. Second, it increases the mechanical force with which material is drawn through the phaco needle. This can decrease the requirement for ultrasound energy.

The unwanted phenomenon of postocclusion surge limits how high the vacuum can be safely set. Following tip occlusion, vacuum quickly rises to the maximum pre-programmed limit. Surge occurs as this occlusion breaks and fluid from the anterior chamber rushes into the tip to equilibrate the lower pressure environment of the aspiration line. A minor degree of surge produces a momentary flicker of iris movement. Severe surge may collapse the chamber.

Postocclusion surge is probably the most common cause of posterior capsule rupture during nuclear emulsification. The amount of nucleus present affects the risk. A mild to moderate degree of surge is of little consequence with enough remaining nucleus shielding the tip. However, as progressively more nucleus is removed, the same amount of surge can cause the posterior capsule to vault into the unguarded phaco tip.

At the same machine settings, nuclear density and the phaco method also affect the amount of surge seen. Because surge results from occlusion break at the maximum vacuum level, tip occlusion is required. This explains why surge may be absent with sculpting, but quite evident with chopping where the phaco tip impales the nucleus during every chop. At the same vacuum setting, surge is often more evident with soft nuclei than with dense nuclei. As fragments are being evacuated, the softer lens material molds to and quickly plugs the phaco tip. Maximum vacuum levels are rapidly and repeatedly attained. In contrast, when brunescent fragments are emulsified, their rigid contours neither conform to nor completely plug the phaco tip (see Figure 9-4). These partial occlusions generate fewer instances of surge because maximum vacuum levels are not reached.

Surge Prevention Strategies

Phaco machine manufacturers have devised numerous strategies for minimizing surge. The goal has been to provide surgeons with the advantages of high vacuum without the dangers posed by surge. One set of strategies addresses infusion. These range from bottle height extenders or irrigation tubing with increased lumen diameter, to forced infusion pumps available with combined anterior-posterior segment machines.

With respect to outflow, so-called *smart* pump technologies have been one of the most important innovations. The Millennium (Bausch + Lomb, Rochester, NY) was the first machine to offer dual linear foot pedal control over

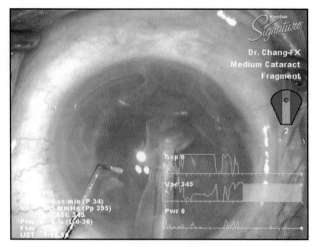

Figure 9-6. For the mobilized fragments, switching to the fragment setting employs the antisurge algorithm (CASE) in conjunction with transversal ultrasound. This effectively prevents postocclusion surge despite an initial and momentarily high vacuum level (395 mm Hg), by reducing the vacuum to 345 mm Hg prior to occlusion break (see far right of the time line). This setting can be used for mobile nuclear fragments once the posterior capsule becomes exposed.

ultrasound and vacuum. Now available with the Stellaris (Bausch + Lomb) and the Signature in venturi mode (AMO), this feature allows the surgeon to lower vacuum just prior to when the occlusion is about to break. The occlusion mode programming of the AMO Sovereign and Signature machines can automate a similar change in pump speed pre- and postocclusion. Latest generation phaco machines use fluid venting to create an entirely closed, bubble-free aspiration system. Using microprocessors to monitor vacuum at remarkably frequent intervals, a dedicated onboard fluidic computer regulates the pump speed in order to minimize surge.

Another approach involves aspiration tubing where reducing the compliance diminishes surge. Virtually all companies have evolved toward stiff-walled, low compliance tubing with narrower lumens that resist collapse.[1] This option may be called *high vacuum* tubing or cassette.

A final set of surge-reducing strategies involve phaco tip design. The overall resistance to outflow is determined by the narrowest caliber lumen in the aspiration system, which is usually the internal diameter of the phaco needle. Micro phaco needles (21- or 20-gauge instead of 19-gauge) reduce surge in this way.[2] The flare tip designs produced by Alcon Laboratories (Fort Worth, TX) improve holding power by pairing a larger diameter tip opening with a narrower shaft.[3,4] Finally, the Alcon advanced bypass system (ABS) tip reduces surge by creating a shunt flow behind the occluded tip.[5] This reduces air-venting, which results in lower compliance of the aspiration system.

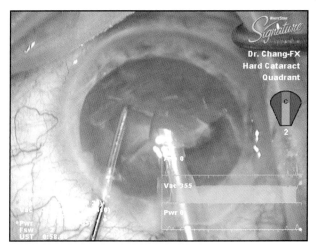

Figure 9-7. Surge test. A fragment is held in foot pedal position 2 until the vacuum limit is reached (355 mm Hg here). As the piece is emulsified and occlusion breaks, the surgeon gauges the amount of surge.

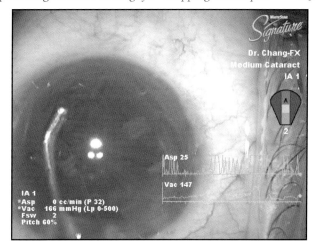

Figure 9-8. A medium level of vacuum grips and holds the cortex. At this moment in time, the surgeon is using linear control of vacuum (range 0 to 500 mm Hg) to achieve a level that grips the cortex (166 mm Hg) without evacuating it through the tip.

Determining the Vacuum Limit Through the "Surge Test"

After becoming familiar with the surge prevention features of their particular phaco system, surgeons should customize his or her individual parameters using the following surge test. To facilitate tip occlusion, a soft-medium density nucleus should be used. One starts with a low flow rate and their preferred quadrant setting, which is the vacuum limit used for quadrant emulsification in divide-and-conquer. With most of the nucleus still present, one holds an impaled nuclear fragment in the center of the pupil until the maximum vacuum setting is reached, identified by a beeping tone (Figure 9-7). Ultrasound is then applied. As the occlusion breaks, one gauges the amount of iris movement caused by any resulting surge. To reduce surge, one can raise the bottle height, decrease the flow rate, or reduce the maximum vacuum setting.

If there is no surge, the vacuum setting is increased by 20% to 25%. By repeating this step, one will eventually discover an unacceptable amplitude of surge. At this point the maximum "safe" vacuum level has just been exceeded; the vacuum limit must be lowered. Slight chamber bounce during the initial chopping maneuvers is tolerable as long as there is enough nucleus present to hold the posterior capsule back. However, as the last pieces of nucleus are removed and the posterior capsule is exposed, surge must be completely eliminated. The surge test teaches the surgeon what vacuum limits can be safely used for each of these steps.

Fluidics for Removing Epinucleus and Cortex

For epinucleus and cortex, the main fluidic objective is being able to aspirate lens material without ensnaring the capsule. Careful control of vacuum is the key. This is best achieved by using linear control of vacuum in foot pedal position 2 (FP2) for these steps. For epinucleus, this can be configured in a dedicated phaco memory setting. A reasonably high flow rate helps to attract material to the tip. However, the resulting rapid vacuum rise time reduces the surgeon's reaction time.

With linear control, one generally uses 3 different vacuum levels during cortical clean-up. When first trying to draw cortex to the tip without catching the capsule, low vacuum is safer. To loosen and strip the cortex, one needs increased vacuum to grasp the cortical "handle" without letting it go. However, excessive vacuum results in premature evacuation of the cortex. A medium level of vacuum that grips but does not ingest the cortex is needed (Figure 9-8). Finally, a high vacuum level safely evacuates the mobilized cortex once the aspirating port is safely facing the cornea and is located in the center of the pupil.

The same vacuum principles apply to aspirating the epinucleus with the phaco tip under linear control. When fishing for the epinucleus peripherally, the vacuum should be kept low (eg, to 50 mm Hg) to prevent aspirating the capsule. To draw the epinucleus centrally, one increases the vacuum hold (eg, 100 mm Hg) to avoid releasing it (Figure 9-9). Maximum vacuum (eg, 200 mm Hg) is used to flip or aspirate the shell once the phaco tip is in the safe, central zone. These sample vacuum settings apply to a 20-gauge phaco tip. Linear control of vacuum in FP2 allows the surgeon to continuously vary the vacuum levels with linear foot pedal control.

OPTIMIZING ULTRASOUND FOR CHOPPING

Ultrasound Power

All machines provide surgeons with linear control of ultrasound power in FP3. This allows one to vary the power according to the density of each nucleus. Many surgeons misunderstand how the machine produces increasingly more power. As the pedal is depressed, it is not the frequency of vibration that changes, but rather the axial stroke length of the oscillating tip. One hundred percent power means that the phaco tip is vibrating back and forth with maximum stroke length. Fifty percent power means that the axial needle stroke is only half as long.

While learning to sculpt, every surgeon recognizes that the higher the power, the better the tip cuts. This is because progressively more cavitational energy is created. However, this creates a corresponding tendency to use excessive power while emulsifying mobile fragments. Contrary to sculpting, the nucleus is not fixated and nuclear emulsification requires aspiration to pull the piece toward the tip. However, the greater the stroke length of the phaco tip, the greater the mechanical repelling force that will be generated. Thus, if one is experiencing poor followability when emulsifying a dense fragment, one should avoid the natural reflex to increase phaco power, which usually exacerbates the chatter. Instead, the counterintuitive response of decreasing power may improve followability by decreasing the repelling force of the tip. Like tuning a radio dial, the surgeon should use the foot pedal to find the most efficient power level (and therefore stroke length). Along the power continuum, this is the "sweet spot" between having too little power to cut and excessive phaco tip stroke length that repels nuclear fragments.

In addition to creating greater repelling force, maximum power levels also generate the most frictional heat and cavitational energy. Lowering the risk of incisional burn and endothelial cell loss are equally important goals of minimizing the ultrasound power level when possible.

Ultrasound Power Modulation

Power modulation refers to how and in what pattern ultrasound is delivered in FP3. Clinically, there are 4 longitudinal phaco power modulations commonly used—continuous mode, burst mode, pulse mode, and hyperpulse

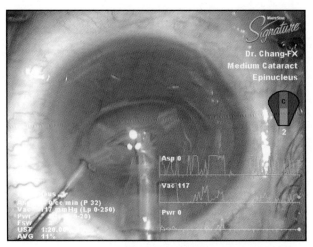

Figure 9-9. Linear control of vacuum in FP2 (range 0 to 250 mm Hg) allows one to find that medium level of vacuum (117 mm Hg) that grips the epinucleus without consuming it. This vacuum level allows the epinucleus to be flipped.

mode. Torsional (OZil, Alcon Laboratories) and transverse (Ellips, AMO) are both nonlongitudinal phaco power modulations. All produce different tissue effects that can either facilitate or impede the phaco objective desired.

Objective 1: Sculpting Efficiency— Continuous Mode

Continuous mode is uninterrupted ultrasound and produces maximum cavitational energy. This mode is typically used for sculpting for this reason. Cavitational waves emanate ahead of the vibrating tip and have the ability to disrupt material with minimal contact from the phaco tip. This is ideal for sculpting grooves where overly deep tip penetration risks contact with the underlying posterior capsule. High power ultrasound can make the deepest lamellae of nucleus seemingly melt in front of the sculpting tip. However, this mode also delivers the most ultrasound heat and energy into the eye. As described in the following section, hyperpulse—if available—can also be used for sculpting. Flow rate must be high enough to scavenge debris and maintain clear visibility (see the sidebar titled, *Pearls for Sculpting Brunescent Nuclei*).

Objective 2: Impaling/Holding Power—Burst Mode

These powerful cavitational waves of continuous ultrasound are a distinct disadvantage when the surgeon is trying to grip tissue with the phaco tip. With a toothpick, a single stab works best to impale a piece of melon. Further wiggling of the toothpick only serves to weaken the purchase. With brunescent nuclei, a continuously vibrating phaco tip tends to core out a small cavity around the tip, eroding the

PEARLS FOR SCULPTING BRUNESCENT NUCLEI

When sculpting a large brunescent nucleus, excessive movement of the nucleus may weaken the zonules. The surgeon must therefore monitor whether excessive nuclear displacement is occurring during sculpting strokes. To address excessive movement, the surgeon should either increase ultrasound power, sculpt along a shallower path, or advance the tip more slowly. The surgeon must also recognize if a murky cloud of fluid appears in front of the tip. If enough retentive OVD admixes with brunescent nuclear material, the resulting sludge-like emulsate might occlude the phaco tip. This will usually occur when ultrasound commences, such as with sculpting. If the tip is completely blocked there can be no fluid outflow, and this will prevent any gravity fed inflow of irrigation fluid. The cessation of all fluid flow alongside a vibrating phaco needle will cause an immediate incision burn. The first warning sign of significant phaco tip occlusion during sculpting may be a cloud of milky emulsate, which is not immediately cleared by the obstructed aspiration line. Seeing this, the surgeon must stop immediately to assess whether there is any clogging of the aspiration line or phaco tip. Finally, with a brunescent lens, it is best to momentarily aspirate any OVD directly above the anterior lens surface prior to commencing sculpting in order to avoid this situation from occurring.

seal. A peristaltic pump cannot generate high vacuum if the tip does not stay embedded and occluded.

Burst mode is a power modality that was first introduced with the Diplomax (AMO). It is now available with most phaco equipment platforms. Burst mode is able to deliver a single momentary pulse of phaco energy.[6,7] Bursts can be delivered individually or in rapid succession via surgeon foot pedal control. By embedding the tip without losing the surrounding tight seal, individual, successive bursts of phaco are ideal for impaling and gripping dense nuclear material for chopping (see Figures 9-2 and 9-3).

Burst mode delivers a fixed level of power that is preset on the machine console (panel control) rather than with the foot pedal. Therefore, this preset power should be varied according to the density of the nucleus. High power burst mode may be dangerous for soft nuclear sections in the bag; it may penetrate too aggressively if the power setting is too high.

Objective 3: Followability—Pulse Mode

The maximal cavitational force of continuous mode is also counterproductive for emulsifying mobile nuclear fragments. "Chatter" refers to the rattling and bouncing movement of nuclear pieces as they alternately contact and separate from the phaco tip. This results from the shifting balance of opposing forces of suction (pump) and repulsion (tip oscillation) acting upon nuclear material. As explained earlier, excessive phaco power and stroke length actually kick nuclear particles away.

In pulse mode, each pulse of phaco, or "ON" time (ON-T), is followed by an equally long pause of "OFF" time (OFF-T). Compared to continuous mode (which is always on), pulse mode interrupts the tip oscillation 50% of the time. Having these rest periods therefore reduces heat and energy delivery by cutting the phaco time in half. In addition, the pump aspiration force competes with the tip repelling force only 50% of the time. Compared to continuous mode, pulse mode improves followability by favorably shifting the balance between these opposing forces at the tip.

Hyperpulse Mode

In 2001, AMO introduced a new power modulation for the Sovereign machine called WhiteStar technology.[8] This author first coined the term *hyperpulse* to convey the ability of dramatically increased pulse frequency to leverage the aforementioned advantages of pulse mode.[9] Alternatively called ultrapulse, micropulse, or microburst, this technology is now offered with the AMO, Alcon, and Bausch + Lomb platforms.[10-17]

Hyperpulse represents a paradigm shift from traditional pulse mode in 2 ways. First, it can be programmed at rates ranging from 30 to 100 pulses per second (pps). It is this rapid interruption and fragmentation of phaco time that reduces heat build-up at the tip. Cadaver studies have demonstrated that even with the irrigation clamped, the heat build-up remains below the clinical threshold for producing a wound burn.[10-13] Most importantly, the pulses of phaco utilize traditional ultrasound with the full power continuum. Thus, there is no functional loss of cutting efficiency with brunescent tissue.

The second major enhancement introduced with hyperpulse was the ability to alter the duty cycle, which refers to the percentage of time that ultrasound is active while in foot pedal position 3. Compared to the uninterrupted ON-T of continuous mode, pulse mode interrupts these "ON" pulses with equally long rest periods of "OFF" time. Duty cycle expresses the percentage of time "ON" and is equal to ON-T divided by (ON-T + OFF-T). The duty cycle for continuous mode is 100% and for pulse mode is 50%, indicating that pulse mode reduces ultrasound delivery by a factor of 2. This is true whether one uses 3 or 6 pps.

In hyperpulse mode, the duty cycle can be further varied by lengthening or shortening the rest periods. For example, following a 6 m/sec phaco pulse with a 12 m/sec rest period creates a 33% duty cycle and 55 pps. A 24 m/sec rest period would create a 20% duty cycle and 33 pps. These settings are a dramatic departure from traditional pulse mode (eg, 4 pps = 125 m/sec pulse followed by a 125 m/sec rest = 50% duty cycle). The overall effect of hyperpulse with duty cycle reduction is to dramatically reduce heat and energy delivery without any loss of cutting efficiency.[13,14,16] This is another way of saying that continuous mode phaco is an inefficient way of delivering far more energy than is necessary to accomplish the task.

Nonlongitudinal Phaco

Arguably the most important advance in ultrasound technology during the past decade was Alcon's torsional phaco.[18-28] Dubbed "OZil," this technology utilizes oscillating, rotational movement of the phaco tip in place of longitudinal strokes. To generate cutting action, a bent tip—such as a Kelman tip or one of several variations—is used. This utilizes mechanical action rather than cavitation to cut nuclear material. Compared to axial tip movement, torsional phaco provides the efficiency of cutting with oscillatory movements in both directions. AMO was the next company to introduce its nonlongitudinal technology and called it transversal ultrasound, or "Ellips," during which an elliptical movement of the phaco tip is created. Because the tip movement traces an ellipse along with some slight longitudinal motion, a straight phaco tip can be employed (see Figure 9-5). There are several major benefits to nonlongitudinal phaco. The ability of the tip to cut throughout its entire cycle of movement improves cutting efficiency and reduces ultrasound time.[18-22] As with a lower duty cycle, this reduction in ultrasound energy reduces heating of the incision.[23,24,28] There is also a dramatic reduction in repelling force associated with a purely axial movement of the phaco tip.[25] As a result, chatter that is normally seen with brunescent fragments is significantly diminished.[19] This not only improves followability, but also lessens endothelial cell trauma caused by particle turbulence at the tip.[18-20] While burst mode is still effective for impaling dense nuclei during chopping, nonlongitudinal phaco is ideal for emulsifying mobile fragments (see Figure 9-6).

Effective Phaco Time

The ability to dynamically adjust phaco power and change power modulations creates tremendous variability in ultrasound delivery during an individual case. Effective phaco time (EPT) attempts to quantify this by expressing what the equivalent phaco time would have been in continuous mode with 100% power. For example, 2 minutes of continuous phaco time (100% duty cycle) using 25% power would give a 30-second EPT (120 s ÷ 4). Switching to pulse mode (50% duty cycle) would have further cut the EPT in half (15 seconds). Hyperpulse with a 33% duty cycle would have cut the EPT by one third (10 seconds).

EPT is primarily affected by the power level used. Since there is no industry-wide standard for measuring stroke length, EPTs cannot be used to accurately compare machine performance from 2 different manufacturers. However, EPT is useful for comparisons within the same system. For instance, EPT will reflect the difference in ultrasound energy used for different grades of nucleus (brunescent versus soft) with different techniques (divide-and-conquer versus chop) and with different power modulations (hyperpulse versus traditional pulse or continuous mode). EPT can also be used to compare the performance of new machines with predecessors from the same manufacturer.

Choosing Phaco
Tips for Chopping

Among the basic options for phaco tips, there are different shapes (straight versus Kelman curved), different calibers (standard 19-gauge versus micro 21- or 20-gauge), and different tip bevel angulations (0, 15, 30, and 45 degrees). There are specialty tips (eg, diamond-shaped tip or Dewey rounded edge tip) that improve cutting ability or alter sharpness as well. Designs to reduce surge, such as the flare tip and the ABS tip, were discussed previously. Each of these different tip configurations may be associated with advantages or disadvantages depending on the situation. However, unlike other parameters such as flow rate, vacuum level, phaco power, and power mode, the tip is the only variable that cannot be easily changed during the case. Therefore, one must compromise in choosing characteristics that might be alternately advantageous or disadvantageous at different stages of the procedure.

Standard Versus Micro Tips

The first consideration is the size of the needle. It is helpful to separately consider the width of the shaft apart from the size of the tip opening. This is because the same shaft size can be paired with a smaller (0-degree bevel) or larger (30-degree tip) area opening in the tip.

Compared to the standard 19-gauge tip, a 20-gauge micro needle has a narrower lumen that restricts flow.[2] The increased fluid resistance reduces surge and prevents material from rushing in as fast compared to a standard diameter needle shaft. Slowing things down in this way helps when one wants to carefully control what enters the tip. This is important during aspiration of the epinucleus or when aspirating the thin, crumbling pieces of soft nucleus in the bag. However, like drinking a milkshake through a cocktail straw, using a micro tip can seem painfully sluggish when large chunks of nucleus need to be evacuated.

The size of the phaco tip opening also influences performance. While 19-gauge phaco needles have larger tip openings than 20-gauge needles, it is also possible to increase the surface area of the tip's mouth by going from a 0- or 15-degree bevel to a 30-degree bevel. A flare tip goes even further in combining the advantages of a large surface area mouth with a narrower shaft.[3,4]

Gripping strength is proportionate to the surface area of the tip opening. At any given vacuum level, a larger mouth provides more holding power than a smaller mouth. A wider opening is also better for followability. Like a larger baseball glove, a big mouth can better catch particles as they tumble toward the tip. Tissue can more readily mold into a larger opening, resulting in quicker occlusion. Thus, chatter and reduced holding power are the liabilities of a smaller tip opening.

There are, however, significant advantages to a smaller-sized mouth. Like a narrower profile spike, a micro tip can more easily penetrate and incise a brunescent nucleus for vertical chop. Because a smaller phaco tip reduces particle size within the emulsate, downstream clogging of the line is less likely. Finally, one also has greater control over what tissue can enter a small tip. Surgeons prefer a 0.3-mm port instead of a 0.5-mm port for cortical aspiration because it is easier to avoid ensnaring the capsule with the smaller opening. The same principle holds for using the phaco tip to aspirate epinucleus or thin nuclear fragments abutting the posterior capsule.

The most impressive advantage of a small tip opening is the ability to occlude the tip with minimal tissue penetration (see Figure 9-6). The larger the tip surface area, the more deeply the entire tip must be embedded to create a vacuum seal. If one is trying to elevate a thin, soft segment of nucleus out of the peripheral bag, this is a disadvantage. If part of the fragment crumbles apart, one may need to penetrate dangerously close to the capsule to occlude the tip. In contrast, a small mouth tip would only need to penetrate superficially before the entire opening is embedded enough to build vacuum. This allows one to pluck soft, thin pieces from the periphery with diminished risk of overpenetration.

Smaller gauge phaco tips reduce the incidence of clogged tubing, more easily penetrate dense nuclei, and are easier to maneuver and occlude. By restricting flow, they reduce surge and prevent overly abrupt tissue aspiration. The smaller tip opening provides greater selective control over what and how much tissue enters the mouth, which is also an advantage. However, these gains in safety come at the expense of reduced holding power and sluggish evacuation of large blocks of nucleus. Each surgeon must therefore prioritize which among these characteristics is most important.

If one uses a 20-gauge phaco needle, one should employ a 30-degree rather than a 0-degree tip. The latter is simply too small an opening when paired with a micro tip. Compared to the parameters for a standard 19-gauge tip, one must raise the aspiration flow rate to offset the more restrictive lumen size. One must also increase the vacuum to compensate for reduced holding power from the smaller tip surface area. Using hyperpulse with reduced duty cycles or torsional or transversal ultrasound can greatly improve the followability that is otherwise compromised by the small tip design. Finally, just as meat is cut into smaller pieces for a child, one should chop the nucleus into smaller fragments to better match the size of the tip. These measures allow surgeons to enjoy the greater safety of smaller phaco tips without noticeably sacrificing speed and efficiency. Of all the variables discussed, going from a standard 19-gauge to a 20-gauge phaco tip may yield the single biggest improvement in posterior capsule rupture rate. The smaller tip is therefore strongly encouraged for residents and surgeons transitioning to phaco chop.

Phaco Tip—Bevel

Besides the aforementioned issues of the surface area of the opening, the bevel design also impacts function.[29] Using hydrophone experiments, William J. Fishkind, MD, FACS has shown that during continuous ultrasound, an exit cone of cavitational micro bubbles streams from the tip in the direction of the tip bevel.[30] During sculpting, a 30-degree tip used bevel up is therefore directing this stream of micro bubbles toward the endothelium. For chopping, as discussed in Chapter 8, orienting the bevel toward the flat surface of the nucleus produces a more rapid occlusion (Figure 9-10). Some surgeons initially impale with the tip oriented bevel down for this reason.[31]

This author prefers to chop with the bevel facing to the right. This is because as the hemisections are laterally separated to propagate and complete the fracture, the phaco tip is always displacing the impaled portion to the right (see Figure 9-3). Angling the bevel to the right takes full mechanical advantage of the longest portion of the tip. During fragment emulsification, particle turbulence is also directed by the bevel. For this reason, it may make sense to emulsify mobile particles with the bevel directed slightly sideways, rather than toward the cornea. As the posterior capsule becomes increasingly exposed, one can turn the bevel toward the cornea so that it is facing away from the capsule.

Fishkind's experiments also show that the curved Kelman tip directs cavitational energy downward, rather than forward. This correlates with the superiority of this tip design for sculpting. However, this sharply curved tip is less well suited for chopping, particularly if the surgeon actively changes the direction of the bevel as described previously.

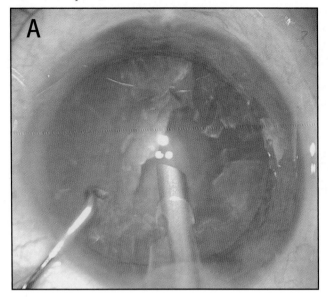

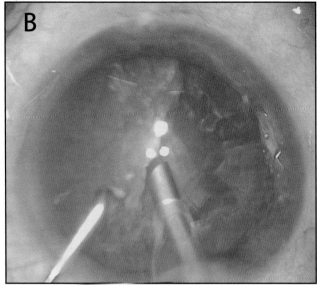

Figure 9-10. Occlusion of a 30-degree beveled tip is more difficult with a bevel aimed (A) away from the nuclear surface, (B) rather than toward the surface.

PHACODYNAMIC GAME PLAN FOR CHOPPING

The following game plan integrates these concepts into a unifying chopping paradigm for a peristaltic pump system. A separate memory setting is used to preset a package of parameters for each of the 4 phacodynamic objectives: sculpting (if needed), impaling/holding power, followability, and chamber maintenance. In addition, the entire set of parameters can be made slightly more or less aggressive according to differing nuclear density. Many machine platforms allow surgeons to preprogram different parameters for each of these memory settings according to nuclear density (Grades 1 through 4), that can then be altered with a single button function.[32]

Sculpting Memory Setting

As discussed in Chapters 4 and 5, sculpting a partial trench or pit is helpful for brunescent nuclei and is a transitional step to pure nonstop chopping. In the sculpting memory setting, one can use either continuous mode or a hyperpulse mode. The power setting should be high enough so that the tip cuts, rather than pushes the nucleus. Cavitation helps in sculpting the deepest lamellae by reducing the requirement for tip penetration. Vacuum should be kept low (but not 0) in order to avoid an abrupt vacuum rise as the tip occludes in the periphery (see Figure 9-1). Flow rate must be high enough to scavenge debris and maintain clear visibility.

Impaling/Holding Power Memory Setting

Burst mode and high vacuum combine to provide a maximally strong purchase of the nucleus. Holding power is helpful for chopping and for elevating the initial fragments out of the capsular bag (see Figures 9-2, 9-3, and 9-4). Since burst mode needs to be set at a high fixed panel power for impaling dense nuclei, the power for burst mode should be lowered for soft-medium nuclei. The highest vacuum level safely attainable (as determined by the surge test) is utilized for this stage. Flow rate is less important because so little tissue is removed.

Followability Memory Setting

Efficient emulsification of mobile, dense fragments requires a higher flow rate. Even though the occlusions are usually partial during this stage, a high vacuum setting still increases the aspiration force which can proportionately lower the amount of ultrasound required. One should therefore increase the flow rate from the preceding setting and decrease the vacuum limit slightly[33] (see Figure 9-6). This offsetting vacuum reduction will prevent an increase in surge due to higher flow. The lower vacuum holding power will still suffice to chop and elevate the residual nucleus (see Figure 9-6).

With respect to power modulation, nonlongitudinal phaco reduces energy delivery and improves followability by minimizing the repelling cavitational forces from the tip. The resulting decrease in chatter and particle turbulence is most noticeable with dense nuclei, particularly if a micro tip is used. To reduce the duty cycle, traditional pulse mode or hyperpulse can be paired with nonlongitudinal phaco.

Chamber Stability/Epinucleus Memory Setting

Even slight postocclusion surge is unacceptable when the posterior capsule is exposed to the phaco needle, so vacuum should be significantly reduced for this step.[33] This allows a slightly higher flow rate to be employed for epinuclear aspiration (see Figure 9-9). Linear control of vacuum in FP2 provides even greater control as the phaco needle is used primarily for aspiration. One can switch to this setting as the final sharp fragments of a dense nucleus are being removed. Alternatively, for very soft nuclei, one can use this setting for the entire case. This is because very soft nuclei more resemble the epinucleus in their consistency and behavior.

MACHINE-SPECIFIC RECOMMENDATIONS

Modern phaco machine platforms offer an ever-expanding array of fluidic and power modulation options that specifically benefit chopping. The availability of so many innovative choices and features creates a double-edge sword. While this permits a degree of phacodynamic customization that was never before possible, it also requires the surgeon to comprehend and preprogram an intimidating number of variables. In other words, such progress comes at the expense of simplicity.

The next 3 chapters are intended to help the reader configure a chopping program for his or her specific phaco machine. Individual chapters cover the 3 most popular machine platforms in North America (in alphabetical order)—the Alcon Infiniti, the AMO Signature, and the Bausch + Lomb Stellaris. These chapters are not intended to be a shopper's guide to buying a new machine. Rather, the goal is to help users understand the unique options available with their machine for chopping and to provide them with a starting point for configuring and later customizing their personal parameters. Although sample programs differ from one machine to the next, each is based upon the principles discussed in the current and preceding chapters.

REFERENCES

1. Wilbrandt HR. Comparative analysis of the fluidics of the AMO Prestige, Alcon Legacy, and Storz Premiere phacoemulsification systems. *J Cataract Refract Surg.* 1997;23:766-780.
2. Davidson JA. Performance comparison of the Alcon Legacy 20000 1.1 mm Turbosonics and 0.9 mm MicroTip. *J Cataract Refract Surg.* 1999;25:1382-1385.
3. McNeill JI. Flared phacoemulsification tips to decrease ultrasound time and energy in cataract surgery. *J Cataract Refract Surg.* 2001;27:1433-1436.
4. Davison JA. Performance comparison of the Alcon Legacy 20000 straight and flared 0.9 mm Aspiration Bypass System tips. *J Cataract Refract Surg.* 2002;28:76-80.
5. Davidson JA. Performance comparison of the Alcon Legacy 20000 1.1 mm Turbosonics and 0.9 mm Aspiration Bypass System tips. *J Cataract Refract Surg.* 1999;25:1386-1391.
6. Fine IH, Packer M, Hoffman RS. Use of power modulations in phacoemulsification. Choo-choo chop and flip phacoemulsification. *J Cataract Refract Surg.* 2001;27:188-197.
7. Badoza D, Fernandez Mendy JF, Ganly M. Phacoemulsification using the burst mode. *J Cataract Refract Surg.* 2003;29:1101-1105.
8. Fine IH, Packer M, Hoffman RS. New phacoemulsification technologies. *J Cataract Refract Surg.* 2002;28:1054-1060.
9. Chang DF. "Can cold phaco work for brunescent nuclei?" *Cataract & Refractive Surgery Today.* 2001;1:20-23.
10. Soscia W, Howard JG, Olson RJ. Bimanual phacoemulsification through 2 stab incisions. A wound-temperature study. *J Cataract Refract Surg.* 2002;28:1039-1043.
11. Soscia W, Howard JG, Olson RJ. Microphacoemulsification with WhiteStar. A wound-temperature study. *J Cataract Refract Surg.* 2002;28:1044-1046.
12. Donnenfeld ED, Olson RJ, Solomon R, et al. Efficacy and wound-temperature gradient of WhiteStar phacoemulsification through a 1.2 mm incision. *J Cataract Refract Surg.* 2003;29:1097-1100.
13. Olson RJ, Kumar R. White Star technology. *Curr Opin Ophthalmol.* 2003;14:20-23.
14. Osher RH, Injev VP. Thermal study of bare tips with various system parameters and incision sizes. *J Cataract Refract Surg.* 2006;32:867–872.
15. Fishkind W, Bakewell B, Donnenfeld ED, Rose AD, Watkins LA, Olson RJ. Comparative clinical trial of ultrasound phacoemulsification with and without the WhiteStar system. *J Cataract Refract Surg.* 2006;32:45-49.
16. Braga-Mele R. Thermal effect of microburst and hyperpulse settings during sleeveless bimanual phacoemulsification with advanced power modulations. *J Cataract Refract Surg.* 2006;32:639–642.
17. Osher RH, Injev VP. Microcoaxial phacoemulsification Part 1: laboratory studies. *J Cataract Refract Surg.* 2007;33:401–407.
18. Liu Y, Zeng M, Liu X, Luo L, Yuan Z, Xia Y, et al. Torsional mode versus conventional ultrasound mode phacoemulsification; randomized comparative clinical study. *J Cataract Refract Surg.* 2007;33:287–292.
19. Davison JA. Cumulative tip travel and implied followability of longitudinal and torsional phacoemulsification. *J Cataract Refract Surg.* 2008;34:986–990

20. Berdahl JP, Jun B, DeStafeno JJ, Kim T. Comparison of a torsional handpiece through microincision versus standard clear corneal cataract wounds. *J Cataract Refract Surg.* 2008;34:2091–2095.

21. Rękas M, Montés-Micó R, Krix-Jachym K, Kluś A, Stankiewicz A, Ferrer-Blasco T. Comparison of torsional and longitudinal modes using phacoemulsification parameters. *J Cataract Refract Surg.* 2009;35:1719–1724.

22. Vasavada AR, Raj SM, Patel U, Vasavada V, Vasavada VA. Comparison of torsional and microburst longitudinal phaco emulsification: a prospective, randomized, masked clinical trial. *Ophthalmic Surg Lasers Imaging.* 2010;41:109–114.

23. Han Y, Miller K. Heat production: longitudinal versus torsional phacoemulsification. *J Cataract Refract Surg.* 2009;35:1799-1805.

24. Jun, B, Berdahl JP, Kim T, Thermal study of longitudinal and torsional ultrasound phacoemulsification: tracking the temperature of the corneal surface, incision, and handpiece. *J Cataract Refract Surg.* 2010. 36: 832-837.

25. Fernández de Castro LE, Dimalanta RC, Solomon KD. Bead-flow pattern: quantitation of fluid movement during torsional and longitudinal phacoemulsification. *J Cataract Refract Surg.* 2010;36:1018–1023.

26. Reuschel A, Bogatsch H, Barth T, Wiedemann R. Comparison of endothelial changes and power settings between torsional and longitudinal phacoemulsification. *J Cataract Refract Surg.* 2010;36:1855–1861.

27. Cionni RJ, Crandall AS, Felsted D. Length and frequency of intra-operative occlusive events with new torsional phacoemulsification software. *J Cataract Refract Surg.* 2011; 37:1785–1790.

28. Vasavada AR, Vasavada V, Vasavada VA, Praveen MR, Johar SR, Gajjar D, Arora AI. Comparison of the effect of torsional and microburst longitudinal ultrasound on clear corneal incisions during phacoemulsification. *J Cataract Refract Surg.* 2012;38:833-839.

29. Frohn A, Dick HB, Fritzen CP. Corneal impact of ultrasound and bevel position in phacoemulsification. *J Cataract Refract Surg.* 2002; 28:1667-1670.

30. Packer M, Fishkind W, Fine IH, Seibel B, Hoffman R. The physics of phaco: a review. *J Cataract Refract Surg.* 2005;2(31):424-431.

31. Joo CH, Kim YH. Phacoemulsification with a bevel-down phaco tip: phaco-drill. *J Cataract Refract Surg.* 1997; 23:1149-1152.

32. Nixon DR. Preoperative cataract grading by Scheimpflug imaging and effect on operative fluidics and phacoemulsification energy. *J Cataract Refract Surg.* 2010;36:242-246

33. Vasavada AR, Raj S. Step-down technique. *J Cataract Refract Surg.* 2003;29:1077-1079.

Please see companion narrated videos on the accompanying Web site at
www.Healio.com/phacochopvideos

10

Optimizing the Alcon Infiniti for Chopping

David F. Chang, MD and Barry S. Seibel, MD

The Infiniti vision system (Alcon Laboratories, Fort Worth, TX) is based on low compliance peristaltic-pump fluidics (Figure 10-1). This surgical system offers 3 different cataract removal technologies: conventional (longitudinal) ultrasound (US), torsional US (commercially known as OZil), and AquaLase. In this chapter we are focusing primarily on the use of torsional US, as it has been the clear preference of Infiniti surgeons. The system also provides a disposable 800 cuts per minute (cpm) 20-gauge and a 2500 cpm 23-gauge anterior vitrectomy cutter.

TORSIONAL ULTRASOUND

One of the most important advances introduced with the Infiniti is torsional phaco called OZil.[1-11] As the name suggests, torsional US achieves cutting by having the US tip move in an ultrasonically oscillating torsional direction (from side to side) about the axis of the phaco needle shaft. This side-to-side movement of the US tip shears the engaged nuclear material. Conversely, longitudinal ultrasound cuts the nucleus using the traditional "jackhammer" movement. One advantage of the side-to-side motion is significantly lower repulsion of the engaged nuclear material

and thus less dependence on elevated vacuum and flow settings to keep the nuclear material at the tip's cutting plane.

The OZil IP, in which "IP" is commercially branded as *Intelligent Phaco* torsional technology, adds a user selectable feature that introduces a short longitudinal pulse when a predetermined vacuum is reached and torsional ultrasound is commanded. The interjection of the short longitudinal pulse at the right moment facilitates the continuous aspiration flow through the ultrasound needle and better positions material at the shearing plane of the tip for optimized cutting. This feature has also been shown to minimize the risk of inadvertent tip occlusion during nuclear emulsification when using flared tips.[10] Therefore, the IP feature is especially important when emulsifying brunescent cataracts.

The surgeon can select both the duration and intensity of the IP longitudinal ultrasound pulse. The 3 IP system adjustable parameters are vacuum threshold, phaco pulse, and longitudinal/torsional ratio (Figure 10-2). For purposes of illustration, assume sample settings of 95%, 10 ms, and 1.0, respectively. The vacuum threshold allows the surgeon to control the vacuum level at which the IP feature is engaged. The 95% percent setting indicates that IP will engage if 95% of the vacuum preset is reached and the user is in foot pedal position 3 (FP3). As an example, if

Chang DF.
Phaco Chop and Advanced Phaco Techniques: Strategies for Complicated Cataracts, Second Edition (pp 111-126).
© 2013 SLACK Incorporated.

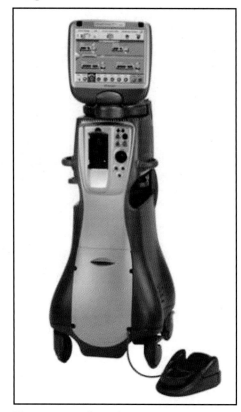

Figure 10-1. Infiniti phaco system.

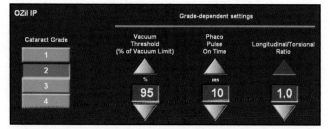

Figure 10-2. Infiniti screen showing torsional IP adjustable parameters.

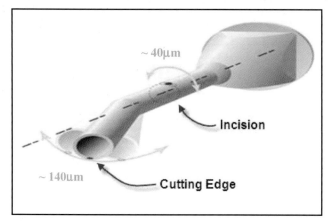

Figure 10-3. Stroke amplification with a bent phaco tip showing the greater radius of cutting edge movement relative to the radius of shaft movement within the incision.

the maximum preset vacuum is set to 400 mm Hg, then IP will engage at 380 mm Hg (95% of 400) when in FP3. The phaco pulse of 10 ms refers to the time duration of the longitudinal pulse. The longitudinal/torsional ratio indicates the magnitude of the longitudinal US power that the pulse would engage at, expressed as a ratio to the active (at the time) torsional amplitude (note that "power" refers to the longitudinal US magnitude, whereas amplitude is refers to the torsional US magnitude). As an example, if the vacuum threshold is triggered and the user is in FP3 with a delivered torsional amplitude of 50%, then the longitudinal pulse will also be delivered at 50% US power (with the default ratio set at 1.0). If the ratio is selected as 0.8, in this example, the longitudinal pulse will deliver 40% US power (50% × 0.8 = 40%).

Torsional ultrasound works best with a Kelman style 22-degree bent phaco tip, which provides a mechanical amplification of the torsional motion generated about the central axis of the phaco needle shaft. Surgeons can select from several different types of bent tips with different degrees of bend and bevel angles, according to personal preference and technique. The benefit of the stroke amplification provided by a bent-style tip is that the surface of the oscillating needle shaft within the incision only moves a fraction of the amount of the tip's cutting edge movement due to the bent tip's greater radius measured from the axis

of rotation (Figure 10-3). This reduction in intraincisional needle movement (and resulting friction) will vary depending on the specific tip used. The Infiniti's calculation of cumulative dissipated energy (CDE) represents the total US energy delivered in FP3 (both phaco and torsional) and approximates a 60% reduction in energy at the incision associated with torsional phaco. CDE is therefore calculated as: (Phaco Time × Average Phaco Power) + (Torsional Time × 0.4 × Average Torsional Amplitude).

ULTRASOUND POWER MODULATIONS

The Infiniti offers several power modulation options including continuous, pulse, and burst modes. Continuous mode delivers US power in FP3 in a continuous, uninterrupted fashion. This simplest of modes can be programmed to come with either fixed or linear control of power in FP3.

Pulse Mode

Pulse mode interrupts continuous US delivery with rhythmic rest periods in FP3. As with continuous mode, the power intensity can be delivered in linear or fixed fashion. There are 2 important parameters related to pulse mode.

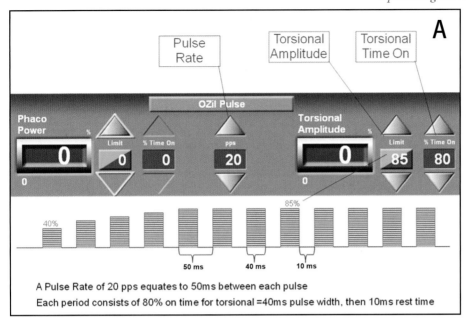

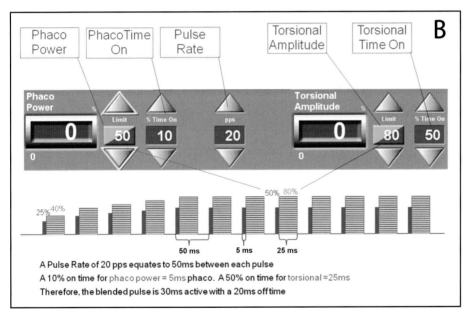

Figure 10-4. Illustration of phaco tip modulation for a 20 pps pulse mode with pure torsional ultrasound. (A) The longitudinal phaco power modulation is on the left side of the settings screen and is set to 0. Torsional phaco modulation is on the right side of the settings screen. The bottom graph shows the linear increase in pulse magnitude as the foot pedal is depressed further in a linear fashion in FP3. As shown on the settings screen, the preset limits in this illustration are 0% for longitudinal phaco power and 85% for torsional amplitude. In the bottom graph, the pulse starts with 40% torsional and gradually increases to the maximum presets of 85% torsional as the pedal is depressed linearly in FP3. (B) The longitudinal phaco modulation is in blue and on the left side of the settings screen. Torsional phaco modulation is in red and is on the right side of the settings screen. The bottom graph shows the linear increase in pulse magnitude as the foot pedal is depressed further in a linear fashion in FP3. As shown on the settings screen, the present limits in this illustration are 50% longitudinal phaco power and 80% torsional amplitude. In the bottom graph, the pulse starts with 25% longitudinal and 40% torsional and gradually increases to the maximum presets of 50% longitudinal and 80% torsional as the pedal is depressed linearly in FP3.

The first is the "pulse rate," which determines how many pulses are delivered per second (pps). The second parameter is duty cycle, which is defined as the ratio of the ultrasound "ON" time (ON-T) to the total time interval while in FP3.

Two pulse mode examples are provided in Figure 10-4. The first example shows a 20 pps setting with pure torsional ultrasound, which delivers 20 pulses in 1 second (Figure 10-4A). This equates to having a pulse occur once every 50 ms (1000 ms/20 pulses). If the duty cycle were set to 50%, then the phaco ON-T would equate to 25 ms during every 50 ms pulse. The 80% duty cycle in the sample illustration means that the phaco ON-T of 40 ms alternates with 10 ms of "off" time (OFF-T) during every 50 ms pulse.

The system also allows both longitudinal and torsional ultrasound to be blended together while in pulse mode, as shown in Figure 10-4B. In this example, a blended application with 10% ON-T for the longitudinal and 50% ON-T for the torsional results in a longitudinal US power duration of 5 ms (10% of 50 ms pulse cycle). The torsional US duration would be 25 ms (50% of 50 ms pulse cycle). Figure 10-4 illustrates these 2 time values as well as how the pulse magnitude increases in a linear fashion (with progressive foot pedal depression in FP3) to the preset limits of 50% longitudinal power and 80% torsional, as discussed in the illustration.

ULTRA CHOPPER THEORY AND TECHNIQUE

Alan S. Crandall, MD

Introduction

There are many strategies available to reduce complications during phacoemulsification. These include chop techniques and power modulations such as OZil IP (Infinity) and Ellips Transversal FX (Signature). There are also devices, such as capsule support systems, capsule tension rings, and capsular dye. However, cataracts that are physically hard (LOCS Grade 4 or worse) can still present significant risk for difficulties such as capsule tears, corneal wound burns, and endothelial cell damage.

There have been many previous attempts to soften hard nuclei with nonphaco technologies. One example was to inject warmed balanced salt solution with the Site phaco system. AquaLase technology and early laser phaco machines shared a similar problem of being ineffective with hard nuclei. Femtosecond lasers are able to aid in these dense cataracts but there are significant cost issues that preclude the use of the laser for all patients, and certainly in third-world situations where hard lenses are extremely common. One could argue that small incision extracapsular techniques should be used in this arena. However, if there is a way to increase the safety factor and maintain the smaller phaco incision, one should consider it. Luis J. Escaf, MD, of South America modified a phaco tip by squeezing or pounding to flatten the tip and used it to "cut" the nucleus.

Instrument Design

The cutting portion of the tip is 3 mm (Figure 10-SB1). The tip can be used with different sleeves to allow for incision size preferences (Figure 10-SB2) and can be used through small incisions (Figure 10-SB3).

Technique

The tip is placed on the phaco handpiece just as a standard phaco tip would be. It is then turned. Once it has been used to score the nucleus, it is removed and a standard tip is put on the handpiece. The goal is to cut thin grooves in the nucleus and to do so with as little nuclear displacement as possible. There is both longitudinal and torsional movement of the tip and one can titrate the 2 movements to maximize the effect. Typically, the author uses surgeon control with 100% maximum available power, which allows good control and sufficient power on demand. Knowing the tip is 3-mm long allows one to carefully go deep centrally. The realization that one does not need to be deep peripherally to prechop the nucleus increases the

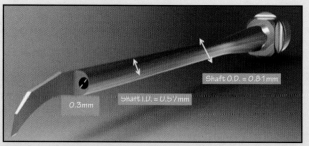

Figure 10-SB1. The design is similar to standard Kelman phaco tip. Figure shows aspiration, hole, and shaft diameter.

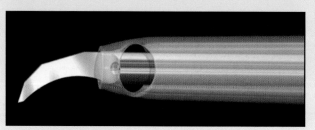

Figure 10-SB2. Any size tubing may be used for incision girth.

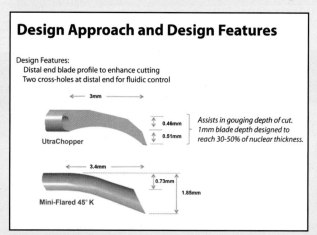

Figure 10-SB3. Although sharp, it is similar to the Kelman tip.

safety of this method. One can make as many grooves as one wants; creating quadrants works well for most lenses. However, with harder lenses the author may cut the nucleus into as many as 6 or 8 pieces. The Akahoshi prechopper (Asico, Westmont, IL) is then used to split the nucleus, while making sure that the fibrotic posterior fibers are completely separated.

Complications

Because the tip moves at ultrasonic speed and is very sharp, there are risks such as iris or corneal incisional burn. The causes of wound burn are no different with the ultra-chopper than with a standard phaco tip. Risk factors include too tight a wound and tip occlusion with viscoelastic. The sharp Ultrachopper tip can cut the iris and the anterior or posterior capsule. Therefore, the surgeon should move the tip slowly and constantly reassess the anatomy by rotating the nucleus as with a divide-and-conquer technique.

Burst Mode

Burst mode provides single bursts of power lasting anywhere from 5 to 500 ms. A 50-ms long burst is a good starting point with a minimum off time of 100 ms. A newer option with the Infiniti is linear burst mode. This gives the surgeon simultaneous linear foot pedal control (in FP3) of both the power and frequency of the bursts. Depressing the pedal further increases phaco power and progressively shortens the "OFF" interval between bursts. Burst mode can be paired with high vacuum whenever the surgeon wants to maximize holding power and purchase. Because the surgeon can preset a different burst power range according to nuclear density and further vary the power with linear foot pedal control, burst can be used at both the softest and the firmest ends of the cataract density spectrum.

Smart Pulse

When the duration of ultrasound pulse in FP3 becomes less than 20 ms, a proprietary algorithm is activated. This is indicated by the Smart Pulse message, which appears on the screen below the power bar. With the Smart Pulse algorithm, US power will be initiated at either 10% or half of the commanded power (whichever is lower) prior to generation of the main power pulse. This low-powered pulse contributes a negligible amount of energy to the procedure, but it allows the computer to determine the optimum operating parameters for the main power pulse, making it more efficient for even the shortest duration of ultrasound.

FLUIDICS

The selected fluidic parameters are important for optimizing surgical efficiency. With a peristaltic pump, the 2 primary fluidic parameters are aspiration flow rate and preset vacuum limit. The aspiration flow rate setting controls the rate at which the material is attracted to the tip. Higher aspiration settings would result in a faster rate of nuclear attraction which translates to faster removal of material. Higher aspiration settings, however, might also momentarily shallow the anterior chamber, produce more anterior chamber turbulence, and consume more irrigation fluid. Surgeons wishing to mimic venturi-like performance would select high aspiration flow rates. It should be noted that most venturi systems do not have separate aspiration flow control and thus produce high flow rates as a result of a given commanded system vacuum.

The vacuum limit varies the force with which the nuclear material is held at the fully occluded tip. For example, for the divide-and-conquer surgeon, a low vacuum setting is preferred for sculpting because holding power is not important at this stage. By comparison, when one disassembles the quadrants or performs nuclear chopping,

higher vacuum settings provide the greater vacuum holding power needed for these maneuvers.

Surge Control

A goal for every modern phacoemulsification system is to maximize chamber stability and minimize postocclusion surge.[12-14] The higher the operating vacuum, the greater the potential degree of surge will be following an occlusion break. One critical characteristic for minimizing postocclusion surge is the system compliance, which correlates with the collapsibility of the aspiration tubing between the handpiece and the peristaltic pump. Systems or tubing with greater compliance will experience greater postocclusion surge and inferior chamber stability when there is an occlusion break at the US tip.[14]

The Infiniti reduces system compliance with an innovative pump design. Instead of wrapping flexible tubing over the pump-roller mechanism, the Infiniti pump features a rigid fluid channel coupled with silicone only at the peristaltic roller contact points. This also improves the machine's ability to accurately monitor vacuum levels within the tubing and to more rapidly adjust the pump speed accordingly. Another fluidic feature is the ability to monitor infusion line pressure via a separate dedicated diaphragm sensor. This sensor will warn surgeons when infusion flow ceases, such as when the irrigation bottle is empty or the irrigation tubing inadvertently becomes detached from the handpiece. The combination of this next generation "smart pump" and the low compliance aspiration system dramatically reduces postocclusion surge. This allows surgeons to safely work at significantly higher vacuum levels than previously possible. The Intrepid Plus tubing incorporates improvements that lower compliance and provide good chamber stability without sacrificing ergonomics.

Consumable Packs

The Infiniti system can be used with 2 types of single-use packs or fluid management systems (FMS). The original Infiniti FMS introduced tubing that provided optimal compliance in the middle to lower vacuum operating ranges. The newer generation Intrepid Plus FMS has a lower compliance aspiration tubing that resists constriction at all vacuum levels. This tubing pack provides better postocclusion surge reduction when higher vacuum levels are employed.

Linear Control of Aspiration Parameters

As discussed in Chapter 9, linear control of vacuum in FP2 is useful for removing the epinucleus when the phaco tip functions more like an irrigation-aspiration (I/A) instrument. Most phaco machines provide the option of having linear control of either aspiration flow or vacuum in FP2. The Infiniti can also provide simultaneous linear vacuum and linear flow control in FP2—a feature that could be called *bilinear*. Some surgeons select this option for epinucleus and cortex removal where the speed and strength of aspiration can be restrained in the periphery (lower flow and vacuum) and then maximized in the safe central zone (higher flow and vacuum) Bilinear aspiration can be programmed in FP2, but not during ultrasound in FP3 (when no linear control of aspiration flow or vacuum is possible). A disadvantage of bilinear control, as described, is that lower flow rates produce slower rise times. For this reason, other surgeons may prefer a fixed flow rate but linear control of vacuum in FP2, as described in Chapter 9.

USER INTERFACE

Like other advanced phaco systems, the Infiniti offers full programmability that can be individualized for different surgeons, different techniques, and different nuclei. Primary control of the system parameters for the Infiniti is via a user-interface touch screen.

Within each program one can configure and name 3 or more phaco memory settings, which the manufacturer calls "steps." These are labeled according to the objective for which they are customized (eg, "sculpt," "chop," "quadrant," and "epi"). For someone transitioning to chopping, the surgeon should program 3 or 4 phaco memory settings using these steps in the appropriate sequence. "Chop" would typically have higher vacuum settings (and correspondingly higher bottle height to counter potential postocclusion surge) than "quadrant." Therefore, a surgeon might use "chop" for vertical chopping and then "quadrant" to aspirate and emulsify the resulting free chopped fragments.

Foot Pedal Controls

The foot pedal has several programmable horizontal and vertical toe switches (Figure 10-5). The various switches in the figure, designated with "none," can be programmed with the exception of the left lateral switch, which is dedicated to reflux. Consider having the right lateral horizontal switch control the procedural steps. When this switch is momentarily activated, the steps advance in a forward order, allowing the surgeon to cycle between the different phaco memory settings. Auditory voice confirmation of the new procedural step setting is given each time there is a change. An additional feature for the foot pedal is the enabling of detents and/or vibration in the transitions between pedal positions to give the surgeon additional feedback.

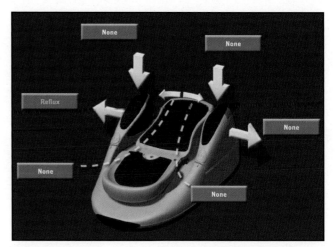

Figure 10-5. Infiniti foot pedal programmability options.

In addition to using these 4 phaco memory settings within each program, one can also vary the settings according to the grade of nucleus (Grades 1 through 4) (see Figure 10-2). While the case is in progress, the machine panel, remote control, or foot pedal can be used to change from a Grade 2 to Grade 3 nucleus, for example. This changes all 4 "step" memory settings to a different set of parameters that are preselected for an appropriate nucleus density. One possible way to utilize this feature is to vary the parameters as follows:

- *Grade 2 settings.* This is used for the default setting. These would represent power and fluidic settings for a soft to medium density nucleus.

- *Grade 3 settings.* These would represent power and fluidic settings for a denser 3+ nucleus. Compared to the Grade 2 settings, they might include higher phaco power and higher vacuum and flow rate.

- *Grade 4 settings.* These would represent power and fluidic settings for an ultra-brunescent nucleus. Higher power, higher vacuum, and a faster rise time might be advantageous for the densest nuclei.

- *Grade 1 settings.* These could be "slow motion" contingency settings for a complicated case, such as one with very weak zonules. They would feature lower aspiration flow and vacuum settings to slow the pace of the procedure. These settings could also be used in the event that phaco is continued following a posterior capsular rent.

The foot pedal can be configured to allow the surgeon to change from one package of nuclear grade settings to another. For example, if the 2 lateral side gates are used to move between the steps (eg, from chop to quad). Pressing the top of the right gate can be used to change between different nuclear grade settings (eg, from Grade 2 to Grade 3).

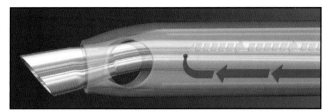

Figure 10-6. ABS ultrasound tip showing irrigation fluid flowing external to the needle (solid arrows) shunting through the 0.18-mm bypass port into the needle (broken arrows).

Ultrasound Tips

Depending on the preferred technique, Infiniti users can choose from a variety of tip configurations including standard, tapered, Kelman, mini-flared, micro tips, Mackool, and mini. Most of these tip configurations are available in the 0.9-mm size, which refers to the diameter at the tip opening. The most commonly used tip with the torsional system is the 0.9-mm 45-degree bevel mini-flared Kelman tip. Another popular tip is the 0.9-mm mini tip (which is actually a 0.8-mm tip). Both tips provide a full 20-degree shaft bent and a sharp 45-degree bevel that is ideal for effective tissue shearing with torsional ultrasound. For surgeons more accustomed to straight ultrasound tips, the Partial 12 degree Kelman bent ultrasound tip may be easier to transition to when adopting OZil for the first time. However, the partial 12 Kelman tips are not as effective for sculpting in hard nuclei. Due to the smaller angle bend, these tips produce a smaller displacement at the shearing plane compared to the full Kelman tip configuration. The resulting reduction in cutting efficiency can be compensated for by increasing the torsional amplitude or the power setting. One must remember, however, that increasing the power generates more frictional heat within the incision.[6,15]

A key benefit of torsional phaco with a bent tip is the reduction of heat generated at the incision when compared to traditional longitudinal phaco. The shaft bend with the Kelman tip results in amplified motion at the shearing plane, but minimal torsional motion of the shaft within the incision. Needless to say, both longitudinal and torsional phaco can produce wound burns if the tip becomes occluded (eg, OVD), but torsional technology provides the advantage of a greater margin of safety with higher phaco powers and tighter incisions.[7]

The Aspiration Bypass System (ABS) ultrasound tips are offered with both the Legacy and Infiniti.[16] The 0.18 mm bypass port opening located on the side of the phaco tip becomes "active" upon tip occlusion (Figure 10-6). At this point, a small amount of flow (4 to 11 cc/min, depending on fluidic settings) starts to pass through the bypass opening so that outflow never ceases during tip occlusion. This supplemental flow through the ABS port during occlusion

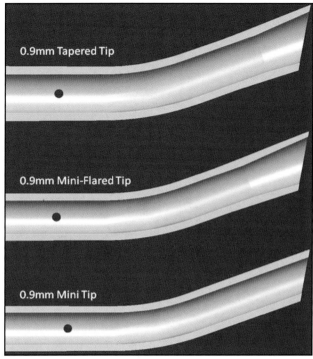

Figure 10-7. Flared tip configurations.

likely cools the tip within the incision under ultrasound load and should improve its thermal safety profile.

The flared ultrasound tip pairs a narrower shaft with a wider tip diameter in order to increase holding power at the tip[17,18] (Figure 10-7). As discussed in Chapter 9, a narrower shaft lumen can reduce surge by slowing the ability of tissue to rush into and through the tip. However, this also slows the aspiration of larger pieces of nucleus. Because reduced tip surface area reduces holding power for any given vacuum setting, the flared tip marries a larger mouth (for improved gripping) with a narrower shaft (for reduced surge).

There are some relative disadvantages to the flared tip design for chopping, however. A larger diameter tip opening means that one must embed the tip more deeply to occlude it. The wider tip profile may also be less conducive to incising into a brunescent lens. Finally, the internal bottleneck within the flared tip can give rise to momentary occlusion with brunescent tissue. Other tip configurations such as the mini-flared, micro tips, tapered, and mini have smaller transitions between the mouth and shaft of the tip. One should therefore choose a tip based on whether having a larger or a smaller "mouth" is more important (see Chapter 9 discussion on pros and cons of smaller or larger diameter tip openings). The tapered tip features a narrow shaft and a slightly wider mouth. This represents a compromise between the classic flared tip design and a purely straight phaco needle.

Figure 10-8. Irrigation sleeve options.

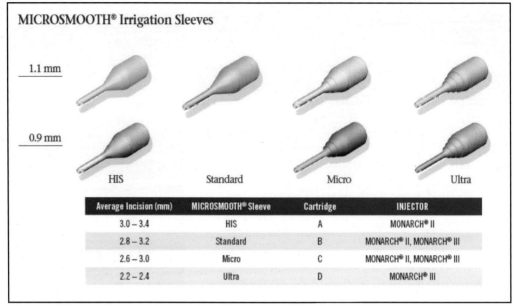

The insulated Mackool tip has specific features designed to reduce the potential risk of an incisional burn. While this tip configuration has merits for sculpting and continuous mode phaco, the use of power modulations such as pulse, burst, and torsional modes for chopping already minimize the risk of wound burn with standard tips.

Infusion Sleeves

The infusion sleeve configuration also affects fluidic performance. Which of the several sleeve options is selected depends on the incision size and the ultrasound tip so as to provide the proper balance of outflow and inflow through the incision (Figure 10-8). Larger diameter infusion sleeves increase irrigation in-flow in order to reduce postocclusion surge and provide better thermal protection.[15] The Ultra Sleeve is designed for incisions measuring 2.2 to 2.4 mm. The Micro Sleeve should be used for incisions measuring 2.6 to 3.0 mm, and the High Infusion Sleeve (HIS) covers incisions measuring 3.0 to 3.4 mm (see Figure 10-8). Certain IOLs might require enlargement of the original phaco incision (eg, from 2.4 to 3.0 mm for a Crystalens). In such situations, the original Ultra Sleeve might need to be changed to a Standard or High Infusion Sleeve to avoid excessive incisional leakage during I/A removal of viscoelastic.

Dynamic Rise

The Infiniti system allows surgeons to vary the slope of the vacuum rise curve by programming the dynamic rise (DR) setting. This feature can be set for either a faster (+) or a slower (-) rate of vacuum rise upon occlusion onset. With the new FMS cassettes, DR does not add much value, and it is recommended that it be set to 0.

SAMPLE SETTINGS

As discussed in Chapter 9, sample settings are meant to serve as a starting point from which surgeons can subsequently customize different parameters based on individual preference and differences in technique. Suggested starting parameters are offered in the following figures for transitioning surgeons according to different phases of stop and chop or pure chopping (Figures 10-9 to 10-16). This is followed by the personal settings of one of the authors (Barry S. Seibel, MD) with an explanation of why certain characteristics were selected for each memory setting. This will illustrate the customizability of fluidic and ultrasound parameters, which should be the eventual goal of all phaco surgeons.

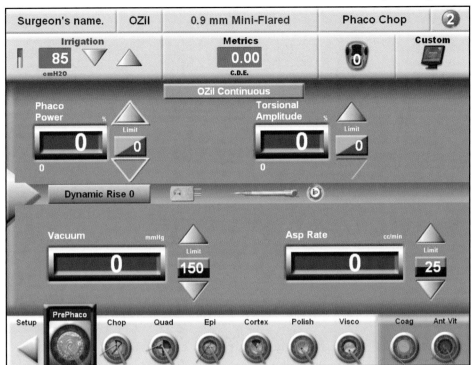

Figure 10-9. Sample PrePhaco setting. The first step, regardless of the phaco method, is to clear working space for the phaco tip. This is one example for such a setting. While the default OZil setting is 20% linear, there is generally no need to apply power during this step. Note that regardless of the phaco machine, it is important to remove some OVD just above the lens to form a fluid filled working space before applying ultrasound.

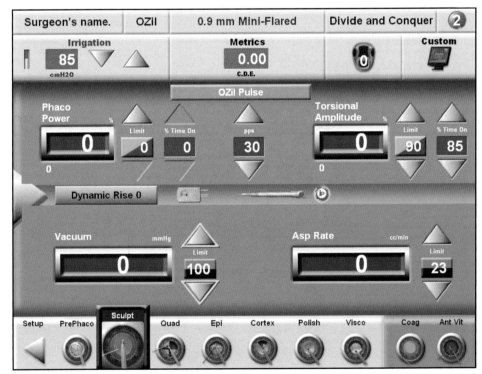

Figure 10-10. Sample settings for sculpting. The OZil handpieces offer 2 energy modes: traditional longitudinal ultrasound and torsional oscillatory phaco. Depending on individual preference, surgeons may use either energy mode for sculpting. Note that sculpting with OZil may be easier using the 45-degree mini-flared Kelman or 45-degree mini tips. Sculpting with partial Kelman tips is generally more difficult. Bottle height—78 to 90 cm H$_2$0; aspiration—20 to 25 cc/min; vacuum—80 to 120 mm Hg. Surgeons may opt for linear, linear with minimums, or fixed control of aspiration and vacuum. Ultrasound (continuous): torsional amplitude 80 to 100%; phaco power 60%. Ultrasound (pulse): torsional power 80 to 100%, 30 pps, 85% ON-T; phaco power 60% or 75% on, 70 pps.

Figure 10-11. Sample chop settings. Surgeons can use a quadrant setting to chop and remove lens fragments, or separately designate a setting for chopping. For the latter, consider using a brief initial power application (eg, burst) to impale the nucleus and to elevate the first lens fragment out of the capsular bag. Bottle height—95 to 110 cm H$_2$0; aspiration—30 cc/min; vacuum—300 to 380 mm Hg. Surgeons may opt for linear, linear with minimums, or fixed control of aspiration and vacuum. Ultrasound (burst)—power: 15% minimum to 45% maximum; 50 to 80 ms ON-T, and 25 ms OFF-T. Torsional (burst): 0% minimum to 75% maximum; 100 ms ON-T, and 10 ms OFF-T. Surgeons may opt for linear or linear with minimums for ultrasound.

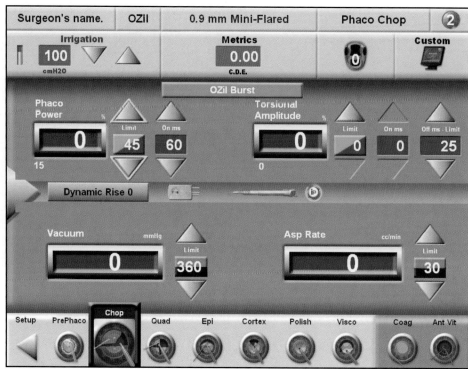

Figure 10-12. Sample quadrant settings. In the quadrant setting, torsional phaco is the optimal choice. High levels of vacuum are not needed with OZil IP due to the reduction in repelling force with torsional phaco. Lower or higher fluidic settings can be selected, depending on personal preference. Bottle height—95 to 110 cm H$_2$0; aspiration—28 to 45 cc/min; vacuum—250 to 380 mm Hg. Surgeons may opt for linear, linear with minimums, or fixed control of aspiration and vacuum. Ultrasound (continuous or pulse [pulse setting 30 pps; 85% ON-T]); torsional amplitude 85 to 100%, 85% ON-T. Surgeons may opt for linear or linear with minimums for ultrasound.

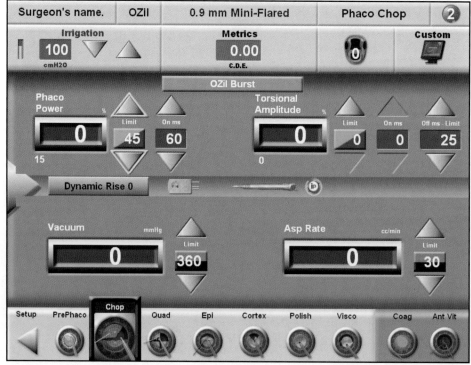

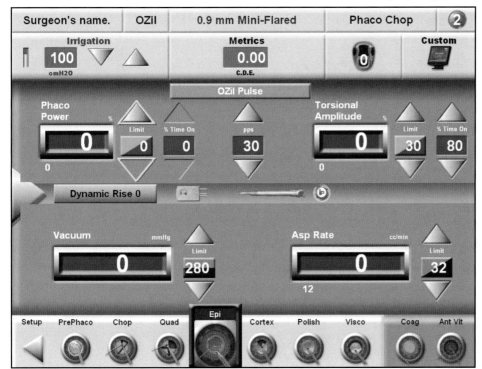

Figure 10-13. Sample epinuclear settings. Bottle height—100 cm H$_2$0; aspiration—23 to 25 fixed or linear with 12 minimum to 32 cc/min maximum; vacuum—250 to 300 mm Hg fixed or linear with minimum vacuum set to 50 mm Hg. Surgeons may opt for linear or linear with minimums for aspiration and vacuum. Ultrasound (pulsed): 20 pps; torsional amplitude 30% linear.

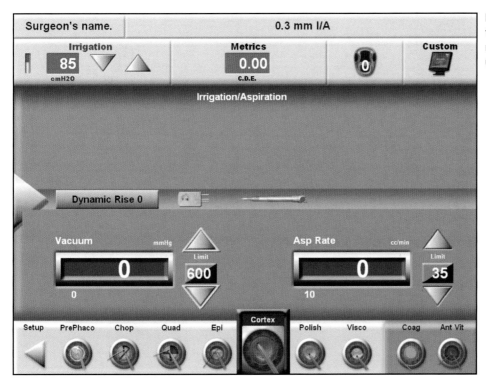

Figure 10-14. Sample I/A settings with a 0.3 mm tip; aspiration—fixed: 30 cc/min; vacuum—linear 30 to 650+ mm Hg.

Figure 10-15. Sample capsule polish settings. Many surgeons may elect to use a silicone or polymer I/A tip for capsule polishing. Flow and vacuum settings should be lowered as with the sample settings.

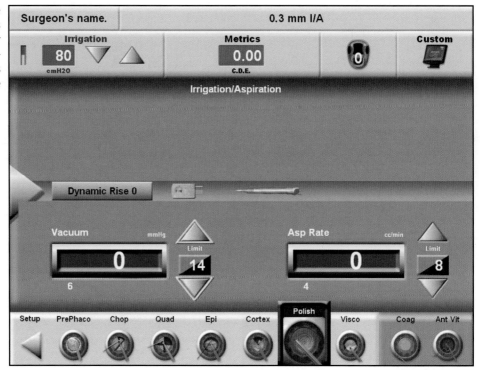

Figure 10-16. Sample OVD removal settings.

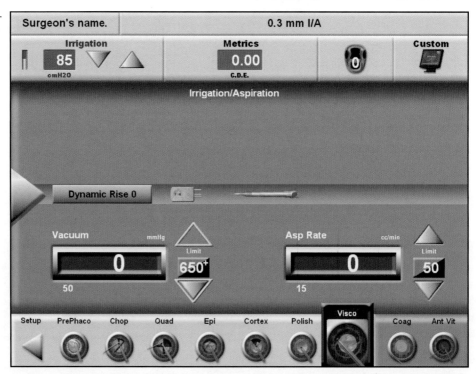

PERSONAL SETTINGS OF DR. BARRY SEIBEL

Notes: Intrepid Plus Tubing, 0.9-mm 30-degree bevel Mini-Flared OZil 12 needle (Figures 10-17 to 10-21).

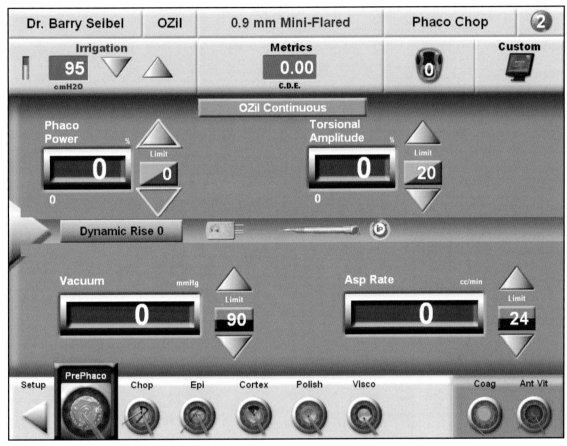

Figure 10-17. Prechop settings. Note upper right corner "2" indicating Grade 2 cataract (medium density). Note the various modes at the bottom of the window, with PrePhaco highlighted to indicate the initial stage of clearing central viscoelastic for fluid turnover as well as removal of anterior epinucleus to expose the endonucleus for chopping. Although only OZil is used at this mode, IP is always engaged to provide longitudinal bursts as needed to help clear occlusions that could otherwise lead to potential incisional burns. Note also that both vacuum limit and aspiration rate are panel (ie, fixed) controlled, not linear, as indicated by the horizontal graphic behind the numbers (as opposed to a diagonal graphic like in the ultrasound settings which indicated linear control). The settings of 90 mm Hg vacuum limit and 24 cc/min aspiration rate are modest but should be sufficient for the stated goals of prephaco, and as such panel control ensures that these parameters are met as soon as FP2 is engaged. Using linear control might risk inadequate amounts of these presets.

Figure 10-18. Seibel Grade 2 chop. This memory setting utilizes high linear vacuum so the surgeon may titrate gripping force to nuclear density after the phaco tip has been appropriately embedded. The panel control of 40 cc/min aspiration rate (note horizontal graphic) ensures a consistent rise time and responsiveness to pedal input when titrating vacuum, as well as brisk followability when phaco-aspirating chopped fragments. Recall that these linear versus panel modulations are relevant only in that pedal position; ie, linear vacuum control is present in FP2 but once FP3 is entered and ultrasound is engaged, the vacuum limit becomes the maximum setting, with the exception of dual linear pedal control as in the Bausch + Lomb Stellaris or AMO Signature. Note that OZil has been increased to 100% linear control for chopping, but is still modulated with IP for longitudinal burst to help clear potential line clogging. Note also the high bottle height to help mitigate postocclusion surge in light of the higher vacuum limit used for chopping.

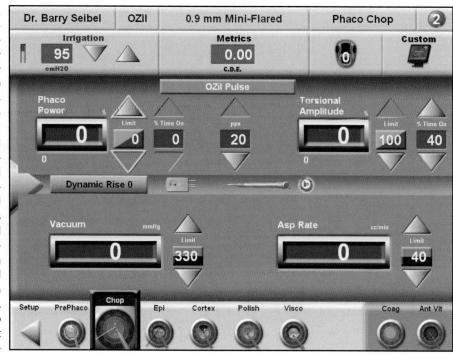

Figure 10-19. Seibel epinuclear settings. Changes for this memory setting include a reduction in ultrasound (OZil) energy, along with correspondingly lower vacuum and aspiration rate settings. In this stage, the surgeon is removing the epinuclear framework that had been keeping the bag formed and somewhat rigid; therefore, there is progressively more danger of posterior capsule trampolining into the aspiration port as more epinucleus is removed. For this reason, the aspiration control has been switched to linear to allow finer modulation of fluidics. Note: for softer nuclei such as mostly PSC cataracts, I will bypass Grade 2 chop and go directly to this epinucleus setting, given the similarity in density between an epinucleus and a softer nuclear sclerosis. A surgeon could alternatively create an additional family of settings for a softer Grade 1 cataract.

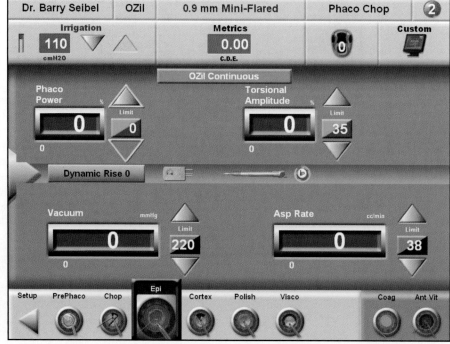

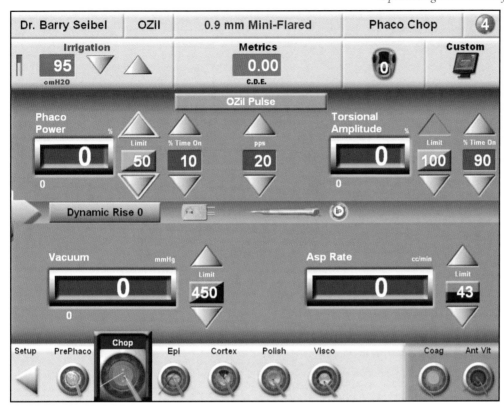

Figure 10-20. Seibel Grade 4 chop. Note the number 4 in the upper right corner of the window. This memory setting is used for dense nuclei that might start to clog the line with Grade 2 settings. The surgeon would be alerted to this condition when hearing an occlusion bell after engaging the cataract with ultrasound that persists even after the aspiration port appears to be cleared and a working space has been formed. The higher vacuum settings along with the addition of longitudinal phaco to OZil will typically clear such clogs with brief engagement of FP3. Note again that pulse modulation as well as IP are maintained through all settings, as they provide potentially greater protection against incisional burns and do not have any clinical disadvantage.

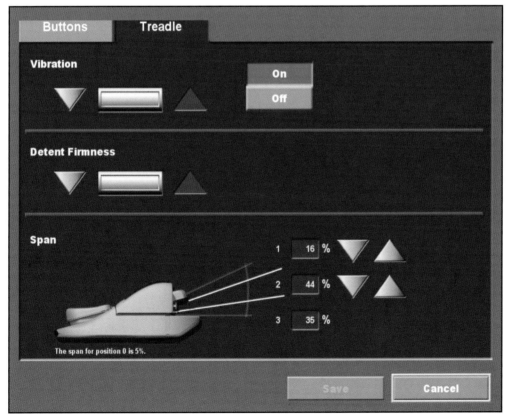

Figure 10-21. Seibel Foot Pedal Settings. Note that both vibration as well as detent firmness have been maximized to give the most surgeon tactile feedback regarding transitions between pedal positions. Recall this is especially important after embedding the phaco tip into a lens with the goal of vacuum fixation for chopping, where the surgeon wants to be in the bottom of FP2 for maximum vacuum grip (assuming sufficient nuclear density) without pressing into FP3 where ultrasonic vibrations would undermine the vacuum's grip.

The authors wish to acknowledge Val Injev and Doug Fanney from Alcon for their input and review of this chapter.

REFERENCES

1. Liu Y, Zeng M, Liu X, Luo L, Yuan Z, Xia Y, et al. Torsional mode versus conventional ultrasound mode phacoemulsification; randomized comparative clinical study. *J Cataract Refract Surg.* 2007;33:287–292.
2. Davison JA. Cumulative tip travel and implied followability of longitudinal and torsional phacoemulsification. *J Cataract Refract Surg.* 2008;34:986–990.
3. Berdahl JP, Jun B, DeStafeno JJ, Kim T. Comparison of a torsional handpiece through microincision versus standard clear corneal cataract wounds. *J Cataract Refract Surg.* 2008;34:2091–2095.
4. Rękas M, Montés-Micó R, Krix-Jachym K, Kluś A, Stankiewicz A, Ferrer-Blasco T. Comparison of torsional and longitudinal modes using phacoemulsification parameters. *J Cataract Refract Surg.* 2009;35:1719–1724.
5. Vasavada AR, Raj SM, Patel U, Vasavada V, Vasavada VA. Comparison of torsional and microburst longitudinal phacoemulsification: a prospective, randomized, masked clinical trial. *Ophthalmic Surg Lasers Imaging.* 2010;41:109–114.
6. Han Y, Miller K. Heat production: longitudinal versus torsional phacoemulsification. *J Cataract Refract Surg.* 2009;35:1799-1805.
7. Jun B, Berdahl JP, Kim T. Thermal study of longitudinal and torsional ultrasound phacoemulsification: tracking the temperature of the corneal surface, incision, and handpiece. *J Cataract Refract Surg.* 2010;36:832-837.
8. Fernández de Castro LE, Dimalanta RC, Solomon KD. Bead-flow pattern: quantitation of fluid movement during torsional and longitudinal phacoemulsification. *J Cataract Refract Surg.* 2010;36:1018–1023.
9. Reuschel A, Bogatsch H, Barth T, Wiedemann R. Comparison of endothelial changes and power settings between torsional and longitudinal phacoemulsification. *J Cataract Refract Surg.* 2010;36:1855–1861.
10. Cionni RJ, Crandall AS, Felsted D. Length and frequency of intra-operative occlusive events with new torsional phacoemulsification software. *J Cataract Refract Surg.* 2011;37:1785–1790.
11. Vasavada AR, Vasavada V, Vasavada VA, Praveen MR, Johar SR, Gajjar D, et al. Comparison of the effect of torsional and micro-burst longitudinal ultrasound on clear corneal incisions during phacoemulsification. *J Cataract Refract Surg.* 2012;38:833-839.
12. Wilbrandt HR. Comparative analysis of the fluidics of the AMO Prestige, Alcon Legacy, and Storz Premiere phacoemulsification systems. *J Cataract Refract Surg.* 1997;23:766-780.
13. Georgescu D, Kuo AF, Kinard KI, Olson RJ. A fluidics comparison of Alcon Infiniti, Bausch & Lomb Stellaris, and Advanced Medical Optics Signature phacoemulsification machines. *Am J Ophthalmol.* 2008;145:1014-1017.
14. Han YK, Miller KM. Comparison of vacuum rise time, vacuum limit accuracy, and occlusion break surge of 3 new phacoemulsification systems. *J Cataract Refract Surg.* 2009;35:1424-1429.
15. Osher RH, Injev VP. Thermal study of bare tips with various system parameters and incision sizes. *J Cataract Refract Surg.* 2006;32:867–872.
16. Davidson JA. Performance comparison of the Alcon Legacy 20000 1.1 mm Turbosonics and 0.9 mm Aspiration Bypass System tips. *J Cataract Refract Surg.* 1999;25:1386-1391.
17. McNeill JI. Flared phacoemulsification tips to decrease ultrasound time and energy in cataract surgery. *J Cataract Refract Surg.* 2001;27:1433-1436.
18. Davison JA. Performance comparison of the Alcon Legacy 20000 straight and flared 0.9 mm Aspiration Bypass System tips. *J Cataract Refract Surg.* 2002;28:76-80.

Figures 10-1, 10-2, 10-3, 10-5 to 10-8, and 10-SB1 to SB3 have been reprinted with permission of Alcon Laboratories, Inc, Fort Worth, TX.

11

Optimizing the AMO Signature for Chopping

David F. Chang, MD

BACKGROUND—PHACO TECHNOLOGY AND THE CHALLENGES OF BRUNESCENT NUCLEI

Continuing advances in phaco technology continue to improve patient outcomes and the safety of cataract surgery. Because phacoemulsification is already such a fast and efficient operation, our greatest need is for new technologies that can expand our margin of safety—particularly in eyes with dense nuclei and weak zonules. Historically, our 3 main safety-related concerns with phacoemulsification have been (1) thermal damage to the incision, (2) endothelial trauma associated with prolonged ultrasound time and particle turbulence within the anterior chamber, and (3) capsular rupture due to postocclusion surge. To appreciate how phaco chop, combined with phacodynamic enhancements, can improve our safety margin with challenging cases, it is important to understand what causes these complications.

Incision burns are most likely to occur with the higher power levels and prolonged ultrasound times needed for brunescent lenses. With traditional longitudinal phaco, increasing the phaco power (linearly in foot pedal position

3 [FP3]) results in a longer axial stroke length of the vibrating phaco tip. In addition to producing more power, this also generates more frictional heat. The thicker nuclear emulsate can admix with a highly retentive ophthalmic viscosurgical device (OVD) to form a viscous "caramelized" plug that clogs the phaco tip or aspiration line. If fluid outflow is blocked, then the gravity-fed inflow of irrigation also ceases. With neither the inflow nor the outflow of fluid to cool it, using continuous mode in a clogged phaco tip will instantaneously burn the phaco incision.

The loss of endothelial cells is also much greater with brunescent nuclei, the size and density of which require increased phaco time and energy for emulsification compared to standard cataracts. In this author's opinion, it is the increased particulate turbulence occurring with brunescent nuclear fragments that most damages and depletes endothelial cells. Rigid nuclear pieces drawn by aspiration to the phaco tip do not mold and conform as well to its opening. This and the added stroke length of higher longitudinal ultrasound power settings (which increases the repelling force) worsen the chatter and turbulence of small nuclear particles within the anterior chamber.

Finally, there are several reasons why posterior capsular rupture is more common with rock hard nuclei. The added rigidity and girth of the nucleus more directly transfers

Chang DF.
Phaco Chop and Advanced Phaco Techniques: Strategies for Complicated Cataracts, Second Edition (pp 127-137).
© 2013 SLACK Incorporated.

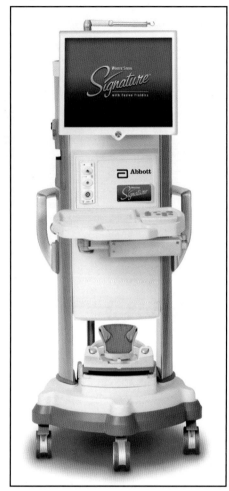

Figure 11-1. WhiteStar Signature Phaco System.

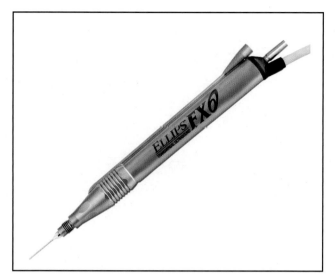

Figure 11-2. The Ellips Transversal FX handpiece with a straight #20 phaco tip (infusion sleeve removed).

ULTRASOUND POWER MODULATIONS

Like its predecessor the Sovereign, the AMO Signature has a dedicated computer that monitors and controls the electrical events that produce ultrasound power. The digitally controlled Ellips FX handpiece, driver circuits, and the control algorithm are engineered to maximize efficiency at the low end of the power continuum (Figure 11-2). This strategy prioritizes the goal of using the minimum amount of ultrasound power possible.

For this reason, traditional power settings (eg, 40% to 60%) may be unnecessarily high. Instead, one should preset the maximum power level at 15% when using Ellips FX mode for Grade 1 to 3+ nuclei. Keeping the maximum setting this low prevents the tendency to use higher power than is required. Lower ultrasound power settings minimize heat, energy delivery, and chatter. In addition, one can better use linear control in foot pedal position 3 to fine tune the optimum power level needed, as discussed in Chapter 9. For example, if that "sweet spot" happens to be somewhere between 5% and 10% power, it will be harder to find if the foot pedal provides a power continuum from 0% to 60%. For brunescent nuclei, the maximum power level should be increased to 35% to 45%. This higher power setting is also recommended for burst mode to facilitate deeper penetration into dense nuclei.

Ellips FX

The OZil Torsional handpiece (Alcon Laboratories, Fort Worth, TX) represents a major advance in phaco technology which replaces the axial movement of a traditional phaco needle with the sideways oscillation of a bent Kelman tip.[1-5] Compared to longitudinal phaco, this dramatically

instrument-related forces to the capsule and zonules, and there is proportionately less of an epinuclear shell to cushion the movements of the endonucleus. We typically maximize vacuum levels to improve holding power in these cases, but this simultaneously increases the risk of postocclusion surge. A lax posterior capsule due to weak or deficient zonules will trampoline more easily toward the phaco tip, making even a minor or momentary degree of surge treacherous.

The WhiteStar Signature System (Abbott Medical Optics [AMO], Santa Ana, CA, Figure 11-1) has a number of unique features that address efficiency, performance, and safety, which Signature users should understand and utilize when performing phaco chop. This chapter will examine the rationale behind these features, and how they can be best applied. The first section will address ultrasound power modulations and phaco tip size. The second section will discuss fluidics and the unique dual pump option available with this platform.

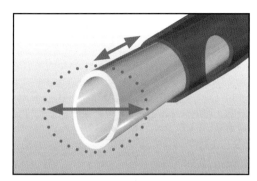

Figure 11-3. Illustration of the phaco tip's transverse elliptical path combined with some longitudinal axial motion in Ellips mode.

improves followability and reduces fragment chatter because pieces of the nucleus are not kicked away. AMO subsequently expanded this concept by blending some longitudinal movement with a transverse elliptical path of the phaco tip (Figure 11-3). Unlike OZil IP, which alternates traditional longitudinal phaco strokes with the torsional tip movement, Ellips generates a continuous 3-dimensional (3D) tip movement whose path essentially traces an ellipsoid (like the shape of an egg). In the 2-dimensional (2D) plane representing a horizontal cross section, the tip moves in an elliptical path. However, adding the axial longitudinal vector creates the 3D ellipsoid path of movement. This simultaneous blending of transverse and longitudinal tip movement offers smoother and more efficient cutting than traditional longitudinal ultrasound.

The lateral elliptical vector of tip movement cuts tissue without the repelling forces associated with pure axial tip movement. As with OZil, this dramatically improves followability of nuclear material and prolongs its contact with the phaco tip. Also similar to torsional phaco, cutting efficiency with lower expended energy results from having the tip cut while moving in both lateral directions. However, in contrast to torsional phaco, which rotates the tip shaft, this elliptical side-to-side movement of the entire tip is able to provide comparable cutting ability with a straight phaco tip. This is my personal preference for phaco chop, because it allows me to constantly redirect the bevel during the different phases of nuclear emulsification.

The longitudinal vector of tip movement with Ellips provides 2 benefits. Continuously blending this axial motion improves the tip's ability to cut dense nuclear material compared to pure lateral movement of the phaco needle. In addition, it prevents the tendency for brunescent nuclear emulsate to clog the tip. Analogous to shaking a ketchup bottle, this axial motion dislodges and keeps lens material moving through the narrow phaco tip shaft. Laboratory research by AMO found that clogging was common with denser nuclei if the tip only moved laterally. As one increases ultrasound "power" with linear foot pedal control in

position 3, both the longitudinal and sideways amplitudes of elliptical tip movement increase. Visualized in 3D, it is as though a larger volume ellipsoid shape is traced by the tip.

Overall, the enhanced followability that characterizes Ellips FX compared to traditional longitudinal phaco is most dramatic and obvious when used on dense nuclei. Thanks to less chatter with brunescent lens material, the reduced endothelial cell trauma is apparent in the form of clearer corneas on postoperative day 1. The improved cutting efficiency also means that lower ultrasound power is needed. This in turn reduces energy emitted into the anterior chamber and reduces the heat generated within the incision. In a comparison of temperature ranges produced by various ultrasound modalities in rabbit eyes, transversal resulted in a much lower temperature range (33.0°C to 37.1°C) compared to longitudinal (36.3°C to 41.1°C) and other modalities.[6] These benefits achieved by significantly reducing axial phaco movement generally render WhiteStar duty cycle reduction (see following discussion) less important when Ellips FX is used.

Burst Mode

Already offered with the AMO Diplomax and Sovereign, burst mode is available with the Signature as well. For impaling the nucleus during chop, single bursts of ultrasound can enhance tip occlusion without coring out surrounding material that produces the desired seal.[7] Of the 3 burst mode options provided, "multi-burst" is this author's preference for chopping. This mode provides 80 millisecond-long bursts of phaco at a fixed power that is preset on the machine panel (eg, 35%). The foot pedal provides linear control of the spacing between successive bursts. Initially, the bursts are separated by pauses measuring 1 second. This allows the surgeon to deliver a single burst at a time. As the foot pedal is depressed further, the successive bursts move closer and closer together until a maximum frequency of 4 bursts per second is reached. Burst mode is used for the "holding power" steps, as outlined in Chapter 9. Although an option exists to have linear control of power with a fixed interval between bursts, this configuration is less advantageous for chopping.

WhiteStar Hyperpulse

Introduced with the AMO Sovereign system in 2001, WhiteStar hyperpulse power modulation was made possible by digital computer control of the ultrasound system and was a significant advance in optimizing power delivery with traditional longitudinal phaco. Shortening the pulse duration increases the frequency of ultrasound pulses, or hyperpulse. In addition, the ability to decrease the duty cycle during pulse mode produces a major reduction in cumulative ultrasound time. For example, continuous ultrasound represents a 100% duty cycle—the tip is continually moving with no rest periods. Setting the hyperpulse mode duty cycle to 25% means that for every second that ultrasound is commanded in foot pedal position 3, the tip is only moving 25% of the time. Each "ON" pulse is alternating with an "OFF" pulse that is 3 times as long. Reducing the duty cycle significantly lessens the production of heat and the total ultrasound energy delivered by an axially moving phaco tip.[8-10] A low duty cycle can virtually eliminate the risk of wound burn.[11] As well illustrated by the American Society of Cataract and Refractive Surgery (ASCRS) award-winning videos of Teruyuki Miyoshi, MD, using ultra-high-speed digital photography, alternating each ultrasonic pulse with rest periods of "OFF" time diminishes the repelling force of the longitudinally vibrating phaco tip. This, in turn, reduces the chatter and turbulence of small lenticular particles at the phaco tip that would otherwise bombard the corneal endothelium.

WhiteStar should be employed when using pure longitudinal phaco, which is still an option with AMO's Signature and Sovereign Compact machines. However, WhiteStar is generally not used with Ellips FX, which is universally preferred by Signature users. The elliptical transversal tip movement already reduces the repelling force and energy/heat generated by pure longitudinal phaco, and interrupting the transversal tip path with frequent rest periods may lessen the cutting efficiency of this power modulation.

MICROPHACO TIPS

Moving from a 19-gauge to a 20-gauge phaco tip is one strategy that all surgeons can use to enhance safety regardless of the brand of phaco machine. As discussed in Chapter 9, this single modification reduces the size of the incision, decreases postocclusion surge, lessens the chance of accidental aspiration of the iris or capsule, and makes it easier to pluck thin or crumbling nuclear fragments from the capsular fornices. The last advantage stems from the fact that the smaller tip becomes occluded without having to penetrate too deeply into the nucleus. The narrower lumen restricts flow, reduces surge, and prevents material from rushing in as fast as through a standard diameter needle shaft. Like using an I/A tip with a smaller opening (0.3 mm compared to 0.5 mm), a microphaco tip provides greater control over what material or tissue is or is not aspirated. Slowing things down in this way helps to guard against snagging the capsule when aspirating epinucleus or thin nuclear pieces abutting the peripheral capsular bag.

Counterbalancing these advantages are several trade-offs. A smaller phaco tip vibrating longitudinally increases nuclear chatter because of its smaller "mouth," and its restricted flow lengthens the time needed to remove a bulky nucleus. The smaller surface area of the tip's opening also reduces the effective holding power for any given vacuum level. Fortunately, followability problems can be solved by chopping the nucleus into smaller pieces and using Ellips FX transversal power modulation (or OZil with the Alcon Infiniti) to virtually eliminate chatter. Improved pump technology enables us to safely use higher aspiration flow and vacuum to compensate for the other factors. It is therefore possible to reap the benefits of a smaller phaco tip regardless of whether performing coaxial or biaxial phacoemulsification; however, using a microphaco tip is the most often overlooked safety modification that surgeons can make. The sample settings at the end of this chapter are meant to be used with a 20-gauge phaco tip.

The AMO Signature system also provides the option of microcoaxial phaco, which can be paired with the smaller tipped cartridge of the AMO Platinum injector system. A 21-gauge phaco tip with a tighter fitting infusion sleeve fits through a 2.1-mm clear corneal incision. Compared to using a 20-gauge phaco tip, the flow rate and vacuum should be increased to compensate for the smaller surface area of the 21-gauge tip opening. By improving nuclear followability, transversal ultrasound seems to negate the increased repelling force associated with smaller phaco tip sizes when using pure longitudinal phaco.

FLUIDICS

In order to not exceed the preset vacuum limit, all peristaltic pump systems require a venting system and a mechanism to sense the vacuum level within the tubing between the pump and the handpiece. Introduced in 1999, the AMO Sovereign and its predecessor, the AMO Prestige, were the first phaco machines to offer a totally closed aspiration system. This is accomplished by using fluid venting instead of air, and by using a different vacuum sensing design. This totally closed system preserves a fluid column that is uninterrupted by any air bubbles. This reduces system compliance and creates a significantly faster and more responsive aspiration system.

Like other modern machines, the Signature utilizes stiff-walled, low compliance tubing to lessen surge. In addition, the Signature uses 2 separate on-board computers to control the pump and the ultrasound functions. A special diaphragm in the tubing cassette allows integrated microprocessors to more directly monitor the vacuum level inside the tubing. What makes this a so-called "smart pump" is that the vacuum is measured dozens of times per second (every 20 ms). This allows the dedicated fluidic computer to more quickly and precisely regulate the pump in order to prevent surge. Experiments in cadaveric eyes by Randall J. Olson, MD were able to measure surge associated with a variety of vacuum levels using different machines with the same experimental eye.[12] These studies have provided

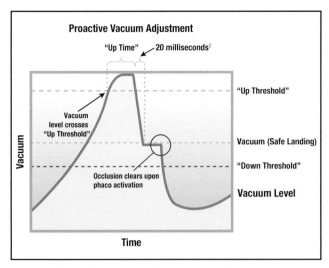

Figure 11-4. Signature antisurge algorithm automatically reduces the vacuum (to level called CASE vacuum) after a predetermined time period (26 m/sec) to minimize surge as the occlusion is broken.

quantitative confirmation of the improved chamber stability that we perceive clinically.

Occlusion Mode

One special feature of the AMO phaco platforms (Sovereign Compact and Signature) is the ability to automatically change both the pump speed (aspiration flow rate) and the power modulation pre- and postocclusion. This option is called occlusion mode and allows one to preprogram different sets of parameters for the periods before and after occlusion of the tip. An onboard fluidics computer senses occlusion according to when the vacuum exceeds a certain threshold level that is specified by the surgeon. This vacuum level is called the occlusion threshold, and is the point at which the desired parameters automatically change.

For example, when using Ellips FX transversal mode to remove free floating chopped nuclear fragments, one can alternate continuous with pulse mode by activating the latter upon tip occlusion. Generally, the elliptical pathway of the phaco tip is so efficient at cutting that there is no need to interrupt it with pulse mode. However, upon occlusion with a free floating fragment, suddenly activating pulse mode to alternate "ON" tip movement with "OFF" pauses may cause the tip to release and re-engage the tissue to promote better followability.

Occlusion mode can also be used to alter fluidic settings, such as to provide a greater margin of safety when aspirating the epinucleus (see sample settings). For example, when the tip is unoccluded, a higher flow rate (32 cc/min) can be used to draw tissue to the tip. Upon occlusion, the flow rate automatically drops (26 cc/min), which immediately slows the rate of vacuum rise. A lower occlusion mode threshold

(eg, 125 mm Hg vacuum, compared to 250 mm Hg for quadrants) causes this slowing to occur earlier. This gives the surgeon more time to move the tip away from the periphery to keep the capsule from being drawn in as well.

There are 2 additional but important safety features of the Signature's Fusion Fluidics pump that should be highlighted: passive automatic reflux and the antisurge algorithm.

Passive Automatic Reflux

Weak zonules significantly increase the likelihood of aspirating a lax posterior capsule during cortical cleanup. All phaco machines provide the option of active fluid reflux, whereby pressing a foot switch reverses flow in the aspiration line. Doing so expels ensnared material, such as the posterior capsule, from the aspirating port. Passive auto reflux is a safety option with both the Signature and the Sovereign that automatically refluxes the port at every transition from foot pedal position 2 to 1. Surgeons instinctively change foot pedal positions in this way as soon as the capsule is aspirated and passive reflux immediately and automatically expels the capsule without having to separately activate a reflux switch. Surgeons should consider selecting this indispensable safety feature for all cases, and it is particularly appropriate for the epinucleus and cortical irrigation-aspiration (I/A) memory settings.

Antisurge Algorithm

The Signature's enhanced fluidics improve chamber stability in even the most challenging cases. Postocclusion surge is still the most common cause of posterior capsular rupture occurring during nuclear emulsification. Postocclusion surge is a particular concern with brunescent nuclei and sharp-edged nuclear fragments. These lenses often have lax or deficient zonules and a thin or absent epinucleus that permits the posterior capsule to trampoline forward as final fragments are removed.

As mentioned previously, AMO machines have historically provided the occlusion mode feature, which allows surgeons to automatically program different ultrasound and fluidic parameters once the phaco tip becomes occluded or unoccluded. However, this author always felt that it would be even safer if the vacuum could be dropped immediately before a break in occlusion. This would allow the surgeon to momentarily harness the benefits of high vacuum levels, but then provide the safety and chamber stability of breaking tip occlusion from a lower vacuum level. In response to this suggestion, AMO's Fusion Fluidics pump technology provides the option of an antisurge algorithm called "CASE" (chamber stabilization environment) that accomplishes this very objective.

When the CASE algorithm is activated, the Signature pump's onboard computer recognizes occlusion and proactively reverses the pump to actively step down the vacuum before the break in occlusion occurs (Figure 11-4). These parameters are all preprogrammed by the surgeon.

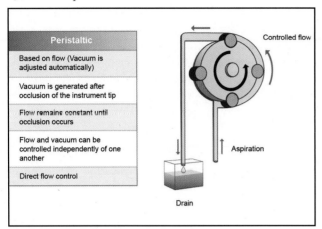

Figure 11-5. Peristaltic pump.

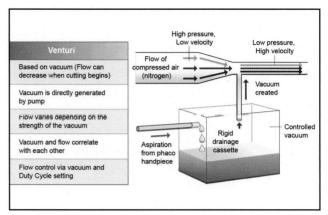

Figure 11-6. Venturi pump.

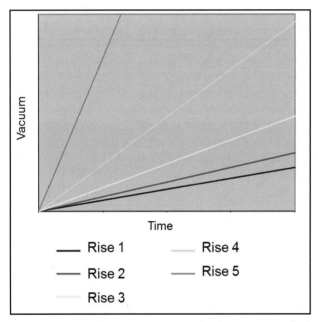

Figure 11-7. Venturi pump rise speeds showing a gradual linear increase in vacuum and flow rate with rise speed "1" (commanded by the foot pedal), compared to a more rapid rise with rise speed "5."

The author uses the CASE antisurge algorithm during emulsification of chopped fragments when breaks in occlusion are happening repeatedly. Like a car's antilock braking system, the pump's antisurge algorithm automates a safety response, automatically reducing the vacuum level after a predetermined interval to prevent surge as the fragments are evacuated from the eye. Indeed, the CASE antisurge algorithm attempts to mimic what an experienced surgeon might do with a dual linear foot pedal once the tip became occluded. After using high vacuum to maximize holding power, the surgeon might next decrease the vacuum with a dual linear foot pedal before delivering enough ultrasound power to clear the phaco tip.

Fusion Dual Pump Technology

Phaco machines generally employ 1 of 2 different pump designs: peristaltic (flow) or venturi (vacuum). With a peristaltic pump, rollers move fluid along a flexible aspiration line to create relative vacuum at the aspiration port whenever complete or partial occlusion occurs (Figure 11-5). The speed at which the wheel of rollers rotates determines the aspiration flow rate and the vacuum rise time.

With a venturi pump, vacuum is generated by the flow of gas or liquid across a port (Figure 11-6). The faster the gas or fluid flows, the higher the resulting vacuum that is created, which causes fluid to be drawn into and through the pump. Vacuum level and aspiration flow rate are interlinked and cannot be controlled independently with a venturi pump. Occlusion of the phaco tip is not necessary in order to generate vacuum and the foot pedal provides direct linear control of the vacuum level. The surgeon can preset the "rise" speed, which is the rate at which the foot pedal commanded linear increase in vacuum and aspiration flow rises over time. For the Signature, a rise speed of "1" produces a gradual slope over time, while a rise speed of "5" produces a much steeper slope (Figure 11-7). As an example, a faster rise speed of "5" can be safely used with I/A (cortical clean-up) to accelerate the response; however, using a slower venturi mode rise speed of "2" would be safer for phaco.

The AMO Signature contains both a true peristaltic and a separate true venturi pump within the same machine (Figure 11-8). Surgeons can therefore select either pump type according to individual preference for each case. The sample parameters listed in the following section are for use with the peristaltic pump, which is recommended for surgeons transitioning to chop. In addition, the AMO Signature positions the separate peristaltic and venturi pumps in parallel, so that a single all-in-one tubing cassette can be simultaneously attached to each of the 2 pumps (Figure 11-9). Using this specially designed dual cassette, the surgeon can actually alternate back and forth between

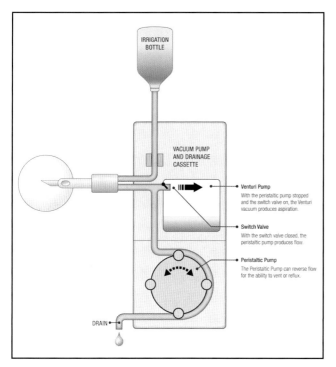

Figure 11-8. The Signature includes separate peristaltic and venturi pumps placed in parallel that can alternately control the aspiration line via a tee connection. With the switch valve closed, the peristaltic pump produces flow. When the switch valve activates, the peristaltic pump stops and the venturi pump produces aspiration.

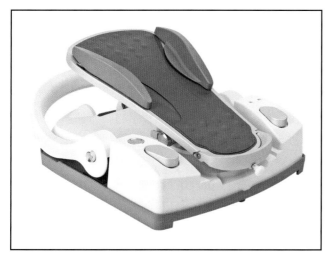

Figure 11-10. Signature programmable wireless foot pedal. Sideways yaw function provides the option of dual linear control with the venturi or peristaltic pump.

the 2 pumps on-the-fly during the same case without any change in tubing or any repriming.

This unique flexibility is accomplished by assigning separate pumps to different programmed memory modes or submodes that are selected and advanced with the wireless foot pedal (Figure 11-10). As the surgeon moves back

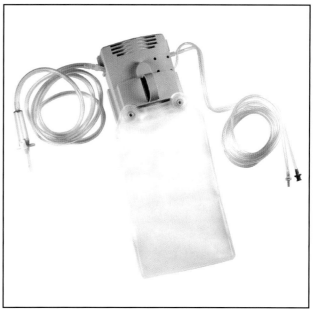

Figure 11-9. Special all-in-one dual cassette to allow on-the-fly switching between the peristaltic and venturi pumps during the same case.

and forth from one memory submode to the next, the machine instantaneously turns off the first pump while simultaneously activating the second. In addition, the Signature foot pedal has a sideways "yaw" functionality that can be configured to provide dual linear function in either the venturi or peristaltic pump mode.

The linear preocclusion vacuum and flow generated by a venturi pump can accelerate the holding and grasping function of the phaco tip to effectively create an instantaneous "rise time." Such speed and efficiency are more noticeable when emulsifying larger masses of nucleus. On the other hand, the immediate and automatic drop in vacuum with peristaltic pumps occurring upon occlusion breaks provides a greater margin of safety when smaller fragments are removed in proximity to an exposed posterior capsule. For example, a surgeon might prefer the venturi pump features for chopping, gripping, and evacuating the first heminucleus. However, switching to the peristaltic pump for the small and mobile fragments from the second heminucleus may afford greater safety as more of the posterior capsule becomes exposed and where instantaneous rise time is not important. As another example, a divide-and-conquer surgeon might employ the peristaltic pump for sculpting, and then switch to the venturi pump for emulsifying bulky quadrants.

Finally, the linked live vacuum and flow of a venturi pump attracts loose material to the phaco tip without having to actually embed the tip opening for occlusion. Therefore, some surgeons may prefer using the venturi pump with linear control for cortical clean-up to draw

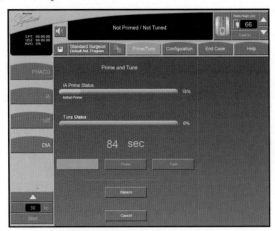

Figure 11-11. Signature set-up touch screen showing 4 major modes: phaco, I/A, vitrectomy, and diathermy.

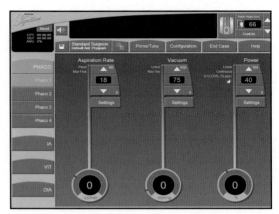

Figure 11-12. Touch screen showing 4 programmable phaco submodes. The surgeon can assign descriptive names to each submode (eg, chop, quad, sculpt, etc).

nearby lens material directly to the tip. With the strong attracting flow of live vacuum, the smaller 0.3-mm opening of the I/A tip (compared to the phaco tip) prevents sucking unwanted structures, such as the posterior capsule, into the tip along with the cortex.

CONFIGURING MEMORY SETTINGS

The Signature allows each surgeon to have multiple personalized phaco programs. For example, there can be a custom program for divide-and-conquer, another for chopping, and another for microcoaxial 21-gauge phaco. Each program has major modes (phaco, I/A, vitrectomy, and diathermy) (Figure 11-11). The surgeon can use one button on the foot pedal to move from one major mode to another (eg, to advance from phaco to I/A). Each major mode can have submode settings. For example, there can be an I/A cortex submode setting with high vacuum, an I/A capsule polishing setting with lower vacuum, and an I/A viscoelastic setting with a higher flow rate. The surgeon can assign any descriptive name to each of the submode memory settings (such as cortex, polish, and viscoelastic).

Surgeons will generally use 4 phaco submode memory settings (Figure 11-12). For the purposes of chopping with the sample parameters listed in the following tables, the author labels the 4 memory settings (1) chop, (2) quadrant, (3) fragment, and (4) epinucleus. The wireless foot pedal allows the surgeon to cycle back and forth between the different memory settings by nudging either of 2 lateral gates (see Figure 11-10). Clicking the right pedal gate advances to the next memory setting in ascending order (1 to 4). Clicking the left pedal gate cycles through the memory settings in reverse order (4 to 1). The surgeon can therefore easily switch back and forth between the chop and quadrant memory settings, for example.

In addition to the stepwise submode settings (each corresponding to a different surgical step), every program also has the ability to vary the entire package of memory settings according to 4 different grades of nucleus. For example, the preprogrammed power and vacuum limit settings can be automatically raised for a 3+ nucleus compared to a 2+ nucleus. For a 4+ nucleus, a sculpting memory setting can be added. One uses a different foot pedal switch to change and cycle between packages of settings according to nuclear density. For example, if a nucleus is denser than anticipated, one can switch from the "soft" to the "medium" nucleus bank of settings. This would result in the phaco power increasing for each of the steps (chop/quadrant/fragment/epinucleus).

Tables 11-1 and 11-2 list sample configurations for chopping using a 20-gauge straight phaco tip with Ellips FX. The first chart lists the author's personal settings when only the standard peristaltic pump is used. The second chart illustrates dual pump settings, when both the peristaltic and venturi pumps are used in different submodes during the same case. Chapter 9 outlines the rationale for these parameters, which merely represent a starting point for someone wishing to set up a chopping program. Individual experience will dictate whether one changes to more or less aggressive settings.

To chop a dense 3+ nucleus, one impales the nucleus using burst mode and high vacuum in the chop memory setting (see Figures 9-2 and 9-3). The quadrant setting is also used to elevate the first few tightly packed fragments out of the bag and to then emulsify them with Ellips FX mode. Transversal ultrasound is used in continuous mode preocclusion. Upon occlusion, pulse mode is activated which allows the tip to momentarily release and reacquire lens material to enhance followability. For horizontal chop, one can alternate back and forth between chop for chopping and quadrant for fragment emulsification. Chopping and elevating the last remaining pieces out of the bag is accomplished with the quadrant setting (see Figure 9-4).

To reduce the risk of surge, the CASE antisurge algorithm is activated by moving to fragment as the smaller mobilized fragments are removed with Ellips FX (see Figure 9-6). This setting is used as more of the posterior capsule becomes exposed (see Figure 9-5). The epinucleus setting provides linear pedal control of vacuum for epinuclear removal (see Figure 9-9). For a brunescent lens, one may choose to start by sculpting a small central crater prior to initiating chopping, as discussed in Chapter 4. The "Hard Cataract" program provides a WhiteStar sculpting mode from which the surgeon can then cycle directly into burst mode chop (see Figure 9-1).

CONCLUSION

Advances in ultrasound and fluidic technology continue to improve our ability to manage the most challenging cataracts. Combining Ellips FX transversal ultrasound and the Fusion Fluidics pump improves safety and efficiency, particularly in demanding cases such as with brunescent nuclei. Although such sophistication comes at the expense of simplicity, understanding and properly configuring our phaco machine can deliver better performance while improving safety.

REFERENCES

1. Liu Y, Zeng M, Liu X, et al. Torsional mode versus conventional ultrasound mode phacoemulsification; randomized comparative clinical study. *J Cataract Refract Surg.* 2007;33:287–292.
2. Davison JA. Cumulative tip travel and implied followability of longitudinal and torsional phacoemulsification. *J Cataract Refract Surg.* 2008;34:986–990.
3. Berdahl JP, Jun B, DeStafeno JJ, Kim T. Comparison of a torsional handpiece through microincision versus standard clear corneal cataract wounds. *J Cataract Refract Surg.* 2008;34:2091–2095.
4. Rękas M, Montés-Micó R, Krix-Jachym K, Kluś A, Stankiewicz A, Ferrer-Blasco T. Comparison of torsional and longitudinal modes using phacoemulsification parameters. *J Cataract Refract Surg.* 2009;35:1719–1724.
5. Vasavada AR, Raj SM, Patel U, Vasavada V, Vasavada VA. Comparison of torsional and microburst longitudinal phacoemulsification: a prospective, randomized, masked clinical trial. *Ophthalmic Surg Lasers Imaging.* 2010;41:109–114.
6. Steen M, Smith T, Raney R, Fishkind W, Gwon A. Thermal comparisons of phacoemulsification ultrasonic modalities. Poster presented at: Association for Research in Vision and Ophthalmology (ARVO); 2009 May 3-7; Fort Lauderdale, FL.
7. Badoza D, Fernandez Mendy JF, Ganly M. Phacoemulsification using the burst mode. J Cataract Refract Surg. 2003;29:1101-1105.
8. Olson RJ, Kumar R. White Star technology. *Curr Opin Ophthalmol.* 2003;14:20-23.
9. Osher RH, Injev VP. Thermal study of bare tips with various system parameters and incision sizes. *J Cataract Refract Surg.* 2006;32:867–872.
10. Fishkind W, Bakewell B, Donnenfeld ED, Rose AD, Watkins LA, Olson RJ. Comparative clinical trial of ultrasound phacoemulsification with and without the WhiteStar system. *J Cataract Refract Surg.* 2006;32:45-49.
11. Soscia W, Howard JG, Olson RJ. Microphacoemulsification with WhiteStar. A wound-temperature study. *J Cataract Refract Surg.* 2002; 28:1044-1046.
12. Georgescu D, Kuo AF, Kinard KI, Olson RJ. A fluidics comparison of Alcon Infiniti, Bausch & Lomb Stellaris, and Advanced Medical Optics Signature phacoemulsification machines. *Am J Ophthalmol.* 2008;145(6):1014-1017.

All figures in Chapter 11 have been reprinted with permission of Abbott Medical Optics, Santa Ana, CA.

Please see companion narrated videos on the accompanying Web site at
www.Healio.com/phacochopvideos

Table 11-1.
CHANG WHITESTAR SIGNATURE SYSTEM SETTINGS—PERISTALTIC PUMP

NUCLEUS GRADE	ASP FLOW RATE (CC/MIN)			VACUUM (MM HG)			POWER (%) Continuous FX except where multiburst or long pulse is noted	
	Submode	Unoccluded	Occluded	Max	OM Threshold*	Antisurge Algorithm (CASE)	Unoccluded	Occluded
Soft	Chop	Panel 22	28	Panel 375	250		Linear 25	Linear 20
	Quad	Panel 34	28	Panel 375	250		Linear 20	Linear 20
	Fragment	Panel 34	26	Panel 325	125		Linear 20	Linear 15
	Epi	Panel 32		Linear 250			Linear 15	
Medium	Chop	Panel 22	28	Panel 395	250		Panel 30 multi-burst	Linear 30 L.P. 6 pps
	Quad	Panel 34	28	Panel 395	250		Linear 25	Linear 30 L.P. 6 pps
	Fragment	Panel 34	26	Panel 395	125		Linear 25	Linear 20
	Epi	Panel 32		Linear 250			Linear 20	
Hard	Chop	Panel 24	30	Panel 410	250		Panel 40 multi-burst	Linear 45 L.P. 6 pps
	Quad	Panel 36	26	Panel 410	125		Linear 35	Linear 30
	Epi	Panel 32		Linear 250	100		Linear 30	Linear 55
	Sculpt	Panel 22		Linear 50			Linear 55	
Peristaltic I/A	Cortex	Linear 28		Linear 500				
	Polish	Linear 10		Linear 10				
	Visco	Linear 50		Panel 500				

* Thresholds (adjustable) determine when occlusion mode activates to change the aspiration rates or power modulation.

Note 1: Peristaltic ramp speed is set for 60 except for "chop" when it is 70.

Note 2: Recommended bottle height is 36 inches.

Table 11-2.
CHANG WHITESTAR SIGNATURE SYSTEM SETTINGS—DUAL PUMP

| Submode | ASP FLOW RATE (CC/MIN) | | | VACUUM (MM HG) | | | POWER (%)
Continuous FX except where multiburst or long pulse is noted | | |
	Pump	Unoccluded	Occluded	Max	Threshold*	Antisurge Algorithm (CASE)	Unoccluded	Occluded	Rise (Venturi)
Phaco									
Chop	Peristaltic	Panel 22		Panel 395	250		Linear 25	No Occl Mode	
Quad	Venturi			Linear 180	250		Linear 20	Linear 30 L/P.	2
Fragment	Peristaltic	Panel 34	28	Panel 395	125		Linear 20	6 pps	
Epi	Peristaltic	Panel 32	26	Linear 250			Linear 15	Linear 20	
I/A									
Cortex	Venturi			Linear 500					5
Polish	Peristaltic	Linear 10		Linear 10					
Visco	Peristaltic	Linear 50		Panel 500					

*Thresholds (adjustable) determine when occlusion mode activates to change the aspiration rates or power modulation.

Note 1: Peristaltic ramp speed is set for 60 except for "chop" when it is 70.

Note 2: Recommended bottle height is 36 inches.

12

Optimizing the Bausch + Lomb Stellaris for Chopping

Louis D. "Skip" Nichamin, MD

Since the introduction of phacoemulsification by Charles D. Kelman, MD in the 1970s, surgeons and industry have partnered to continuously improve the safety and efficacy of this vital and frequently performed procedure.[1-3] A core component to this process has been the improvement in phaco technology, promoting refinements in fluidics, along with an ongoing reduction and reliance on ultrasound energy. In addition, incremental reductions in incision size have led to increased surgeon control of the intraoperative milieu, safer outcomes given a decreased opportunity for wound leak and infection, and enhanced refractive outcomes. Recently, the term *microincision cataract surgery* (MICS) has emerged and generally refers to incisions in the range of 2 mm or less. Bausch + Lomb (Rochester, NY), with the development of their Stellaris Vision Enhancement System, has been one of several industry leaders in this area by providing surgeons with the technology to perform lens-based procedures through incision sizes of 1.8 to 2.2 mm. The features of this system are described in the following paragraphs.

STELLARIS SYSTEM DESIGN

The Stellaris is an advanced microsurgical system that had as its design goals the reduction of incision size, improvement upon the fluidic balance between aspiration and infusion forces through the smaller phaco tips used for MICS, optimized delivery of modulated ultrasound energy for improved control of cutting dynamics, and improved ergonomics for both surgeon and operating room staff. Though capable of enhancing a sleeveless biaxial technique (utilizing separated infusion, an approach more widely used outside of the United States) this platform specifically permits the use of a traditional coaxial technique.

The general housing unit of the Stellaris system is more compact than earlier machines and has a relatively small footprint (Figure 12-1). A user-interface computer, which includes a large 19-inch display, touch screen, and graphical user interface, facilitates quick responses to commands given by the foot controller. A modular system design permits upgrades as future technologies emerge.

Chang DF.
Phaco Chop and Advanced Phaco Techniques: Strategies for Complicated Cataracts, Second Edition (pp 139-142).
© 2013 SLACK Incorporated.

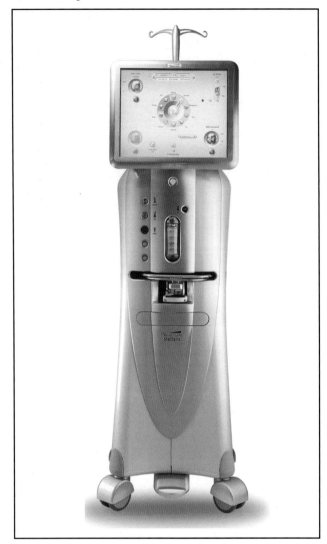

Figure 12-1. The Stellaris Vision Enhancement System.

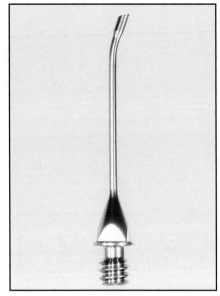

Figure 12-2. Stellaris 1.8-mm MICS needle.

STELLARIS SYSTEM FLUIDICS

The system's StableChamber fluidics have been designed to minimize surge and promote a stable anterior chamber by balancing fluid inflow and outflow through smaller phaco tips—specifically while using a 1.8-mm MICS needle (Figure 12-2) at high vacuum settings up to 600 mm Hg.

Surgeons may customize the Stellaris system based on their personal fluidics preference by choosing an advanced flow module (AFM)-based or a vacuum-fluidics module (VFM)-based StableChamber system.

FLOW-BASED FLUIDICS

The AFM is a software-controlled, positive-displacement peristaltic pump system. It allows a surgeon to configure a single pump system to work in a flow or vacuum mode and choose flow and vacuum levels suitable for each step of surgery. Vacuum thresholds, rise times, and duration at high vacuum before powering down can all be set by the surgeon depending on individual needs.

The AFM was designed to dampen postocclusion surge, a troublesome phenomenon frequently seen on earlier peristaltic pump systems. The MICS needle has been designed to limit flow while providing optimal purchase of nuclear material. A small cassette with stiffer, narrow tubing and low dead volume is used to prevent deformation of aspiration tubing caused by rise in vacuum.

VACUUM-BASED FLUIDICS

The VFM is an electric system that does not require external compressed gases. Outflow stability is enhanced using StableChamber flow-restrictive tubing (Figure 12-3), with a micromesh filter that helps to reduce clogging of the aspiration line, thereby further helping to maintain flow at a constant level while enabling higher vacuum levels. Surge suppression and more precise fluidics control are achieved through advanced software, sensors, and actuators that monitor and regulate the vacuum level at a high frequency. When coupled with proper surgical technique, stable fluidics and reduced postocclusion surge may reduce endothelial cell loss.

DIGIFLOW

The DigiFlow option affords a more automated means (as opposed to gravity-fed control of bottle height) by which

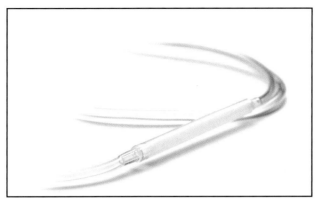

Figure 12-3. StableChamber tubing.

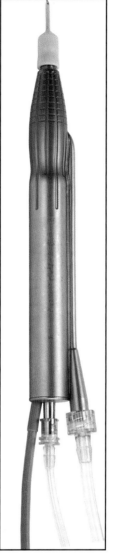

Figure 12-4. Stellaris Attune handpiece.

infusion pressure may be controlled through air pressurization of the infusion bottle, thereby potentially further minimizing intraocular pressure fluctuation during surgery. By dampening such changes, DigiFlow permits higher rates of steady, uninterrupted infusion, thereby balancing the higher vacuum settings that are commonly being used for MICS surgery. In a comparative case series conducted to evaluate the safety and efficacy of gas-forced infusion (air pump) in uncomplicated coaxial phacoemulsification, 76% of surgeons found more stable chambers with the DigiFlow System compared to gravity feed.[4,5]

ATTUNE ENERGY MANAGEMENT SYSTEM

The Attune Energy Management System has been designed to allow for efficient cataract removal while minimizing phaco energy. It permits customization of multiple aspects of the ultrasound pulse, including pulse duration and interval, and the advanced waveform modulation allows for the setting of a variable wavefront duration and depth. These features may lead to better nuclear fragment followability, reduction in heat generation, and increased phaco efficiency.

A redesigned Stellaris Attune handpiece (Figure 12-4) is driven with 6 piezoelectric crystals (rather than the usual 4). It operates at 28.5 kHz—a lower frequency than many other systems—theoretically leading to less heat generation and maximum cavitation for enhanced nuclear emulsification at a given power setting. The Attune handpiece incorporates a longer needle stroke length and consistent ultrasound resonance to ensure optimum cutting and cavitation. The handpiece is smaller, lighter, and narrower in diameter than earlier models and is balanced to reduce the pull of the attached cable and thereby minimize hand fatigue. The handpiece infusion connector has a Luer lock mechanism to prevent the irrigation tubing from inadvertently coming off during surgery.

STELLARIS DUAL LINEAR FOOT PEDAL

Stellaris system's foot controller has 4 programmable buttons and a center foot pedal. The foot pedal operates with both pitch (up and down) and yaw (side to side) travel, so it can control 2 user-selected linear functions simultaneously. The foot pedal interfaces with Bausch + Lomb's Custom Control Software, vacuum and flow sensors, and computer algorithms to help the surgeon control fluidics and optimize chamber stability. Although the foot controller can be connected to the Stellaris system by a physical cable, one of its features is wireless operation using Bluetooth technology. Alternatively, a larger user-friendly touch screen interface allows for switching between modes and adjustment of fluidics and phaco power settings.

PERSONAL EXPERIENCE WITH CHOPPING

Like many surgeons, I personally employ both the traditional and vertical quick-chop techniques throughout a given case. The vertical quick-chop is particularly useful in creating the initial cleavage planes, obviating the need to make a peripheral excursion beneath the anterior capsular rim. Following creation of several division planes, fragments may then be more easily aspirated by passing the chop instrument around the segment's periphery and subdividing them utilizing a horizontal chop maneuver. Central sculpting is only performed on rock-hard cataracts in order to weaken the core of the nucleus prior to chopping.

Without a doubt, chopping's popularity has grown due to its inherent efficiency, and once the technique is mastered along with optimization of the chosen phacoemulsification equipment, it provides enhanced safety as a nuclear disassembly technique.

MACHINE SETTINGS

- Needle: 1.8-mm coaxial MICS (trapezoidal incision of 1.7 to 1.9 mm)
- Sculpting (only performed on rock-hard nuclei): Ultrasound = 0 to 45% linear, continuous power
  - Vacuum = 0 to 200 mm Hg
  - Infusion = Air pressure 60 mm Hg, bottle height 70 cm

- Chopping (includes epinuclear removal): Ultrasound = 0 to 35% linear with microburst of 4 m/s duration and 4 m/s off interval
  - Vacuum = 0 to 600 mm Hg
  - Infusion = Air pressure 80 mm Hg, bottle height 70 cm
- Cortex removal (45-degree bent irrigation and aspiration with silicone sleeve, 0.35-mm port)
  - Maximum vacuum = 0 to 600 mm Hg, air pressure 55 mm Hg, bottle height 60 cm
  - Minimum vacuum = 0 to 50 mm Hg, air pressure 43 mm Hg, bottle height 60 cm
  - Capsule polish = 0 to 10 mm Hg, air pressure 43 mm Hg, bottle height 60 cm

REFERENCES

1. Kelman CD. Phaco-emulsification and aspiration. A new technique of cataract removal. A preliminary report. *Am J Ophthalmol.* 1967;64(1):23-35.
2. Kelman CD. Phaco-emulsification and aspiration. A progress report. *Am J Ophthalmol.* 1969;67(4):464-477.
3. Kelman CD. Phaco-emulsification and aspiration. A report of 500 consecutive cases. *Am J Ophthalmol.* 1973;75(5):764-768.
4. Wallace RB. Evaluation of a pressurized infusion system to replace or augment gravity feed of fluid during cataract surgery. Paper presented at: ASCRS Symposium on Cataract, IOL and Refractive Surgery; April 10-13, 2010; Boston, Mass.
5. Wallace RB. Gravity feed gets upgraded. *Ophthalmology Times.* 2010;35:SU6249.

All figures in Chapter 12 have been reprinted with permission of Bausch + Lomb, Rochester, NY.

SECTION III

Femtosecond Laser Nuclear Prechopping

13

Femtosecond Laser Nuclear Fragmentation (LenSx Platform)

Robert J. Cionni, MD

Since the beginning of phacoemulsification, numerous techniques for safe and efficient nucleus removal have developed. Initial techniques involved maneuvers designed to "bowl-out" the dense core of the nucleus. The remaining outer nucleus portion was then tilted or flipped forward to complete its emulsification.[1,2] Though these techniques accomplished the task, they remained somewhat challenging and many surgeons opted to abandon phacoemulsification and fall back to extracapsular methods for nucleus removal. Additionally, these techniques required significant manipulation of the entire nucleus, which led to complications such as zonular dialysis, posterior capsule rupture, and corneal decompensation from excessive endothelial cell loss.

More recently, surgeons have developed techniques to fracture and divide the nucleus to allow for easier manipulation, lowering the risk of complications and improving efficiency, especially for the denser cataracts.[3-5] These techniques include divide-and-conquer, vertical chop, horizontal chop, prechop, and numerous variations of these.

The advent of femtosecond laser use at the time of cataract surgery now challenges us to devise new strategies for nucleus fragmentation in order to make cataract surgery even safer and more predictable. This chapter will focus on the development of lens fragmentation techniques developed for the femtosecond laser. Although the author's experience has been limited to the LenSx femtosecond laser (Alcon Laboratories, Fort Worth, TX), similar techniques will likely be available for each system with some variations expected based on hardware and software differences. Even now, software changes are allowing for more versatility in lens chop patterns and therefore, in time, the author is certain surgeons will find even these most current techniques obsolete.

FEMTOSECOND LASERS

Before discussing specific techniques for nucleus fragmentation using the femtosecond laser, we must briefly describe how the laser accomplishes this task.

A femtosecond laser can be focused very precisely to any depth in the lens or the cornea. A femtosecond laser (originally developed by Kurtz, Juhasz, et al) was commercialized in 2001 for creation of the corneal flap for LASIK.[6] This procedure, pioneered by the company IntraLase, similarly revolutionized LASIK with an all-laser approach that eliminated many of the most frequently occurring complications with the manual technique for flap creation.

Chang DF.
Phaco Chop and Advanced Phaco Techniques: Strategies for Complicated Cataracts, Second Edition (pp 145-150).
© 2013 SLACK Incorporated.

Technical requirements for a femtosecond laser to operate in the lens and capsule are entirely different from any other commercially available laser for corneal surgery today. These new femtosecond lasers require a different laser engine, optical delivery system, and hardware. Very high quality image-guidance systems are required to enable the surgeon to visualize all anatomical features of the anterior segment in 3D. Innovative software enables the surgeon to plan all treatment patterns and execute with micron-level laser precision.

At this writing, only the LenSx Laser System is FDA cleared and commercialized for all of the following indications in cataract surgery:

- Fragmentation of the lens
- Anterior capsulotomy
- Corneal incisions, including arcuate incisions

The femtosecond laser energy results in the formation of gaseous bubbles as it photodisrupts tissue. With femtosecond LASIK flap creation, these bubbles frequently form an opaque bubble layer (OBL) that can limit visualization. During creation of corneal incisions with the femtosecond laser for cataract surgery, similar OBL may form. Bubbles are also created during capsulotomy and lens chop. Factors that can affect the degree of bubble formation include the following:

- Energy level
- Spot size
- Spot spacing
- Degree of lens/eye tilt with docking
- Capsulotomy size
- Chop diameter
- Number of chops
- Cylinder diameter
- Number of cylinders
- Lens thickness and depth of lens fragmentation treatment

The bubbles from the capsulotomy form under the anterior capsule and in the anterior chamber, coming to rest against the corneal endothelium. These bubbles can limit visualization, decrease the ability for the laser to effectively fragment the nucleus, and can stimulate pupillary constriction as they migrate anteriorly near the pupil margin. It is best to flush these bubbles out of the anterior chamber with viscoelastic prior to beginning phacoemulsification in order to improve visualization during the procedure.

Bubbles also form during femtosecond laser lens fragmentation, which can further decrease visualization and may increase intralenticular pressure. These bubbles tend to remain within the capsular bag and therefore cannot be flushed out with viscoelastic. Overaggressive

hydrodissection combined with an already pressurized capsular bag could encourage a posterior capsule rupture. One goal for the surgeon, therefore, is to minimize bubble formation while at the same time maximizing laser fragmentation effect. In general, by limiting laser treatment to zones where the effect is most needed, surgeons can maximize laser effect while minimizing bubble formation. Additionally, by utilizing the minimum power level needed to achieve the desired effect, surgeons can also decrease unwanted bubbles. For example, with a typical Grade 2 to Grade 3 cataract densities, program a 2-chop (4 segment) setting instead of a 3- or 4-chop setting. Surgeons have also found that by reducing the lens chop diameter to 4.7 mm from 6.0 mm, bubble formation is reduced, yet the lens chop effect is not. Additionally, as long as the capsulotomy diameter is set larger than the chop or cylinder settings, the anterior extent of fragmentation can be brought quite far anteriorly so that many of the fragmentation-induced bubbles can escape into the anterior chamber where they are flushed peripherally with a viscoelastic agent. As a surgeon gains more and more experience with femtosecond laser cataract surgery, he or she will also learn to optimize energy levels and fragmentation patterns based on cataract grade and type to more efficiently fragment the nucleus while minimizing bubble formation.

LENS FRAGMENTATION PATTERNS

Lens fragmentation patterns may vary depending on manufacturer. Several patterns have already been utilized including chops, cylinders, and cubes. The author's personal experience is limited to the cylinder and chop patterns available on the LenSx femtosecond laser.

Cylindrical Fragmentation

The cylinder pattern allows the surgeon to effect a single cylinder or numerous cylinders of various diameters in the lens nucleus (Figures 13-1 and 13-2).

Cylindrical fragmentation induces softening of the center of the cataract. After aspirating the fragmented central cylinder, the surgeon is essentially left with a "bowled-out" nucleus. The remaining peripheral nucleus and epinucleus can then be manipulated anteriorly for final emulsification. Some surgeons have found the cylinder softening program to help significantly when performing nucleus flip techniques. If the nucleus is soft enough, the peripheral portions can be simply aspirated as they collapse centrally. Still, if the nucleus is quite soft to begin with as is found in most refractive lens exchange patients, the cylindrical fragmentation does not add much benefit while at the same time inducing considerable gaseous bubbles that reduce red reflex and overall visualization.

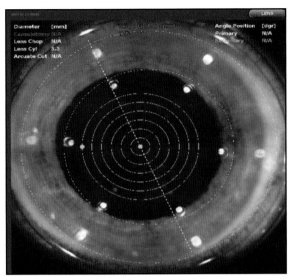

Figure 13-1. The cylinder cut pattern is designed to soften the central nucleus.

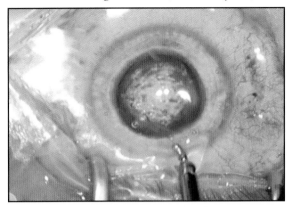

Figure 13-2. The LenSx femtosecond laser has softened the central nucleus in preparation for lens removal. (Reprinted with permission of Stephen G. Slade, MD, FACS.)

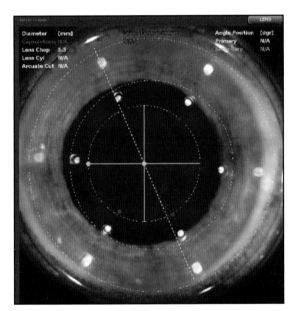

Figure 13-3. The 2 chop pattern divides the nucleus into 4 segments.

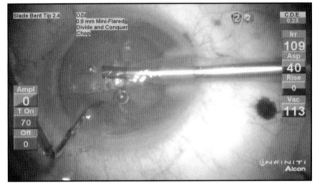

Figure 13-4. Once the femtosecond laser has divided the nucleus into 4 quadrants, each quadrant can be manipulated anteriorly for emulsification. (Reprinted with permission of Stephen G. Slade, MD, FACS.)

Chop Fragmentation

This program allows the surgeon to effect 1, 2, 3, or 4 chops of specifically set diameters through the center of the nucleus. The result are 2, 4, 6, or 8 segments, respectively (Figures 13-3 and 13-4).

Use of chop alone provides a nice separation of nuclear segments. Following confirmation of a complete capsulotomy and gentle hydrodissection, the lens chops are propagated peripherally and posteriorly using either a prechopper or the phacoemulsification tip and a second nucleus manipulator.

The segments still need to be brought centrally and anteriorly using a combination of second instrument manipulation and the vacuum of the phaco tip. This movement is somewhat impeded by the apical portions of each segment as in manual divide techniques. The 3-chop (6 segment) program allows for easier segment manipulation than a 2-chop (4 segment) technique.

Combining Chop and Cylindrical Fragmentation

The initial commercial software version provided the ability to divide the nucleus in either chop-like segments or in cylinders but not both together. Newer software allows for a combination of lens chop and lens cylinders fragmentation (Figure 13-5). The central cylinder, in effect, severs the apical portion of each segment and, since it is a

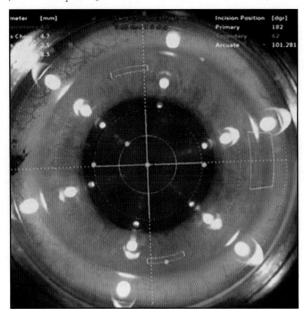

Figure 13-5. The video screen image of the 2-chop/single cylinder setting.

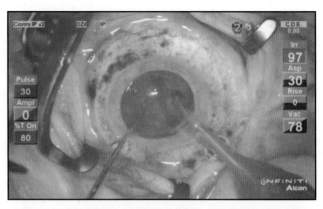

Figure 13-6. A Cionni nucleus manipulator and the 45-degree miniflare Kelman phaco tip are used to propagate the laser separation peripherally and posteriorly. Notice the empty central "well" created by the central cylindrical laser fragmentation, which creates space for nuclear segment manipulation.

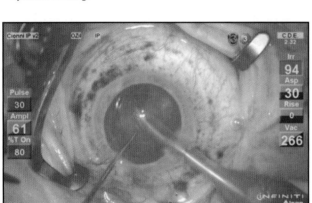

Figure 13-7. Removing the central apical portions of the nucleus segments first allows the more peripheral segments to move centrally more easily with the emulsification tip.

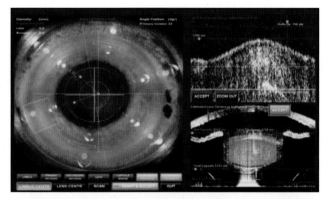

Figure 13-8. Setting the chop depth to the level of the nucleus/epinucleus interface (yellow arrow) helps to eliminate a residual epinuclear bowl while maintaining a safe distance from the posterior capsule (purple arrow).

small diameter cylinder, it adds very little time and very few bubbles to the procedure. By combining chop with cylindrical cuts, the apical portion can then be aspirated as emulsification first begins, thereby creating space for easier segment manipulation (Figure 13-6). Using a hybrid chop and cylinder approach, the author has never found it easier to bring each segment into the phaco tip (Figure 13-7).

Additionally, this technique rarely leaves an epinuclear bowl to deal with as long as the laser is set as deep as the anterior portion of the epinucleus, as detailed by the shaded yellow area of the lens fragmentation optical coherence tomography (OCT) scan.

The OCT is taken along the greatest angle of tilt. The yellow shaded area indicates the area of lens fragmentation for chop and cylinder incisions (Figure 13-8). Note the high density line (yellow arrow), indicating the interface between nucleus and epinucleus. The goal is to reach this line within the shaded area without hitting the posterior capsule (purple arrow). A tilted dock makes this task more difficult.

CURRENT TECHNIQUE

The following describes the author's preferred techniques for femtosecond laser cataract surgery lens fragmentation at the time of this writing. The author prefers a 2-chop (4 segment) combined with one central small cylinder. For dense cataracts, 4 cylinders and 3 chops are preferred.

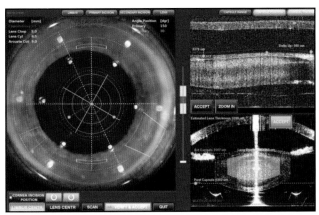

Figure 13-9. This case demonstrates excellent docking procedure with the limbus perfectly centered on the patient interface. The circle scan produces a uniform anterior capsule surface depth around the entire circumference.

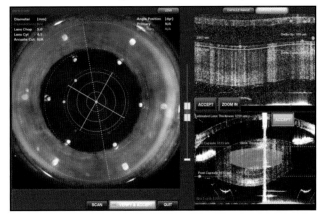

Figure 13-10. In this case, the eye is tilted slightly superiorly. The circle scan shows a nonuniform anterior capsule depth, shallowest at about 300 degrees, and deepest at about 120 degrees. A cross-sectional scan is performed at this axis, indicated by the white dotted line.

LENS FRAGMENTATION SETTINGS

With the current software the author has settled into the following settings:

- Lens 2 Chop Diameter—4.7 mm

- Lens 1 Cylinder Diameter—2.5 mm

The capsulotomy diameter is set at 4.9 mm to be slightly larger than the lens fragmentation. By doing so, the shaded lens fragmentation area can be brought up into the anterior portion of the lens without damaging the residual anterior capsular rim. This allows bubbles that form during lens fragmentation to escape anteriorly in order to improve red reflex visualization and to decrease intralenticular pressure and capsular bag expansion. A flat dock allows for maximal lens fragmentation while a tilted dock limits the anterior and posterior extent of lens fragmentation in order to avoid damaging the anterior and posterior capsules (Figures 13-9 and 13-10).

The laser procedure takes less than 1 minute of treatment time and about 3 minutes of surgeon time in the laser room. The patient is then taken into the intraocular operating room where the eye is prepped and draped per routine cataract surgery. After opening the incisions and instilling an ophthalmic viscosurgical device (OVD), the capsulotomy is confirmed complete before proceeding to hydrodissection. Aggressive hydrodissection is discouraged until some of the bubbles present within the capsular bag can be evacuated by gently depressing one pole of the nucleus. Hydrodissection can be carried out with minimal fluid, using a Chang Cannula (Katena Eye Instruments, Denville, NJ). A partial fluid wave is directed under the anterior capsule rim until it reaches the bubbles located along the posterior capsule. Gentle yet firm pressure on the opposite pole of the nucleus dissects the bubble and fluid around the remainder of the lens, allowing both to escape

into the anterior chamber. The lens nucleus can then be rotated freely.

The phaco tip (a 45-degree miniflare Kelman) is placed at the central "well" created by the small central cylinder fragmentation and this central portion emulsified and aspirated first. Doing so creates a generous space in which the phaco tip and a nucleus chopper/manipulator (Cionni Nucleus Manipulator; Crestpoint, St. Louis, MO) can be placed to grasp and propagate the fragmented segments peripherally and posteriorly. Each segment, one at a time, is thus separated and brought centrally within this space for easy emulsification. The epinucleus typically follows the last segment into the phacoemulsification tip.

LENS DENSITY AND FEMTOSECOND LASER LENS FRAGMENTATION

The author has been impressed with the femtosecond laser's ability to penetrate through dense nuclear cataracts as long as a decent red reflex can be attained (Figure 13-11). As the laser fragments the denser cataract, one will notice the bubbles appear more yellow in color and petaloid in appearance as the dense nature of the cataract prevents the bubble from assuming a round shape. Typically, the laser fragmentation markedly simplifies the dense cataract phacoemulsification procedure. However, the author has been less impressed by the completeness of the nuclear fragmentation in some cases, indicating a need to adjust energy levels, spot sizing, and/or spacing settings relative to the nuclear density. As surgeons learn more about the effect of energy level, spot size, and spot spacing the author is certain that even very dense cataracts will fragment effectively for easier emulsification.

Just as the femtosecond laser cannot deliver energy well through bubbles, it also cuts poorly through opaque media such as corneal scars, white cortical spokes, and opalescent lenses. Therefore, for white intumescent lenses, surgeons perform corneal incisions and capsulotomies but segment the nucleus with manual techniques.

LenSx integrated OCT images the posterior capsule even in dense cataracts.

CONCLUSION

Techniques to divide the lens nucleus have markedly improved surgeons' ability to safely and efficiently remove the cataractous lens. The advent of femtosecond laser use to fragment and divide the nucleus prior to phacoemulsification is further improving one's ability to increase safety and efficiency during cataract surgery. As it is still early in this new and exciting era of cataract surgery, the author is confident that surgeons will see continued improvements developing rapidly over the next few years.

REFERENCES

1. Kratz RP, Colvard DM. Kelman phacoemulsification in the posterior chamber. *Ophthalmology.* 1979;86(11):1983-1984.
2. Maloney WF, Dillman DM, Nichamin LD. Supracapsular phacoemulsification: a capsule-free posterior chamber approach. *J Cataract Refract Surg.* 1997;23(3):323-328.

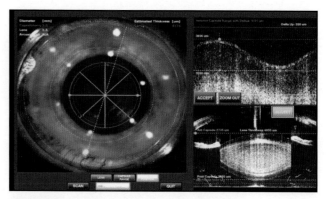

Figure 13-11. LenSx integrated OCT images the posterior capsule even in dense cataracts.

3. Gimbel HV. Divide and conquer nucleofractis phacoemulsification: development and variations. *J Cataract Refract Surg.* 1991;17(3):281-291.
4. Vasavada AR, Raj SM. Multilevel chop technique. *J Cataract Refract Surg.* 2011;37(12):2092-2094.
5. Park JH, Lee SM, Kwon JW, Kim MK, Hyon JY, Wee WR, Lee JH, Han YK. Ultrasound energy in phacoemulsification: a comparative analysis of phaco-chop and stop-and-chop techniques according to the degree of nuclear density. *Ophthalmic Surg Lasers Imaging.* 2010;41(2):236-41.
6. Ratkay-Traub I, Juhasz T, Horvath C, et al. Ultra-short pulse (femtosecond) laser surgery: initial use in LASIK flap creation. *Ophthalmol Clin North Am.* 2001;14(2):347-55:viii-ix. Review.

14

Femtosecond Laser Nuclear Fragmentation (LensAR Platform)

Louis D. "Skip" Nichamin, MD

The application of femtosecond laser technology to the field of lens-based surgery may represent one of the most important advances since Dr. Kelman's introduction of phacoemulsification and the adoption of small incision surgery. This laser technology offers the ability to improve the accuracy and reproducibility of several crucial steps in cataract surgery including the performance of the capsulorrhexis, lens fragmentation, and incision creation, thereby leading to a safer and more effective surgery.

LensAR (Orlando, FL) is one of several companies developing such a laser system. LensAR was the second company in the United States to receive FDA approval to perform anterior capsulotomy and has subsequently received approval for lens fragmentation, and should receive approval for corneal incisions in the very near future. The first such company to be granted approval for these surgical steps was LenSx, now a division of Alcon. At the time of this writing, OptiMedica has received FDA clearance for capsulotomy, fragmentation, and corneal incision creation and Technolas Perfect Vision is also developing similar technologies.

The LensAR laser system was designed with the goal of being able to perform high accuracy ultra-short pulse laser cutting of corneal and lens tissue in concert with a new and advanced 3-dimensional (3D) imaging system,

permitting exact delivery of laser energy to vital structures within the anterior segment. This proprietary measuring system, referred to as "3D-CSI," is one of the distinguishing features of this laser system from other platforms that use optical coherence tomography (OCT); its name derives from the use of a confocal structured illumination scanning transmitter that enhances 3D reconstruction accuracy. The ultra-high resolution infrared imaging system has lateral (x, y) and longitudinal (z) pixel resolution of approximately 10 μm, thereby locating and defining the position of anterior and posterior surfaces within the eye. This very high contrast optical system thus generates distinct anatomical edges for detection of key ocular surfaces and the application of the laser energy and cutting of tissue. These high contrast images are then linked to automated software algorithms that provide a 3D reconstruction of the anterior eye through optical ray tracing, which allows for determination and execution of 3D laser treatment without significant surgeon intervention (Figure 14-1). Biometric data are also calculated and any lens tilt is quantified and displayed in the reconstruction screen (Figure 14-2).

A key feature of the 3D-CSI technology is the ability to rapidly image the entire anterior segment from the posterior surface of the lens to the top of the nonapplanated corneal surface with 1 high resolution image

Chang DF.
Phaco Chop and Advanced Phaco Techniques: Strategies for Complicated Cataracts, Second Edition (pp 151-155).
© 2013 SLACK Incorporated.

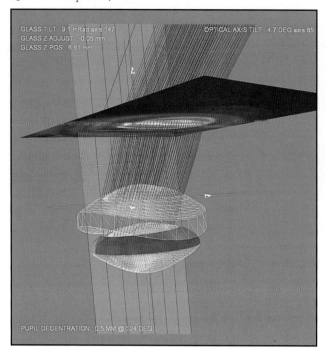

Figure 14-1. Three-dimensional reconstruction utilizes a minimum of 3 images for ray tracing to produce a 3D representation of the eye including all key surfaces.

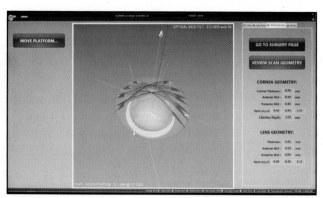

Figure 14-2. During 3D reconstruction, key biometric data are calculated and displayed on the right hand screen. Lens tilt is quantified in both extent and axis and displayed at the top right of the center screen.

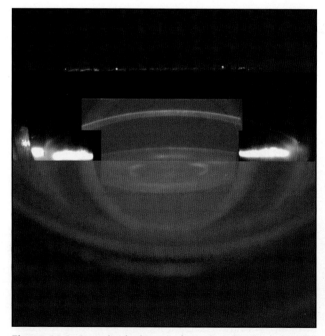

Figure 14-3. An individual image from the 3D-CSI camera. All surfaces can be clearly identified.

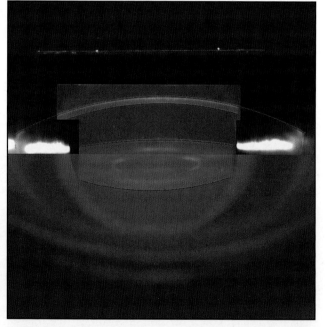

Figure 14-4. Once all images are collected, the software runs a sophisticated edge detection algorithm and automatically detects anterior and posterior cornea and anterior and posterior lens.

(Figure 14-3), obviating the need to combine separately scanned images. The high contrast images allow the software to automatically determine the key ocular surfaces for the surgeon to review (Figure 14-4). The accuracy of the laser system is felt to be further enhanced because image scanning is accomplished directly in the coordinate system of the treatment laser using sophisticated algorithms

for distortion compensation and calibration. Due to the differential scanning and integration rates, the scanned 3D-CSI transmitter is less sensitive to bulk lens scatter and can effectively image the highest grade cataracts, a task that can prove difficult for conventional OCT used in the other

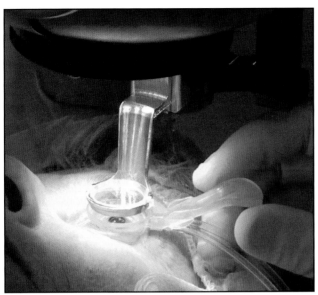

Figure 14-5. The fluid-filled, no corneal contact patient interface in situ. The docking arm is controlled by a joystick and docked to the suction ring.

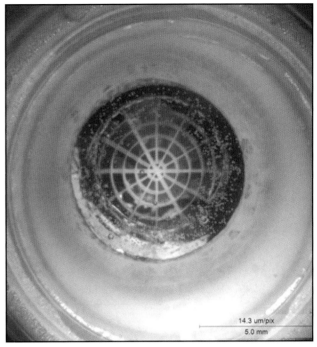

Figure 14-6. Phacofragmentation pattern with radial "chop" cleavage planes.

femtosecond cataract systems. In addition, fine structural details of the lens may be captured with the potential for automatic grading of cataract opacity and density, making it possible in the future to create automatic fragmentation algorithms that are selected based on a 3D volumetric scattering assessment.

The LensAR patient interface has been designed around a nonapplanating suction fixation device, which preserves the natural anatomy of the anterior segment (Figure 14-5). This interface is composed of a miniature water bath filled with a balanced salt solution that cancels the optical power of the cornea without touch from a curved or flat glass surface. Astigmatic corrections may benefit from this type of touch-free interface.

This laser platform has been designed to be operated in either a separate laser room outside the surgical theater or within the operating room itself. Because the treatment head provides a wide range of motion, the laser may be positioned over the patient's eye either in superior or temporal orientation. The system can measure and then apply the laser cutting component and then be automatically retracted, allowing the surgery to be completed using the surgeon's standard operating microscope.

Studies evaluating the laser's ability to enhance the performance of the capsulorrhexis showed a mean deviation from intended diameter of 0.18 mm for the laser treated patients, compared to 0.46 mm for patients receiving a manually performed rhexis.[1] Analysis of residuals to determine consistency of shape was 0.003 mm for the laser capsulotomies and 0.02 mm for the continuous curvilinear capsulorrhexis. It is now widely accepted that a laser capsulotomy produces a far more predictable and

regularly shaped capsular opening that may impact refractive outcomes, reduce posterior capsular opacification, and potentially augment the function of future accommodative lens technologies. Similar reports of improved accuracy and circularity have been published on the LenSx system[2] and the OptiMedica system.[3]

With the LensAR laser system, over 90% of capsulotomies were reported as free floating and needed no manual manipulation to separate them from the remaining capsule.[4] This is attributed to the imaging system and 3D reconstruction, which allows lens tilt to be detected and included within the capsulotomy pattern. This allows the pattern to also be tilted to match the tilt of the lens. This ensures that the capsulotomy cuts symmetrically, avoiding tags that can lead to radial tears. The consistency of the capsulotomy is demonstrated in the greater predictability of effective lens position (ELP). In a contralateral eye study, the proportion of cases being on or very close to the target postoperative refractive outcome were significantly closer to the intended outcome for laser capsulotomy eyes. At 6 months after surgery, 59% of cases with a laser capsulotomy were within 0.25 D of target compared to 26% with manual capsulorrhexis.[5]

During the development of the fragmentation patterns, 3 approaches were originally assessed during early clinical work. At the suggestion of David F. Chang, MD, a series of radial chop lines were designed to create cleavage planes along which phaco chop approaches could be applied (Figure 14-6). When these modified algorithms were assessed in a randomized trial, it was found that one

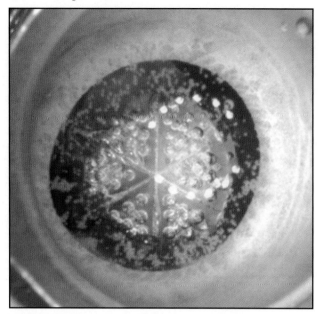

Figure 14-7. The spheres pattern, which, in a hard nucleus, prevents engagement of the nucleus by the phaco tip.

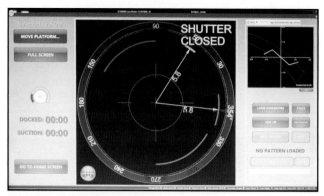

Figure 14-8. The corneal incision planning screen. The position of the CCI and paracentesis can be moved via the touch screen and the distance from the corneal center is displayed while they are moved. The geometry of the incision is shown on the left screen. Arcuate LRI incisions can be added and positioned via the software. A reticule is provided to offset the patterns if cyclorotation is evident from marks previously placed on the cornea or at the limbus when the patient was sitting up.

such pattern was more effective across all cataract grades than the others. In particular, it was found that cutting the nucleus into very small pieces was counterproductive, as segments would tend to break off individually, preventing meaningful engagement of the lens with the phaco tip (Figure 14-7).

For the chop surgeon, these patterns are configurable to fit with his or her preferred disassembly approach; personal experience has confirmed that laser-assisted chopping is effective and improves efficiency even on dense nuclei, as demonstrated during recent studies in Peru. Proper phaco settings and use of fluidics remain important considerations, as with traditional manual chop techniques.

Data from lens fragmentation studies have shown a marked decrease in the amount of energy needed during phacoemulsification. Most recent data suggest that reductions in cumulative dissipated energy (CDE) of up to 100% are possible with low-grade cataracts (Grades 1 and 2), with only aspiration needed in many cases.[6] Recent data gathered by Dr. Harvey Uy of the Philippines have shown that laser fragmentation of harder grades of cataract are associated with reductions in CDE of 66% in Grade 3 and over 55% in Grades 4 and higher.[7] Aspiration has only been achieved in some cases of Grade 4 cataracts. Analysis of clinical results presented at the 2010 Association for Research in Vision and Ophthalmology (ARVO) meeting showed that there was a trend toward faster visual recovery with laser treated cases, as well as lower levels of anterior segment inflammation following cataract surgery using laser lens fragmentation.[8]

Data presented at the annual meeting of the American Society of Cataract and Refractive Surgery (ASCRS) in 2012[9] suggested some benefit to laser surgery in reducing endothelial cell loss, although the differences were not statistically significant.

Work on corneal incisions is ongoing and it is likely that laser astigmatic incisions will prove to be more consistent and predictable than manual relaxing incisions, which will further enhance refractive outcomes. While some systems already have clearance for this indication within and outside of America, no data on effectiveness in treating astigmatism have yet been presented.

The precision and reproducibility of penetrating incisions will likely result in greater wound integrity with less chance of incisional leakage, thereby potentially reducing infection rates.[10] LensAR has developed a finite element analysis model of the cornea so that the best treatment algorithms can be assessed and refined prior to patient treatments. The treatment-planning screen is shown in Figure 14-8, where the location of clear corneal incision and paracenteses can be moved to meet the individual patient and surgeon requirements. The architecture of the proposed clear corneal incision is shown within the planning screen window. Limbal relaxing incisions can also be planned for location, arc length, and depth.

Though financial and logistical issues may present initial challenges to the adoption of femtosecond laser-based surgery, the inherent benefits of this remarkable technology will undoubtedly spur on its acceptance and widespread use within the field of cataract and implant surgery.

References

1. Tackman RN, Kuri JK, Nichamin LD, Edwards K. Anterior capsulotomy with an ultrashort-pulse laser. *J Cataract Refract Surg.* 2011;37:819-824.
2. Nagy Z, Kranitz K, Takacs AI, Mihaltz K, Kovacs I, Knorz M. Comparison of intraocular lens decentration parameters after femtosecond and manual capsulotomies. *J Refract Surg.* 2011;27:564-569.
3. Friedman NJ, Palanker DV, Schuele G, et al. Femtosecond laser capsulotomy. *J Cataract Refract Surg.* 2011;37:1189-1198.
4. Anon. Data submitted to the FDA K120214. LensAR Laser System User Manual; Orlando, FL; 2012.
5. Edwards KH, Hill WE, Uy HS, Schneider S. Improvement in the achievement of targeted post-operative MRSE with laser anterior capsulotomy matches the theoretical model. Paper presented at: The Association for Research in Vision and Ophthalmology Annual Meeting; May 2012; Ft. Lauderdale, FL.
6. Uy HS, Krueger RR, Edwards KH, Frey R, Schneider S. Commercially available systems: LensAR laser system. Chapter 16. In: *Refractive Laser Assisted Cataract Surgery* (ReLACS). New York, NY: Springer; 2013.
7. Schneider S, Uy HS, Edwards KH, Olmstead RT, Teuma V, Bott S. Reduced laser pulse width improves cutting efficiency in laser refractive cataract surgery. Paper presented at: The Association for Research in Vision and Ophthalmology Annual Meeting; May 2012; Ft. Lauderdale, FL.
8. Edwards KH, Frey RW, Tackman RN, Kuri JV, Quezada N, Bunch T. Clinical outcomes following laser cataract surgery. Paper presented at: The Association for Research in Vision and Ophthalmology Annual Meeting; May 2010; Ft. Lauderdale, FL.
9. Packer M, Uy H, Schneider S, Edwards K. Changes in endothelial cell density in a large cohort of patients undergoing laser refractive cataract surgery. Paper presented at the annual meeting of the ASCRS. Chicago 2012.
10. Masket S, Sarayba M, Ignacio T, Fram N. Femtosecond laser-assisted cataract incisions: architectural stability and reproducibility. *J Cataract Refract Surg.* 2010;36(6):1049.

15

Femtosecond Laser Nuclear Fragmentation (Catalys Platform)

Barry S. Seibel, MD

The foundation of phaco chop is a fundamental understanding of the machine technology and microsurgical maneuvers that underlie and permeate the procedure and its variations. In addition to this essential phacodynamic basis of knowledge and attendant manual skill set, there has been a significant new addition to our technological armamentarium that holds the potential to significantly enhance the safety, precision, and reproducibility of several steps of the procedure. Femtosecond laser-assisted cataract surgery, as introduced in 2011, has applications for the main and auxiliary corneal incisions, corneal arcuate incisions, capsulotomy, and cataract softening and segmentation. OptiMedica (Sunnyvale, CA) has one of the longest track records in this technology space, pioneering a cohesive platform that can significantly enhance cataract surgery in general and phaco chop in particular.

In order to better appreciate how femtosecond laser technology works for cataract surgery, it is helpful to highlight its distinctions from femtosecond corneal refractive surgery (eg, IntraLase [Abbott Medical Optics {AMO}, Santa Ana, CA] for flap creation in laser-assisted in situ keratomileusis [LASIK] surgery).

PLAN, ENGAGE, VISUALIZE AND CUSTOMIZE, TREAT

The OptiMedica Catalys femtosecond cataract laser system has distinctive approaches to the 4 basic elements attendant to this procedure: (1) planning the procedure in advance of the actual procedure; (2) engaging, or docking, the eye to the laser optics; (3) visualizing and customizing the preplanned treatment based on that visualization; and (4) treating with core laser and algorithms optimized for cataract surgery. The first element, planning, draws on insights gained from early cases in which it was observed that numerous elements of the procedure did not vary from case to case and many other elements varied predictably. For example, the planned capsulotomy diameter will typically be consistent for a given lens implant, based on the goal of having a consistent overlap of the optic by typically 0.5 mm in order to help achieve a consistent effective lens position without tilt. Similarly, a given lens density may typically lend itself to one particular laser fragmentation pattern from the many available. Naturally, the eye being

Chang DF.
Phaco Chop and Advanced Phaco Techniques: Strategies for
Complicated Cataracts, Second Edition (pp 157-161).
© 2013 SLACK Incorporated.

treated will typically have the same clock-hour incision sites (right eye versus left eye, assuming that the surgeon is not moving the incisions based on the steep axis), and a given phaco system will typically call for the same incision dimensions for ideal fluidic sealing and ergonomics. All of these consistencies logically led to a planning protocol prior to patient treatment that is template based and, along with an icon-based graphic user interface (GUI), allows a time-efficient and cohesive way of preparing each patient for the actual laser procedure.

The second step involves actual docking of the operative eye to the laser in order to accurately align and calibrate both the diagnostic imaging modality as well as the therapeutic femtosecond beam. Unlike the relatively more simple optics of a corneal refractive femtosecond laser, the Catalys must image a much greater volume of the eye, not only the anterior cornea as with a corneal laser but also the posterior cornea out to the limbus as well as the anterior chamber and complete depth of the crystalline lens. Furthermore, the therapeutic femtosecond beam must be accurately registered to these deeper anatomic structures for precise cutting. Rigorous early trials by OptiMedica involved curved solid interfaces similar to those used in corneal refractive surgery, with the idea that the curve would better approximate the corneal curvature without the distortion attendant with the flat applanation plate used by the IntraLase.[1] However, with enough vacuum engaged to fixate the globe, it became apparent during these early trials that the curved interface still distorted the cornea as noted on optical coherence tomography (OCT) images of posterior corneal folds. The fixed curve interface did not perfectly fit the myriad of potential compound corneal curvatures of the patient population, and even on those corneas that had a similar curve a slight misalignment of engagement and docking could still produce such corneal folds. The suboptimal imaging as well as inconsistent laser cutting was felt to be secondary to the diagnostic and therapeutic beams traversing these corneal folds and being diffused and/or deflected.

At the expense of missing an opportunity to be first to market, OptiMedica abandoned the curved docking interface in favor of developing an innovative Liquid Optics Interface that engaged the perilimbal conjunctiva and sclera with vacuum and had only balanced salt solution touching the cornea to produce an undistorted optical interface. The result was a tremendous improvement in both imaging as well as therapeutic efficacy, such as skip areas of capsulotomy cutting becoming the exception rather than the relatively common occurrence that existed with the curved interface.[2] A further significant advantage was a much lower induced intraocular pressure (IOP) increase with docking due to less globe distortion; the curved interface produced an IOP increase of 80 mm Hg compared to a less than 20 mm Hg increase with the Liquid Optics Interface. The new design with a perilimbal vacuum annulus also allowed a much wider field of view than the curved corneal interface, an appropriate and necessary adaptation from just corneal to whole anterior segment surgery in order to visualize the entire limbus for accurate placement of cataract incisions; the Liquid Optics Interface has a 13.5-mm clear aperture.

With the eye now firmly but safely docked, the third step for femtosecond cataract surgery is accurate visualization of the anterior segment structures, modifying any of the preplanned settings as appropriate based on this visualization, and then registering the therapeutic laser beam accordingly. Unlike a dedicated corneal femtosecond laser, which has to only aim the laser relative to its docking plate (ie, a raster pattern of spots all 120 µm posterior to the corneal epithelium/applanation plate to give a 120-µm-thick flap) in a diameter 9.5 mm or smaller, a cataract femtosecond laser must be able to image the entire thickness and diameter of the cornea out to the corneoscleral limbus to facilitate accurate placement of main and auxiliary cataract incisions as well as peripheral corneal relaxing incisions of a precise percentage depth of the entire corneal thickness. Furthermore, the anterior and posterior lens capsule must be measured across an anterior chamber depth that varies from patient to patient. The anterior capsule must be precisely imaged to help ensure a complete capsulotomy without skip areas but without excessive laser energy anterior and posterior to the capsule. Furthermore, the posterior capsule must be precisely imaged to allow the creation of an accurate safety buffer below which the laser will not fire to prevent inadvertent posterior capsule rupture.

Equally important to anterior segment raw imaging by OCT is processing and mapping of these images by a process known as Integral Guidance, which is analogous to a physician inspecting a retinal OCT and cognitively identifying the internal limiting membrane, the retinal pigment epithelium, the normalcy of the foveal contour, etc. The correlate in femtosecond cataract surgery is identification of the anterior and posterior corneal and lens margins, pupillary margins, and also a mathematically extrapolated capsular bag fornix/perimeter (Figures 15-1A and 15-1B). This mapped architecture is then integrated with treatment plans that were preselected by the surgeon prior to docking, such as the size and centration of the capsulorrhexis and the placement of the corneal incisions. These treatment plans are template based with an intuitive GUI that is time efficient from 2 important perspectives: it (1) allows much work to be done prior to docking the patient (Figure 15-2A) and (2) automatically applies these templates to the mapped surfaces to save the surgeon further time when the patient is docked (Figure 15-2B), compared to competing machines that require the surgeon to manually identify and map surfaces such as the posterior cornea and anterior and posterior lens capsules. Any fine-tuning of the preselected plans is also time efficient via the same intuitive GUI used in the predock phase, such as slightly changing the position of the

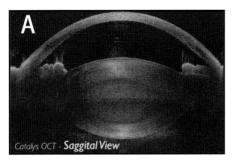 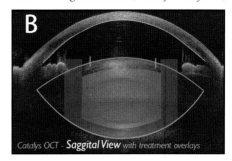

Figure 15-1. (A) High resolution anterior segment imaging utilizing Liquid Optics Interface. Note smooth contours of anterior and posterior lens and corneal surfaces, limbus to limbus. (B) Integral Guidance algorithms map anterior and posterior corneal and lens surfaces, enabling accurate placement of lens treatment (green) as well as a safety "no-laser" zone (red) designed to protect the iris and posterior capsule.

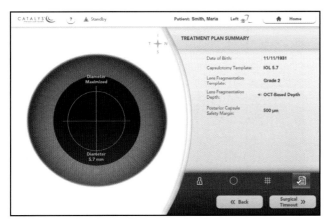 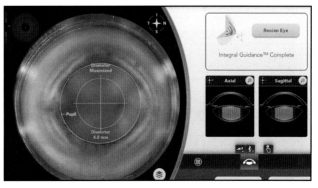

Figure 15-2. Template-based planning enhances time-efficiency and accuracy. Simple and effective Graphic User Interface (GUI) ergonomically enables rapid surgeon visualization and modification of laser patterns.

corneal incisions relative to the visually observed position of the corneoscleral limbus.

The final phase of femtosecond cataract surgery involves actual photodisruptive laser treatment of the target tissues. Although related to a corneal refractive laser (eg, IntraLase), the Catalys laser has been optimized from its origin to be more effective at cataract surgery, specifically being able to deliver larger spot sizes and energy pulses that result in larger shock waves that better disrupt the crystalline lens as compared to a purely corneal laser. A significant difference in the 2 laser platforms is the numerical aperture, which corresponds to the beam divergence angle from the focal point. The IntraLase uses a corneal optimized numerical aperture that is higher than the lens and capsule-optimized beam of the Catalys. Extensive testing indicates that the Catalys's lower numerical aperture (larger spot size) still gives excellent corneal results for main, auxiliary, and astigmatic relaxing incisions but is superior to the higher numerical aperture (smaller spot size) for lens/capsule applications. The end result of the Catalys plan–engage–visualize and customize–treat protocol is a globe with corneal and capsule incisions more precise than any possible manually, plus a lens that has a lower effective nuclear density (requiring less ultrasound energy) as well as preplaced fracture lines that promise to expand the safety and efficacy of phaco chop techniques to an ever larger group of surgeons and patients.[2-4]

The lens-disruption aspect of the Catalys augments lens emulsification in general as well as chopping in particular. The general aspect utilizes various laser spot patterns designed to diffusely destabilize the crystalline structure of the nucleus, lowering its effective density and thereby decreasing the need for ultrasound (Figure 15-3A). The specific chopping application of femtosecond laser technology involves placing spots in planar patterns that predefine the plane that will be chopped, thereby decreasing both the vacuum required for stabilization as well as the mechanical force required for the chopping instrument. In other words, the lens is weakened in the plane that will be traversed by the chopper so that the surgeon will not have to exert as much force when translating the chopper through the lens in this plane (Figures 15-3B and 15-4C). This represents a similar ideology to Takayuki Akahoshi's concept of prechopping but with much greater ease of use as well as precision for the surgeon.[5]

Figure 15-3. (A) Top view of lens segmentation and (B) lens softening patterns for treatment using the Catalys Laser System. (Reprinted with permission of OptiMedica.)

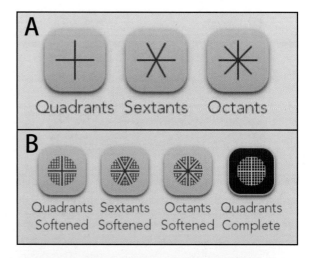

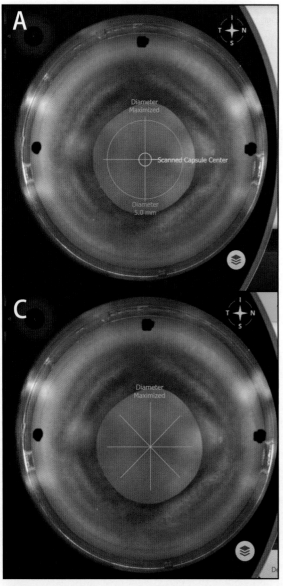

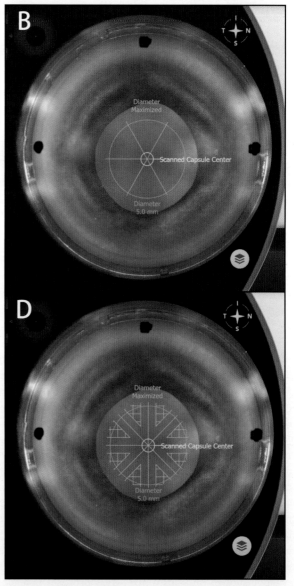

Figure 15-4. Note how lens treatment pattern (green) is greater in diameter than the capsulorrhexis. This is possible because of a 500-micron safety margin between the anterior capsule and the anterior lens treatment margin, as enabled by the Catalys Integral Guidance System. Note also that A, B, and C use lens division only, while D additionally uses a lens softening grid. However, the softening pattern is constrained to allow denser nuclear material for the phaco tip to engage and grip when dividing the nucleus along the laser division lines.

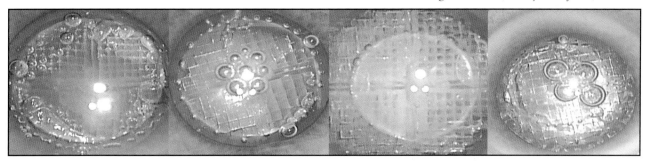

Figure 15-5. Lens softening grids function to lower the effective density of the cataract, enabling lower need for ultrasound, in many cases a greater than 95% reduction. (Reprinted with permission of H. Burkhard Dick, MD, FACS.)

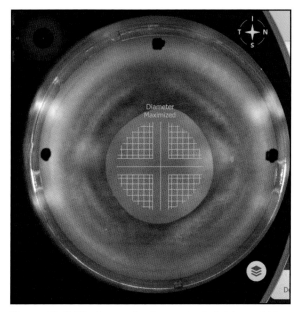

Figure 15-6. The lens softening and subdivision grid has a diameter maximized for the pupil size, utilizing a safety zone of 500 microns between the treatment grid and the pupil margin, as determined by Integral Guidance. This lens treatment diameter can be greater than the capsulorrhexis diameter because of the similar 500 micron safety zone between the anterior capsule and the anterior limit of the lens treatment zone.

The interaction of the 2 femtosecond lens treatments (lens softening and prechopping plane creation) must be considered. For example, combining an extensive lens softening pattern with a chopping pattern (Figures 15-4D, 15-5, and 15-6) can make it difficult to achieve a strong grip with the embedded phaco needle because the laser-softened

nuclear material may tend to deform and aspirate into the aspiration port without transmitting the vacuum's gripping force effectively for counterfixation against the chopping instrument's force. This is more of a problem for vertical chopping techniques than for horizontal methods in which the chopper may be carefully dissected to the nuclear periphery with minimal vacuum and then drawn toward the phaco needle with even less need for vacuum as the nucleus is trapped between the converging instruments, as opposed to vertical chopping, which utilizes the chopper at right angles to the phaco grip, thereby requiring the higher level of vacuum (see Chapter 8, Understanding the Phacodynamics of Chopping). Therefore, when performing vertical chop maneuvers, the surgeon may wish to use a more limited lens softening program, especially in the central nucleus where the phaco needle will be embedded.

REFERENCES

1. Talamo J, Vukich J, Gooding P, Friedman N, Koch DD. Clinical performance of patient interfaces for laser cataract surgery. ASCRS 2012. Chicago.

2. Abell RG, Kerr NM, Vote BJ. Catalys femtosecond laser-assisted cataract surgery compared to conventional cataract surgery. *Clin Experiment Ophthalmol.* 2012;10.

3. Conrad-Hengerer I, Hengerer FH, Schultz T, Dick HB. Effect of fs laser fragmentation on EPT in cataract surgery. *J Refract Surg.* 2012;28(12):879-883.

4. Conrad-Hengerer I, Hengerer FH, Schultz T, Dick HB. Effect of femtosecond laser fragmentation of the nucleus with different softening grid sizes on effective phaco time in cataract surgery. *J Cataract Refract Surg.* 2012;38(11):1888-1894.

5. Akahoshi T. The Karate Prechop Technique. *Cataract and Refractive Surgery Today.* 2002;2:63-64.

SECTION IV

Complicated Cases and Complications

STRATEGIES AND MANAGEMENT

16

Capsulorrhexis
Sizing Objectives and Pearls

David F. Chang, MD

The capsulorrhexis, or continuous curvilinear capsulotomy (CCC), is generally considered the single most important step in cataract surgery and provides numerous surgical advantages.[1] A continuous capsular edge renders the capsular bag more resistant to tearing during surgery. Like an elastic waistband, the capsulorrhexis will stretch, not tear, in response to mechanical surgical forces.[2,3] In contrast, a radial capsulorrhexis tear becomes the focal weak point toward which the mechanical forces exerted upon the capsule are now concentrated. Sufficient force can cause an errant capsulorrhexis tear to extend further radially until it wraps around the equator into the posterior capsule.[4,5] Thus, failure to achieve an intact capsulorrhexis not only precludes the benefits, but also increases the risk of posterior capsular rupture.

A continuous edge is necessary to perform cortical cleaving hydrodissection, and it facilitates cortical clean-up and placement of both haptics into the capsular bag. It also converts the anterior capsule into a contingency platform for intraocular lens (IOL) support should the posterior capsule tear. Because the overall length of many foldable IOLs will be too short for the ciliary sulcus, capturing the optic of a 3-piece IOL with the capsulorrhexis is the best way to assure good IOL centration in this situation.

CAPSULORRHEXIS SIZE

The postoperative advantages of a properly sized capsulorrhexis are equally important. As the capsular bag contracts, a continuous capsulotomy edge prevents pea-podding or escape of either haptic.[6-11] Asymmetric capsular forces resulting from an eccentric CCC can cause delayed optic decentration. Continuous circumferential overlap of the IOL optic edge will produce a capsular shrink wrap effect whereby the posterior capsule is kinked by the optic edge—a major factor in the prevention of posterior capsule opacification[12-15] (Figure 16-1). By sharply indenting the posterior capsule, the optic edge creates a mechanical barrier that blocks lens epithelial cells from migrating behind the lens optic.[16] Capsulorrhexis overlap may also help to reduce positive optic edge dysphotopsias as the anterior capsule opacifies over time. Finally, such continuous overlap of the optic edge is the only way to attain consistency in the axial IOL position from case to case. Being able to accurately predict this effective lens position is a critical factor in calculating the proper IOL power for emmetropia.[17-19] Achieving these advantages is all the more critical for multifocal and presbyopia correcting IOLs.

Chang DF.
*Phaco Chop and Advanced Phaco Techniques: Strategies for
Complicated Cataracts, Second Edition* (pp 165-172).
© 2013 SLACK Incorporated.

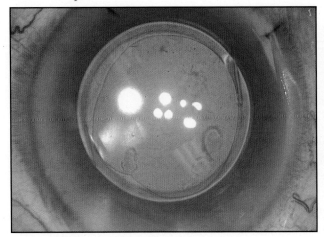

Figure 16-1. Ideal capsulorrhexis size with complete circumferential overlap of IOL edge.

It follows that a capsulorrhexis whose diameter extends beyond the optic edge in some or all areas forfeits these advantages. Posterior lens epithelial cell (LEC) migration will occur in any region where the posterior capsule is not kinked by the optic edge.[16] Slight optic decentration may result from asymmetric capsular contractile forces over time. Finally, as the posterior capsule tenses postoperatively, it may displace the optic slightly more anteriorly wherever it is not restrained by a taut capsulorrhexis edge, resulting in a myopic shift.

SMALL DIAMETER CAPSULORRHEXIS—DISADVANTAGES

What are the disadvantages of a capsulorrhexis diameter that is too small? During phacoemulsification, a smaller capsulorrhexis is much more likely to be torn by the chopper tip or shaft or incised with the phaco tip. Surgeons should take a mental "snapshot" of the capsulorrhexis shape and diameter upon its completion, because its visibility will be subsequently lost following hydrodissection and nuclear rotation. This allows the surgeon to mentally picture the edges of the capsulorrhexis during the emulsification step. Aspirating the anterior epinucleus prior to starting phaco also facilitates this. Using bimanual instrumentation for cortical clean-up may overcome the specific hurdle of aspirating the subincisional cortex with a small diameter capsulotomy.

In addition to impeding surgical steps, a small diameter CCC may create postoperative problems as well. The increased load of lens epithelial cells on the back of the anterior capsule can increase inflammation and cause anterior capsular fibrosis and opacification and excessive contraction of the capsulorrhexis and capsular bag.[20-22] This can lead to zonular damage, dehiscence, or optic decentration.[23-26] Anterior capsular fibrosis and contraction

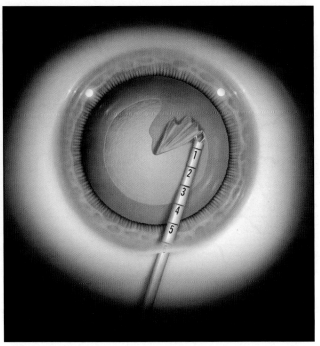

Figure 16-2. Seibel Rhexis Ruler allows measurement of capsulorrhexis diameter. (Reprinted with permission of MicroSurgical Technology.)

is much more likely with silicone than with hydrophobic acrylic optic material.[26] With sufficiently weakened zonules, visually significant capsulophimosis or subluxation of the bag-IOL complex can occur.[21,27,28] Besides secondary capsulorrhexis enlargement, other techniques to reduce capsular contraction include aspiration of lens epithelial cells beneath the anterior capsule and Nd:YAG anterior capsule relaxing incisions.[29,30] Excessive anterior capsular opacification can impair ophthalmoscopic visualization of the peripheral retina and even become visually significant for the patient.[31] Finally, excessive overlap of the nasal optic edge with a capsulorrhexis may be a cause of temporal pseudophakic negative dysphotopsia.[32]

Given the importance of attaining a proper capsulorrhexis diameter, it is ironic that until recently this is one of the only cataract surgical steps that has not been improved through the use of new technology. Most of us continue to employ the "low tech" method of a manual tear performed with a needle and/or forceps whose intended diameter is estimated visually. Individual variability in corneal magnification and in anterior segment and pupil diameter makes it difficult to precisely size the capsulorrhexis. Parallax occurring with movement of the globe makes it difficult to judge the symmetry and centration of the evolving capsulotomy. One of the most appealing advantages of a femtosecond laser capsulotomy is the ability to consistently create a centered capsulotomy of a precise diameter.[33-37] Other methods include the use of corneal markers or capsule forceps with etched millimeter markings to gauge size (eg, Seibel Rhexis Ruler, MicroSurgical Technology [MST], Bausch + Lomb) (Figure 16-2).

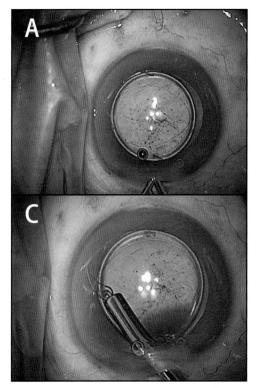

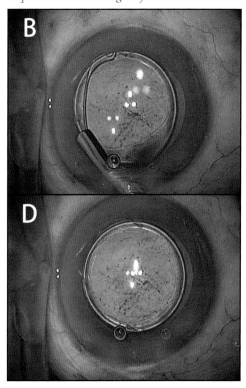

Figure 16-3. A round capsulorrhexis that becomes oval following 3-piece IOL implantation indicates weak zonules. (A) The normal capsular stretching force of the haptics is not counterbalanced by circumferential zonular traction, which results in ovalization of the capsulotomy. (B, C) A capsular tension ring (CTR) can be inserted after IOL implantation if zonular laxity becomes apparent due to capsulorrhexis ovalization. The evenly distributed, outward stretching force of the CTR reduces focal stress on the zonular apparatus. (D) This restores the initial round shape of the capsulorrhexis.

SECONDARY CAPSULORRHEXIS ENLARGEMENT

This chapter addresses manual capsulotomy techniques, where my personal strategy is to plan on performing a 2-stage capsulorrhexis when necessary. As I make the primary capsulorrhexis, I try to err on the small side because the diameter can always be enlarged, but not reduced. I take a moment to assess the appropriateness of the CCC diameter after implantation of the IOL. Frequently, the size and centration are fine, but it is surprising how often the CCC is slightly eccentric to the center of the optic. Sometimes, a perfectly round CCC becomes ovoid following implantation of the IOL due to the directional stretch of the stiff 3-piece haptics. Significant ovalization may indicate zonular laxity and insufficient centrifugal tension in the areas perpendicular to the haptic axis (Figure 16-3).

In either of these situations, or if the overall diameter is too small, I enlarge the capsulorrhexis by first making an oblique cut with scissors and then grasping the resulting flap with capsule forceps (Figure 16-4). The cut should be oblique, rather than radial, to better incline the resulting flap to tear in a circumferential direction. The flap is then maneuvered with capsule forceps under a generous amount of ophthalmic viscosurgical device (OVD). Curved Uthoff-Gills capsulotomy scissors with blunt tips (Katena K4-5126) have the perfect shape for creating an initial curved cut to either side of the phaco incision (see Figure 16-4B and 16-4C). In some cases, I only trim a part of the remaining anterior capsular rim where it is excessively wide (Figure 16-5). Other times, I may retear the entire 360-degree circumference of the opening (see Figure 16-4 and Figure 17-12). If the pupil is small enough to conceal the optic edge, it can be locally retracted with a Lester hook (Figure 16-6) or by maneuvering a Malyugin ring (see Figure 21-6).

The safest time to enlarge the capsulorrhexis is after insertion of the IOL. This is true regardless of whether a capsular tension ring is inserted as well. Executing the second stage enlargement is generally easier than the primary capsulotomy for several reasons. Following removal of the cataract, the red reflex is improved and there is no convexity to the anterior capsule to promote downhill radial extension of the tear. The optic provides a perfect visual template for resizing the CCC diameter. Finally, in cases of weak zonules, the presence of stiff 3-piece PMMA haptics or a capsular tension ring increases outward tension on the capsular bag, which improves control over the direction of

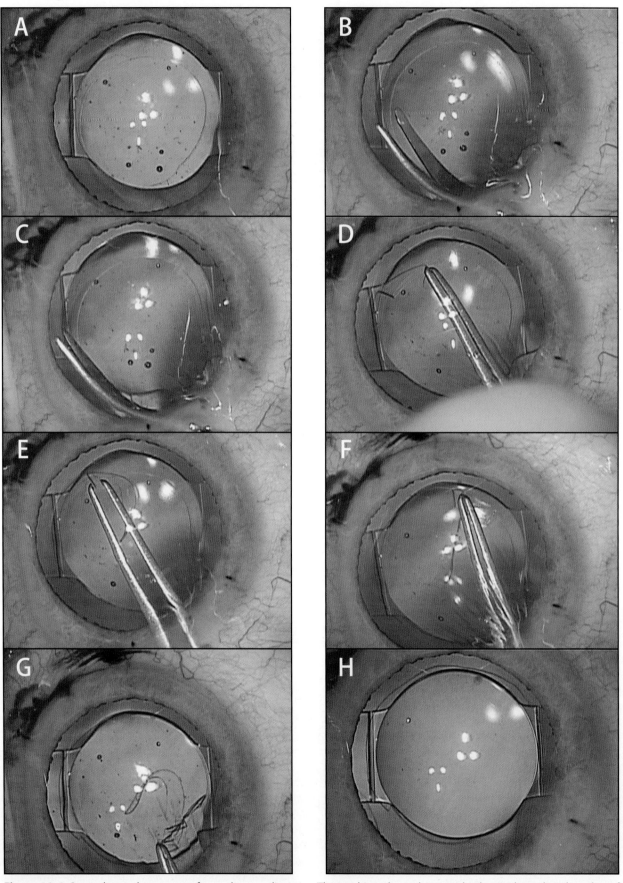

Figure 16-4. Secondary enlargement of capsulotomy diameter. The goal is to have the capsulorrhexis aligned at the edge of the Crystalens optic. (A) After IOL implantation, the capsulorrhexis edge is determined to be too small. (B, C) Uthoff-Gills curved capsule scissors are used to make an oblique cut at one edge. (D-H) This is used to create a new flap that is continually regrasped to complete a secondary enlargement of the capsulotomy.

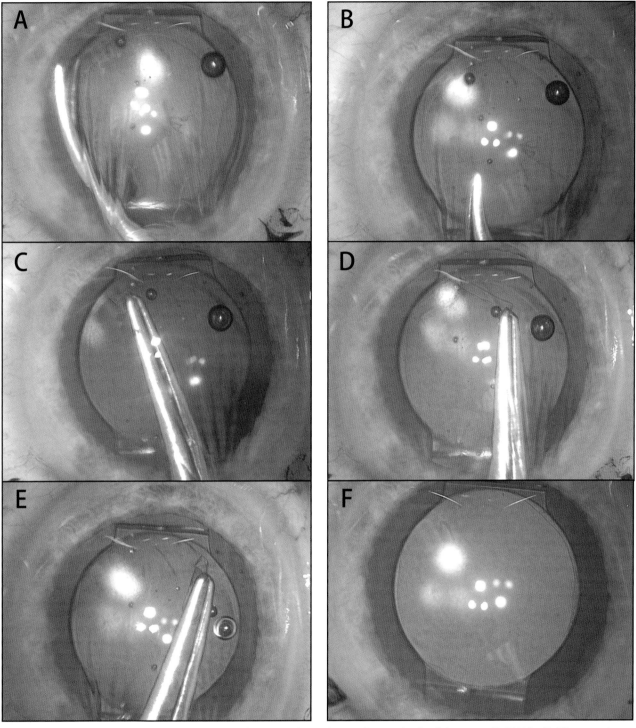

Figure 16-5. The capsulorrhexis is asymmetric with too much overlap on the nasal side of the optic. (A, B) Uthoff-Gills curved capsule scissors are used to make an oblique cut at one edge. (C-F) The nasal side of the capsulorrhexis is secondarily enlarged with capsule forceps, creating the proper and symmetric size.

the anterior capsular tear. It is reassuring that, should the tear escape peripherally, the risk of a posterior wraparound tear is negligible because all of the most forceful surgical steps have been completed. However, the IOL should not be rotated in the presence of a single anterior capsular tear for this reason.

Although enlargement of a small diameter capsulorrhexis is not absolutely necessary in most cases, I would encourage the mastery of this technique. With multifocal IOLs, achieving a symmetric capsulorrhexis that completely overlaps the optic edge is particularly important. There is even less margin for CCC diameter error with

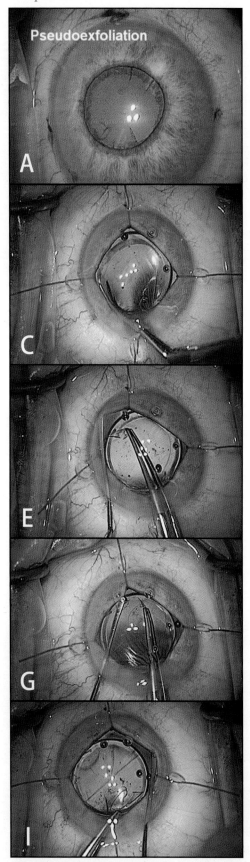
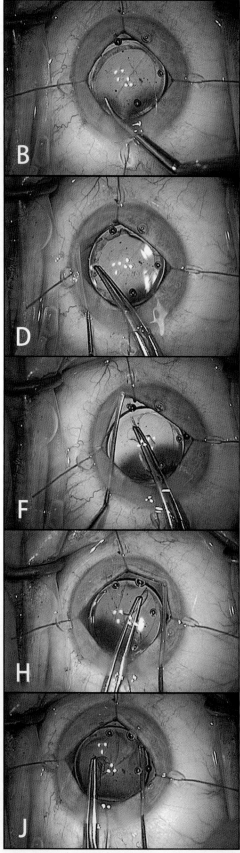

Figure 16-6. (A) Case of pseudoexfoliation with a small pupil. (B, C) After IOL implantation, the capsulorrhexis appears small. Uthoff-Gills curved capsule scissors are used to make an oblique cut at one edge. (D-J) While using a Lester hook to retract the pupil margin, the new capsulotomy edge is widened just beyond or at the edge of the optic. This minimizes the tendency for capsulorrhexis contraction in the setting of progressive zonulopathy.

accommodating IOLs, such as the Crystalens (Bausch + Lomb) (see Figure 16-4). Excessive variability in CCC diameter will have a greater impact on effective lens position for a hinged IOL design. With dynamic accommodating designs, such as the AMO Synchrony IOL, too large a CCC diameter may allow the anterior optic to partially protrude through the capsulotomy. Too small an opening may cause capsulophimosis or excessive capsular fibrosis that can strain the zonules, stiffen the bag, and incapacitate the accommodative mechanism. Initially erring on the small side, with the option to enlarge when and where necessary, is a reliable way to consistently attain a perfect sized capsulorrhexis diameter manually.

Finally, comfort with this secondary enlargement maneuver is important if one is having difficulty steering the flap during the primary capsulorrhexis. Whether the cause is poor visibility, patient movement, a shallow chamber, or weak zonules, one can make a smaller diameter opening in order to increase control and to reduce the risk of a peripheral extension. The Brian Little Tear Out Rescue Maneuver (see Chapter 17) should be mastered and can be used to improve control or rescue an escaping tear. Because of the long-term importance of a properly sized capsular opening, the surgeon should secondarily enlarge a small diameter capsulorrhexis following IOL insertion when the surgical conditions are more favorable.

Special Indications for Capsulorrhexis Enlargement

There are 2 clinical situations in which it may be advantageous to enlarge the capsulorrhexis diameter out to or beyond the IOL optic edge, also known as "all off." Uveitic eyes with preoperative posterior synechiae will have a strong tendency to develop iris adhesions to the anterior capsular edge postoperatively (see Figure 21-2). Iris bombé with full circumferential pupil seclusion and secondary angle closure glaucoma can occur and be refractory to YAG or surgical iridectomy. Some have suggested placing the IOL in the ciliary sulcus in uveitic patients so that the optic will prevent posterior synechiae from developing to the capsulorrhexis edge.[38] As a better alternative, secondarily widening the capsulorrhexis following IOL insertion should accomplish this goal while preserving the immunologic advantages of bag sequestration of the lens (see Figure 21-2F and 21-2G).

A second situation in which a larger than usual capsulorrhexis is advantageous is with weakened zonules. Because capsulorrhexis contracture is countered by centrifugal zonular tension, significant capsulophimosis always indicates severe zonular laxity. Capsulorrhexis contracture, in turn, further dehisces and weakens the zonules and increases the risk of late bag-IOL dislocation with pseudoexfoliation.[24,27,28] Therefore, leaving a small diameter capsulorrhexis in an eye with weakened zonules is particularly objectionable. Hayashi and coworkers have shown that diabetic eyes are also more prone to anterior capsule contraction and fibrosis.[31]

Because a larger diameter capsulorrhexis will have far less of a tendency to contract, the author's personal preference is to secondarily enlarge the capsulorrhexis diameter out to the edge of the optic in weak zonule cases (see Figure 16-6). This is done after insertion of the IOL because of the enhanced control and visibility cited earlier. In pseudoexfoliation eyes where a CTR is not deemed necessary, the author will still secondarily enlarge the capsulorrhexis diameter to reduce the zonular weakening potential of capsular contraction over time. This rationale and strategy are discussed further in Chapter 24.

References

1. Gimbel HV, Neuhann T. Development, advantages, and methods of the continuous circular capsulorhexis technique. *J Cataract Refract Surg.* 1990;16:31-37.

2. Assia EI, Apple DJ, Tsai JC, Lim ES. The elastic properties of the lens capsule in capsulorhexis. *Am J Ophthalmol.* 1991;111:628-632.

3. Krag S, Thim K, Corydon L. Strength of the lens capsule during hydroexpression of the nucleus. *J Cataract Refract Surg.* 1993;19:205-208.

4. Aasuri MK, Kompella VB, Majji AB. Risk factors for and management of dropped nucleus during phacoemulsification. *J Cataract Refract Surg.* 2001;27:1428-1432.

5. Lu H, Jiang YR, Grabow HB. Managing a dropped nucleus during the phacoemulsification learning curve. *J Cataract Refract Surg.* 1999;25:1311-1312.

6. Wasserman D, Apple DJ, Castaneda VE, et al. Anterior capsular tears and loop fixation of posterior chamber intraocular lenses. *Ophthalmology.* 1991;98:425-431.

7. Pollock WS, Casswell AG. Decentration of the posterior chamber lens implant: a comparison of capsulorhexis with endocapsular surgery. *Eye.* 1994;8:680-683.

8. Assia EI, Legler UF, Merrill C, et al. Clinicopathologic study of the effect of radial tears and loop fixation on intraocular lens decentration. *Ophthalmology.* 1993;100:153-158.

9. Assia EI, Legler UF, Apple DJ. The capsular bag after short- and long-term fixation of intraocular lenses. *Ophthalmology.* 1995;102:1151-1157.

10. Ram J, Apple DJ, Peng Q, et al. Update on fixation of rigid and foldable posterior chamber intraocular lenses. Part I: elimination of fixation-induced decentration to achieve precise optical correction and visual rehabilitation. *Ophthalmology.* 1999;106:883-890.

11. Tappin MJ, Larkin DF. Factors leading to lens implant decentration and exchange. *Eye.* 2000;14:773-776.

12. Ravalico G, Tognetto D, Palomba M, et al. Capsulorhexis size and posterior capsule opacification. *J Cataract Refract Surg.* 1996;22:98-103.

13. Hollick EJ, Spalton DJ, Meacock WR. The effect of capsulorhexis size on posterior capsular opacification: one-year results of a randomized prospective trial. *Am J Ophthalmol.* 1999;128:271-279.

14. Ram J, Pandey SK, Apple DJ, et al. Effect of in-the-bag intraocular lens fixation on the prevention of posterior capsule opacification. *J Cataract Refract Surg.* 2001;27:367-370.

15. Auffarth GU, Golescu A, Becker KA, Volcker HE. Quantification of posterior capsule opacification with round and sharp edge intraocular lenses. *Ophthalmology*. 2003;110:772-780.

16. Nishi O, Nishi K, Wickstrom K. Preventing lens epithelial cell migration using intraocular lenses with sharp rectangular edges. *J Cataract Refract Surg*. 2000;26:1543-1549.

17. Cekic O, Batman C. The relationship between capsulorhexis size and anterior chamber depth relation. *Ophthalmic Surg Lasers*. 1999;30:185-190.

18. Norby S. Souces of error in intraocular lens power calculation. *J Cataract Refract Surg*. 2008;34:368-376.

19. Hill WE. Intraocular lens power calculations: are we stuck in the past? *Clin Exp Ophthalmol*. 2009;37:761-762.

20. Hansen SO, Crandall AS, Olson RJ. Progressive constriction of the anterior capsular opening following intact capsulorhexis. *J Cataract Refract Surg*. 1993;19:77-82.

21. Davison JA. Capsule contraction syndrome. *J Cataract Refract Surg*. 1993;19:582-589.

22. Joo CK, Shin JA, Kim JH. Capsular opening contraction after continuous curvilinear capsulorhexis and intraocular lens implantation. *J Cataract Refract Surg*. 1996;22:585-590.

23. Hayashi K, Hayashi H, Nakao F, Hayashi F. Anterior capsule contraction and intraocular lens decentration and tilt after hydrogel lens implantation. *Br J Ophthalmol*. 2001;85:1294-1297.

24. Hayashi H, Hayashi K, Nakao F, Hayashi F. Anterior capsule contraction and intraocular lens dislocation in eyes with pseudo-exfoliation syndrome. *Br J Ophthalmol*. 1998;82:1429-1432.

25. Michael K, O'Colmain U, Vallance JH, Cormack TG. Capsule contraction syndrome with haptic deformation and flexion. *J Cataract Refract Surg*. 2010;36:686-689.

26. Werner L, Pandey SK, Escobar-Gomez M, et al. Anterior capsule opacification; a histopathological study comparing different IOL styles. *Ophthalmology*. 2000;107:463-471.

27. Jahan FS, Mamalis N, Crandall AS. Spontaneous late dislocation of intraocular lens within the capsular bag in psuedoexfoliation patients. *Ophthalmology*. 2001;108:1727-1731.

28. Chang DF. Prevention of bag-fixated IOL dislocation in pseudo-exfoliation. *Ophthalmology*. 2002;109:1951-1952.

29. Tadros A, Bhatt UK, Karim MNA, Zaheer A, Thomas PW. Removal of lens epithelial cells and the effect on capsulorhexis size. *J Cataract Refract Surg*. 2005;31:1569–1574.

30. Hayashi K, Yoshida M, Nakao F, Hayashi H. Prevention of anterior capsule contraction by anterior capsule relaxing incisions with neodymium:yttrium-aluminum-garnet laser. *Am J Ophthalmol* 2008;146:23-30.

31. Hayashi H, Hayashi K, Nakao F, Hayashi F. Area reduction in the anterior capsule opening in eyes of diabetes mellitus patients. *J Cataract Refract Surg*. 1998;24:1105-1110.

32. Masket S, Fram NR. Pseudophakic negative dysphotopsia: surgical management and new theory of etiology. *J Cataract Refract Surg*. 2011;37:1199-1207.

33. Nagy Z, Takacs A, Filkorn T, Sarayba M. Initial clinical evaluation of an intraocular femtosecond laser in cataract surgery. *J Refract Surg*. 2009;25:1053-1060.

34. Naranjo-Tackman R. How a femtosecond laser increases safety and precision in cataract surgery? *Curr Opin Ophthalmol*. 2011;22:53-57. Review.

35. He L, Sheehy K, Culbertson W. Femtosecond laser-assisted cataract surgery. *Curr Opin Ophthalmol*. 2011;22:43-52. Review.

36. Nagy ZZ, Kránitz K, Takacs AI, Miháltz K, Kovács I, Knorz MC. Comparison of intraocular lens decentration parameters after femtosecond and manual capsulotomies. *J Refract Surg*. 2011;27:564-569.

37. Kránitz K, Takacs A, Miháltz K, Kovács I, Knorz MC, Nagy ZZ. Femtosecond laser capsulotomy and manual continuous curvilinear capsulorrhexis parameters and their effects on intraocular lens centration. *J Refract Surg*. 2011;27:558-563.

38. Holland GN, Van Horn SD, Margolis TP. Cataract surgery with ciliary sulcus fixation of intraocular lenses in patients with uveitis. *Am J Ophthalmol*. 1999;128:21-30.

Please see companion narrated videos on the accompanying Web site at
www.Healio.com/phacochopvideos

17

Conquering Capsulorrhexis Complications

David F. Chang, MD

There are 5 general conditions that increase the risk of a radial capsulorrhexis tear. They are poor visibility, unexpected eye movement, anterior chamber shallowing, elevated intralenticular fluid pressure (intumescent white lens), and increased capsular elasticity and "pseudo elasticity." These conditions may arise either because of poor surgical technique or because of predisposing ocular anatomy or pathology. Understanding the mechanisms by which these factors lead to a radial tear is the key to avoiding this complication.

Poor Visibility

A bright red reflex and clear visibility are important in order to control the flap and to monitor the direction of the tear as it develops (Figure 17-1A-D). Delayed recognition of a peripherally escaping tear may preclude any chance to redirect it in time. Ocular causes of a poor red reflex include tear film debris, decreased corneal clarity, small pupils, anterior cortical opacity (anterior spokes or white cataract), nuclear brunescence, and vitreous opacities such as asteroid hyalosis or hemorrhage. Errors in surgical technique may also compromise visibility. Excessive drying can cloud the corneal epithelium. Poor irrigation fluid runoff may submerge the cornea. Clumsy instrument maneuvers might induce cornea striae or displace the globe out of

optimal microscope alignment. Finally, excessive downward pressure from the cystotome tip will penetrate and stir up the epinucleus. The resulting cystotome tracks cause focal disturbance of the red reflex right in the area where the base of the anterior capsular flap inserts (Figure 17-1E).

When difficulty with the capsulorrhexis is encountered, surgeons should continually optimize the microscope focus, the corneal tear film, and eye positioning so as to maximize the red reflex. The surgeon should increase the microscope zoom when necessary. For microscopes with separate coaxial and oblique illumination beams, the red reflex can be enhanced by using only the coaxial system, as described in the sidebar titled, *Optimizing the Red Reflex*. This eliminates the back light scatter from the sclera, limbus, and any corneal or anterior cortical opacity. Finally, trypan blue dye can be utilized if the red reflex is absent or compromised. Techniques for capsular dye staining are described in the following paragraphs.

Unexpected Eye Movement

The potential for eye movement is characteristic of topical anesthesia or the unintended consequence of a poor regional block. A sudden unanticipated head or eye movement as the capsular flap is being maneuvered may cause a peripheral radial tear. Patients must be appropriate

Chang DF.
Phaco Chop and Advanced Phaco Techniques: Strategies for Complicated Cataracts, Second Edition (pp 173-194).
© 2013 SLACK Incorporated.

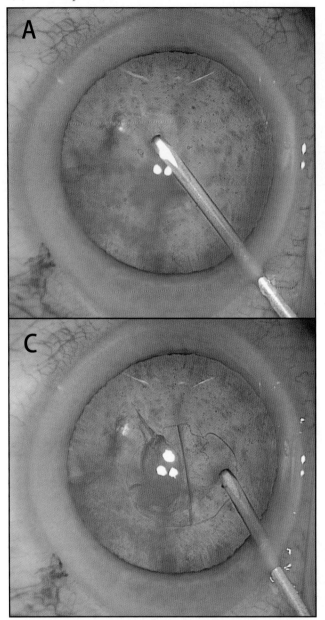

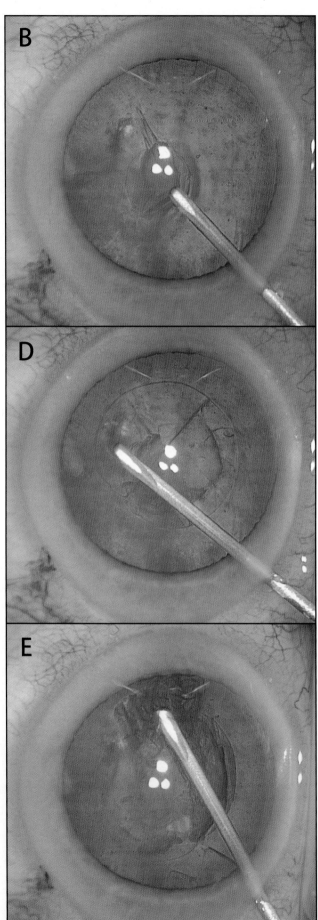

Figure 17-1. (A) Cystotome capsulorrhexis is initiated by puncturing centrally with a bent #25 needle, (B) tracing the shape of a "C" to create a small flap, (C) folding the flap over, and (D) using forceps or a cystotome to pull it. When manipulating the flap with the cystotome, care must be taken not to stir up the underlying cortex by over-penetrating with the needle tip. (E) The cystotome was used to deliberately stir up the epinucleus and cortex nasally to demonstrate focal loss of the red reflex in the exact area where the flap is located.

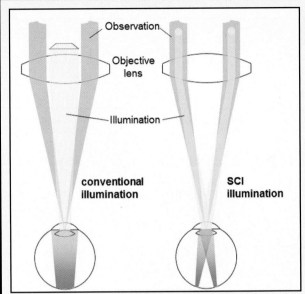

Figure 17-SB1. A comparison of conventional illumination beam (2 degrees offset from viewing axis) and SCI in which each ocular has its own coaxially aligned illumination beam. (Reprinted with permission of Carl Zeiss.)

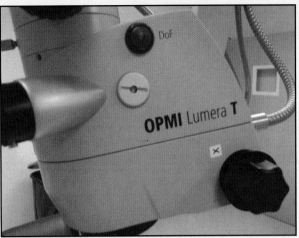

Figure 17-SB2. Autoclavable knob allows surgeon adjustment of oblique illumination beam shutter.

OPTIMIZING THE RED REFLEX

Anterior segment surgeons are not accustomed to thinking of the operating microscope as an "instrument," but increasing clinical experience with the Zeiss Lumera has enabled a better understanding of certain user options with dual illumination source microscope systems. In 2007, Zeiss introduced a new illumination system with their Lumera operating microscope. Compared to their OPMI systems featuring a single light beam, the Lumera actually splits the light source into three separate illumination beams. The traditional single OPMI illumination beam is aligned 2 degrees off of a truly coaxial viewing alignment (Figure 17-SB1). This near-coaxial orientation provides the red reflex familiar to all surgeons, and yet provides enough of an oblique lighting angle to produce minor shadows around structures. The latter are necessary to highlight depth and contrast, providing 3-dimensional (3D) detail of nuclear fragments or a sculpted nuclear trench.

The Lumera provides the surgeon with 2 separate illumination beam angles that can be separately switched off or combined together in differing proportions. The first is a 6-degree oblique *field* illumination, while the second is a separate *coaxial* illumination beam. The latter is subdivided into 2 separate coaxial light paths that are individually aligned with each microscope ocular (see Figure 17-SB1). Retroillumination is thereby maximized because each ocular's optical path has its own dedicated zero degree light source—a system that Zeiss calls *stereo coaxial illumination* (SCI).

The oblique beam can be limited by progressively reducing the aperture of a shutter through which it must pass. A side-mounted "shutter" knob with an autoclavable cover allows the surgeon to adjust the relative brightness of these 2 illumination components (field versus coaxial) during surgery (Figure 17-SB2). A tactile detent locates the knob setting where both beams are delivered at maximal intensity. Rotating the shutter knob in one direction gradually decreases the intensity of the oblique field component while the coaxial illumination is kept 100% open. Adjusting in the opposite direction turns off the coaxial light while maintaining the field illumination. This adjustment knob therefore allows surgeons to vary and customize the proportions of oblique and coaxial light illuminating the eye. Most surgeons will select a single adjustment setting that blends the 2 illumination sources in a preferred proportion to provide both an excellent red reflex and visualization of depth and contrast. Although the surgeon might gradually increase the overall microscope illumination intensity intraoperatively using a foot pedal button, there would generally be no need to adjust this shutter setting during routine cases.

When ocular conditions render a poor red reflex, however, the following shutter algorithm can significantly improve surgical visualization (Figure 17-SB3):

- **Step 1.** Perform the incision using a standard setting which combines coaxial and oblique illumination (Figure 17-SB3A).

- **Step 2.** Prior to the capsulotomy step, turn the oblique illumination beam completely off with the manual shutter knob, leaving the solitary coaxial beam 100% open (Figure 17-SB3C).

- **Step 3.** Use the foot pedal button to increase the coaxial beam brightness so as to compensate for the missing oblique component and intensify retroillumination.

(continued)

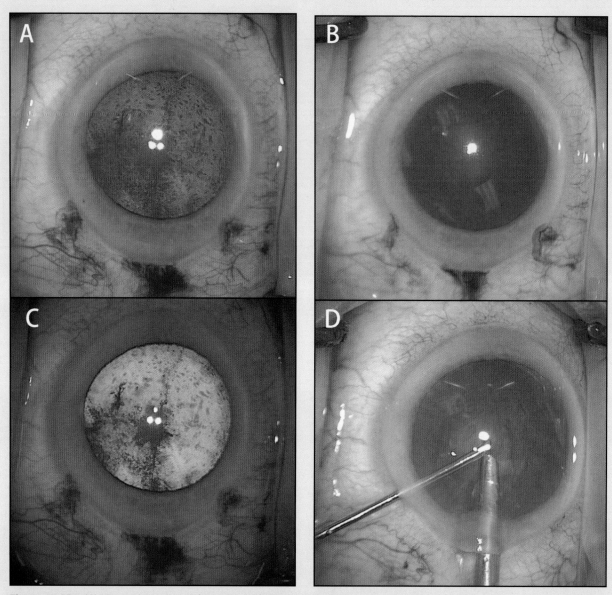

Figure 17-SB3. (A) Microscope view with combined field and SCI. (B) Microscope view with oblique illumination only (coaxial illumination turned off). There is almost no red reflex. (C) Microscope view with coaxial illumination on, but oblique field illumination turned off to enhance red reflex. (D) Microscope view with both coaxial and oblique field illumination restored for nuclear emulsification.

This eliminates oblique light reflecting off of the ocular structures that would otherwise visually wash out the red reflex intensity. The result is a noticeably brighter "Jack O'Lantern" red reflex that provides vastly improved retroillumination in the setting of a brunescent lens, anterior cortical spokes, corneal opacity or edema, small pupils, and vitreous opacities, such as asteroid hyalosis or hemorrhage. This maneuver makes it evident that corneal problems such as striae, band keratopathy, arcus senilis, dystrophic opacities and graft interfaces not only decrease transmission of the retroillumination, but reflect enough backscattered light to effectively wash out

the red reflex intensity. Perform the capsulorrhexis, hydrodissection, and hydrodelineation with this setting (Figure 17-SB3C).

- **Step 4.** Following hydrodelineation and rotation of the nucleus, the red reflex is typically lost. At this point, it becomes very difficult to visualize surgical depth and the contours of nuclear fragments with a coaxial beam only, and one should turn the oblique illumination source back on (Figure 17-SB3D). This maneuver highlights the importance of oblique lighting in allowing us to appreciate 3D depth.

(continued)

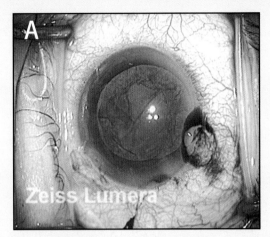 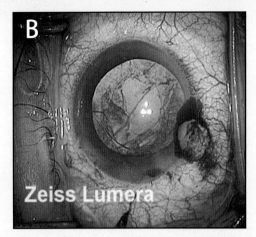

Figure 17-SB4. Microscope view (A) before and (B) after oblique field illumination is turned off to enhance red reflex and view of the posterior capsular tear.

- **Step 5.** Use the foot pedal button to decrease the overall brightness to compensate for adding back the oblique component beam. Complete nuclear emulsification and the remainder of the case.

Steps 2 and 3 can also be taken whenever there is a desire to enhance the red reflex as much as possible, such as when visualizing a posterior capsular tear (Figure 17-SB3). Finally, the coaxial light component can be independently switched off with the shutter adjustment knob in order to reduce light transmission to the retina during times when a red reflex is not required. During anterior segment surgery, such situations might include suturing of an incision and surgical steps involving the conjunctiva or sclera, such as dissecting a trabeculectomy flap.

The ability for the surgeon to independently employ solitary oblique or coaxial illumination, to blend these components in different proportions, and to vary the type of lighting as the case evolves is a new and welcome feature. This enables anterior segment surgeons to change and customize the surgical illumination according to the varying needs of different surgical steps and different eyes (Figure 17-SB4). As discussed, the specific recommendation is to vary the lighting mix using the aforementioned algorithm for those cases where the red reflex is poor.

Other microscopes employ different strategies to enhance the red reflex. The LuxOR with Illumin-i technology (Alcon) employs dual, collimated, zero-degree light beams that overlap at the focal point to provide a large "sweet spot." The light beams remain collimated because the objective lens is placed above the illumination system in the optical head. Using a larger diameter beam enhances contrast and helps create a 3D view, and makes pupil centration and alignment less of an issue compared to microscopes with a smaller illumination beam.

candidates for topical anesthesia; using appropriate levels of sedation and communication should enhance cooperation. For uncooperative patients or those with an excessive squeezing reflex, a retrobulbar or peribulbar block should be considered to better immobilize the eye. Fixation is improved under topical anesthesia by avoiding excessive microscope light intensity, which can induce squeezing. During the capsulotomy, the assistant should moisten the cornea in a manner that avoids startling the patient. One way to eliminate the need for an assistant to manually wet the cornea during surgery is to lubricate it in the following manner (Figure 17-2). The surgeon first smears a few streaks of a dispersive ophthalmic viscosurgical device (OVD) such as sodium chondroitin sulfate (Viscoat), Amvisc Plus, sodium hyaluronate 3% (Healon EndoCoat), or Occucoat onto the corneal surface (Figure 17-2A). Adding several drops of balanced salt solution will create an even, but viscous wetting layer that will resist evaporation and provide superb clarity (Figure 17-2B).

ANTERIOR CHAMBER SHALLOWING

The natural anterior convexity of the equatorial lens tends to steer any capsular tear toward the periphery. The shallower the chamber, the more convex the anterior capsule becomes, and the more the tear tends to run radially "downhill." The direction of the tear is most easily controlled if the anterior capsule surface is flat.

A shallow anterior chamber may be the natural result of a small globe, narrow angles, or an intumescent lens. Severe zonular laxity may result in an unexpectedly shallow chamber despite a normal axial length. A common cause of anterior capsule convexity is intraoperative shallowing

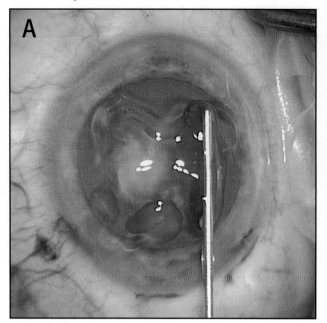 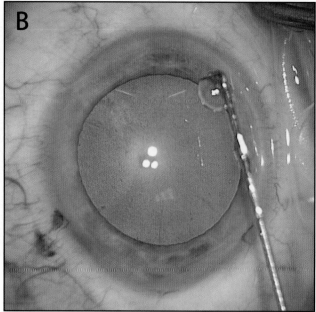

Figure 17-2. Improvement of corneal clarity by (A) spreading dispersive OVD on the surface and (B) placing several drops of saline.

of the anterior chamber caused by fluid or OVD escaping through the wound. Excessive instrument pressure on the posterior incision lip will burp the anterior chamber due to momentary wound gape, and the surgeon should interrupt the capsulotomy step to redeepen the chamber with OVD when necessary.

Because it creates more of a mass effect, a maximally cohesive OVD is better able to flatten the anterior capsule convexity compared to a dispersive OVD. However, the latter better resists being burped out through the incision. The soft-shell technique devised by Steve A. Arshinoff, MD, FRCSC, combines the complementary advantages of each type of OVD by placing the cohesive agent directly over the anterior capsule and blocking the incision with the dispersive OVD[1] (Figure 17-3). Sodium hyaluronate 2.3% (Healon 5) is a maximally cohesive and viscoadaptive OVD that combines both of these desirable characteristics in a single agent.[2,3]

INTUMESCENT WHITE LENS

Because of liquefied cortex, these cataracts create the dual challenge of an absent red reflex and higher intracapsular hydrostatic pressure that tends to forcibly extend a capsular tear peripherally.[4-8] (Cases 1-3: Figures 17-4 to 17-8). An initial anterior capsular puncture that explodes into a bi-directional radial tear creates the so-called "Argentinean flag sign"—so named because of the blue-white-blue striped appearance of such a tear in a trypan blue stained anterior capsule (see Figure 17-4). Not all white lenses are equally prone to this complication. It is often in

younger patients that the lens becomes the most swollen due to cortical liquefaction because the endonucleus is much smaller in these lenses. The resulting hyperosmotic gradient creates an elevated intracapsular fluid pressure. After the capsule is first punctured, a cloud of milky fluid may emanate further, compromising visibility (see Figure 17-7B). One must counterbalance this elevated intracapsular fluid pressure with enough cohesive OVD in order to prevent abrupt radialization of the initial capsular puncture or tear (see Figure 17-5G). Another strategy with an intumescent cataract is to first decompress the lens with a very small puncture or tear to allow lens fluid to escape. It is also possible to aspirate some liquefied cortex with a bevel down needle to further decompress the lens.[4]

With the larger nuclei characteristic of white lenses in older eyes, there is proportionally less liquefied cortex and less likelihood of elevated intracapsular pressure. However, one must be aware that intracapsular liquefied cortex trapped posteriorly will still tend to propel the nucleus forward. This in turn creates a strong tendency for the anterior capsule tear to veer radially (see Figure 17-7F). In addition to adequately pressurizing the anterior chamber with a cohesive OVD, making a smaller diameter capsulorrhexis will help to maintain control over the developing tear with white cataracts[4,8] (see Figures 17-5K-L and 17-7C-M). The capsulorrhexis diameter can always be secondarily enlarged following IOL insertion[8] (see Figure 17-8).

Capsular Dye

By permitting visualization of the anterior capsule in the absence of a good red reflex, capsular dye represents

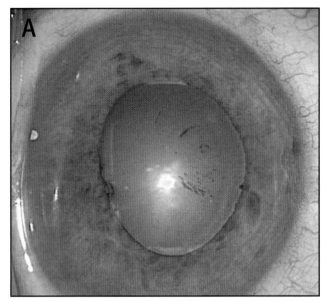 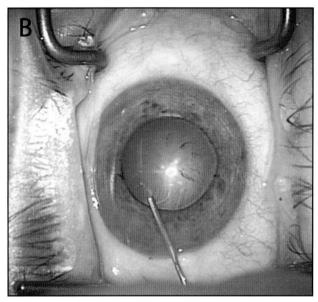

Figure 17-3. (A) Soft shell viscoelastic technique in an eye with a small pupil and crowded anterior segment. Prior laser iridotomy is visible to the left. (B) Dispersive viscoelastic, such as Viscoat, is used to coat the corneal epithelium.

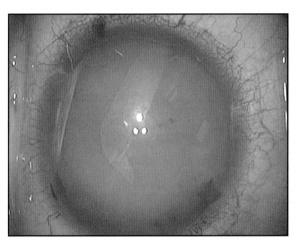

Figure 17-4. Case 1. White intumescent lens in a 16 year old. As soon as the capsulotomy was initiated with a cystotome, high intralenticular pressure caused abrupt and immediate radial extension of the tear.

one of the most important advances in the management of complicated cataracts.[7,9-21] Indocyanine green and trypan blue dyes are both safe and effective. Safety does depend on the specific dye and the formulation, however. Endothelial decompensation requiring corneal transplantation has been reported from using methylene blue dye to stain the capsule,[22] and toxic anterior segment syndrome (TASS) has been reported from using noncommercially formulated trypan blue dye.[23]

In 2000, this author reported the first clinical comparison of ICG and trypan blue.[11] Both agents render the capsule visible against the stark contrast of white cortex. However, trypan blue provides a significantly darker and more intense staining of the capsule.[11,12,14-17] (see Figures 17-5 and 17-6) This is particularly helpful when dealing with a mature brunescent nucleus or when other factors, such as corneal edema, are present. In addition, trypan blue provides a more persistent staining of the anterior capsule. This greatly facilitates nuclear emulsification in mature white and brown lenses, where poor visibility of the capsulorrhexis edge makes it more likely to be torn with the phaco tip or chopper (see Figures 17-7N and 17-7O). Several studies have shown that trypan blue decreases elasticity of the anterior capsule.[24,25] However, this does not appear to decrease the resistance of the capsular edge to tearing.[26]

There are several different capsule staining techniques. Minas Coroneo, MD, MS, MSc, FRACS, FRANZCO pioneered the use of trypan blue and holds the patent for its use in eye surgery. He prefers to inject the dye solution directly into the anterior chamber before washing it out. This produces a reasonable degree of anterior capsule staining. Takayuki Akahoshi, MD has described mixing ICG with viscoelastic for use as a single injection. Marques and Osher described first injecting Healon 5, and then layering a small amount of saline directly over the anterior lens capsule.[18] This creates a thin potential fluid space overlying the anterior lens capsule into which trypan blue can be placed, without creating an opaque mixture of OVD and dye (see Figures 17-6D-F).

Horiguchi and Melles described the technique of injecting capsular dye after first filling the anterior chamber with air to avoid excessive dilution of the dye[9,10] (see Figure 17-6B). Several drops of dye from a tuberculin syringe are placed directly onto the anterior capsule surface through a 30-gauge cannula (see Figures 17-6C-E). The dye is then irrigated away, the anterior chamber is filled

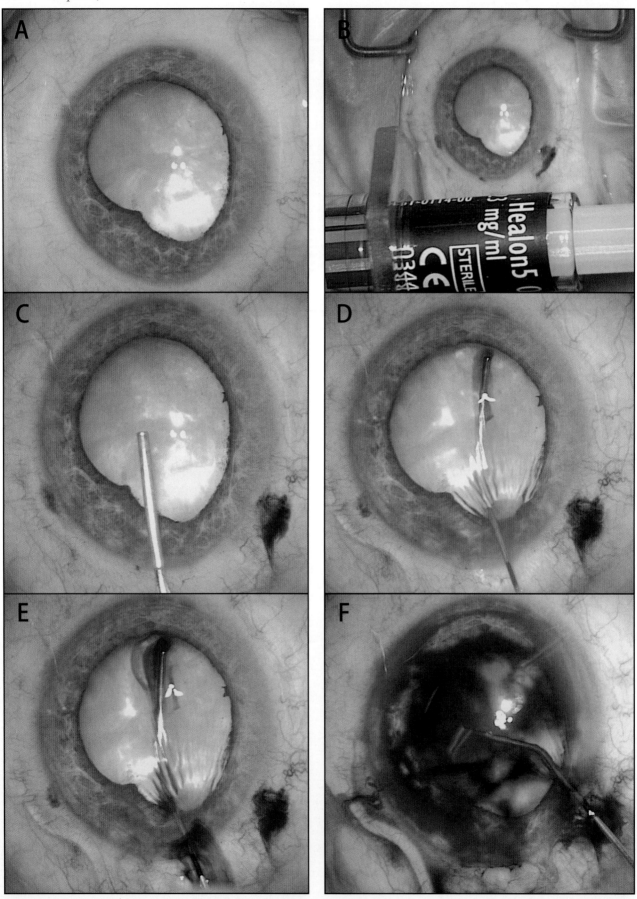

Figure 17-5. Case 2. (A) White intumescent lens. (B, C) Healon 5 is used to inflate, but slightly under-fill the anterior chamber. (D, E) Using a 30-gauge cannula, Vision Blue (DORC) dye is injected onto the anterior capsule surface just beneath the corpus of Healon 5 so that (F) a puddle of dye separates the OVD from the capsular surface.

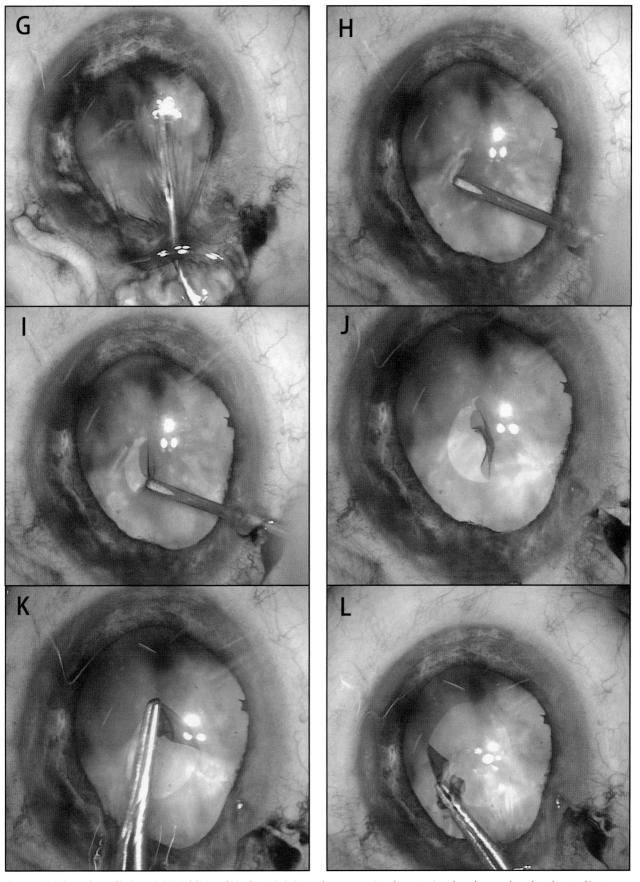

Figure 17-5 (continued). Case 2. (G) Additional Healon 5 is injected to pressurize the anterior chamber so that the elevated intracapsular pressure is counterbalanced. (H) This prevents abrupt radialization of the initial cystotome puncture, (I, J) and allows controlled creation of a curved flap. (K, L) Because of the higher risk of a radial tear, the capsulorrhexis diameter is kept on the small side as it is completed with forceps.

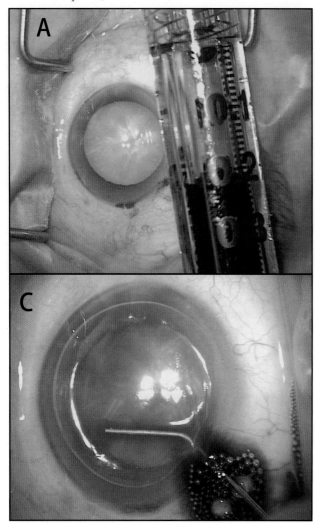

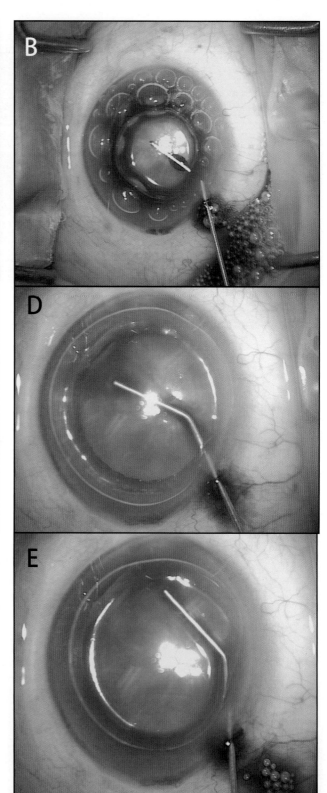

Figure 17-6. Case 3. (A, B) White intumescent lens stained with trypan blue beneath an air bubble. (C-E) Although the bubble meniscus tends to displace dye from contacting the central anterior capsule surface, the cannula is used to contact and paint the capsule by allowing dye to pool alongside it due to capillary action.

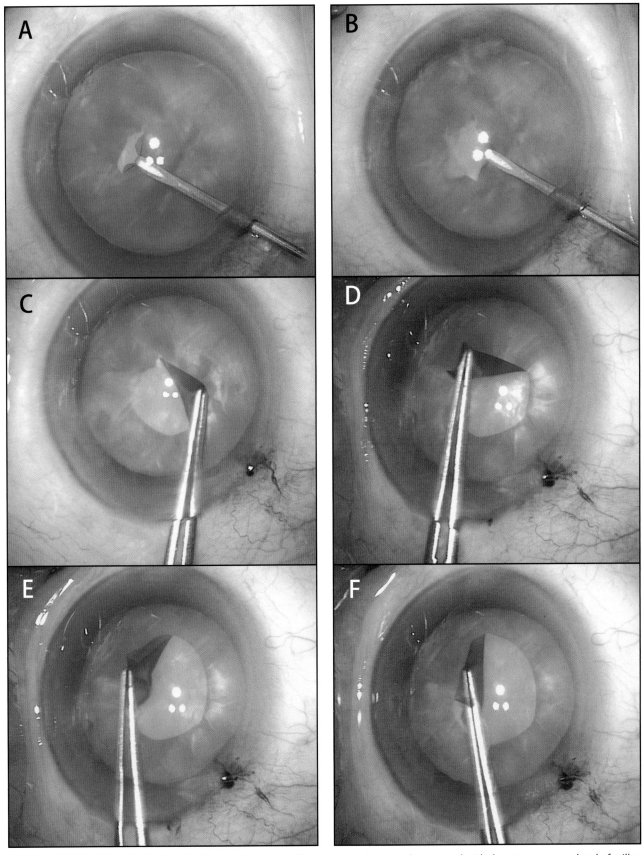

Figure 17-7. Case 3. Brian Little Tear Out Rescue Maneuver. (A) As soon as the capsule is incised with the cystotome, a cloud of milky cortex is released. (B) Note the milky cortical debris overlying the nasal pupil. (C-E) The flap is advanced with forceps with excellent visualization afforded by the intense trypan blue capsule staining. Because of the higher risk of a radial tear, the diameter is kept on the small side. Due to intralenticular pressure, the tear wants to escape radially. (F) The tear is veering away from the direction of the forceps tip vector.

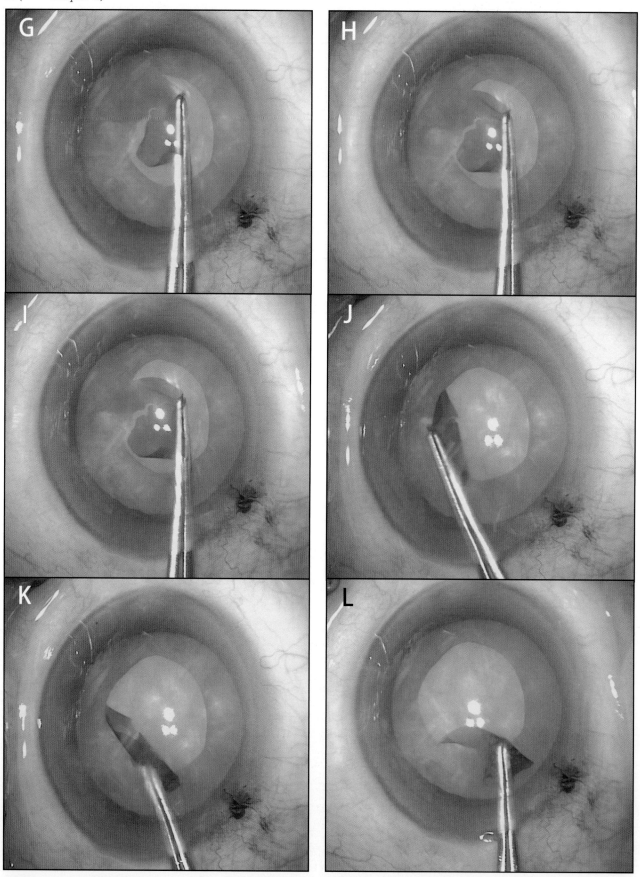

Figure 17-7 (continued). Case 3. Brian Little Tear Out Rescue Maneuver. (G-I) Using the Little Maneuver, the flap is folded back and traction is applied in order to turn the tear centripetally inward. (J-M) Once control is re-established, the flap is pulled forward again to complete the capsulotomy.

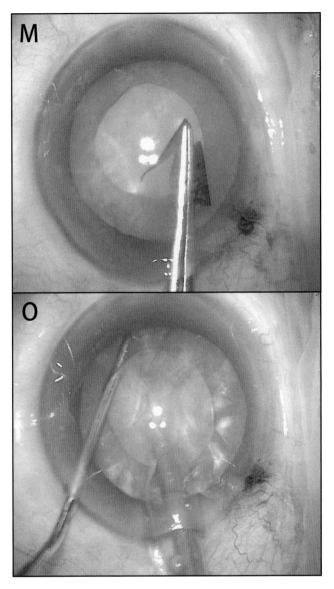

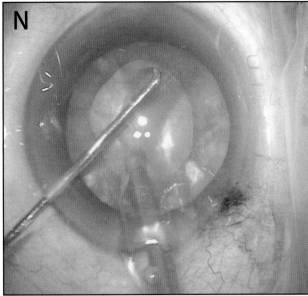

Figure 17-7 (continued). Case 3. Brian Little Tear Out Rescue Maneuver. (N, O) The intense and persistent staining achieved with trypan blue permits visualization of the anterior capsule during phaco chop.

INCREASED CAPSULAR ELASTICITY AND "PSEUDOELASTICITY"

The more elastic a material is, the more difficult it is to control how it tears. As an example, latex is more difficult to tear accurately than paper. As one attempts to tear an elastic material, it first stretches before abruptly splitting. Because of the rebound energy, the resulting tear is overly rapid and tends to slingshot away from, rather than toward, the grasping instrument. Because pediatric anterior capsules are very thin and elastic, the flap tends to spiral outward and is very difficult to control[27] (Figures 17-9 and 17-10). Likewise, the adult posterior capsule has less tensile strength and is thinner and more elastic than the anterior capsule. It behaves more like the pediatric anterior capsule, and accomplishing a posterior capsulorrhexis is very challenging for this reason. Finally, some adult anterior capsules are very thin, and behave in this way. As these anterior capsules tear, the edges are rough, rather than smooth (Figure 17-11).

Lacking sufficient circumferential tension, a capsule that is not taut will also exhibit elastic behavior. As the surgeon pulls on the capsulorrhexis flap, the peripheral anterior capsule should remain immobile if the zonules are strong enough to keep it taut. This facilitates precise control over the ensuing direction of the tear. Weak zonules fail to keep the anterior capsule taut, giving rise to a situation that the author calls *capsular pseudoelasticity*[28] (Figure 17-12). Although the anterior capsule is of normal adult thickness it behaves as though it is thin and elastic because of insufficient zonular traction. Because the lax and pliant peripheral

with OVD, and the capsulotomy is performed in the usual manner (see Figure 17-7). One drawback of this technique is that the air bubble meniscus displaces the dye from contacting the center of the anterior capsule. The author uses an air bubble, but then strokes the cannula slowly back and forth across the central anterior capsular surface (see Figure 17-6C-E). Capillary action causes dye to pool alongside the cannula shaft, assuring prolonged capsular contact. This method results in darker capsular staining compared to the classic air bubble or direct injection techniques, and allows one to exchange the air bubble with a fresh OVD injection to provide a maximally clear view of the capsule.

Capsular dye should be considered whenever difficulty with anterior capsule visualization is anticipated. It can even be applied after the capsulorrhexis has been initiated. This is because both dyes preferentially stain the capsule, but not the cortex. Finally, capsular dye is a useful teaching aid when first learning to perform a capsulorrhexis, or for when transitioning to horizontal phaco chop.

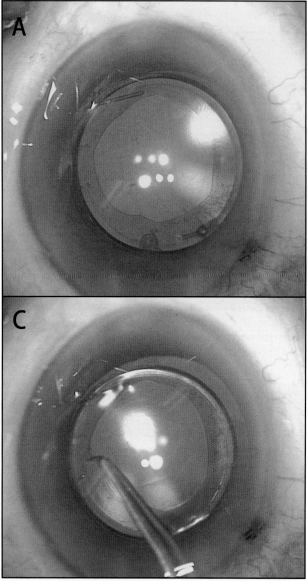
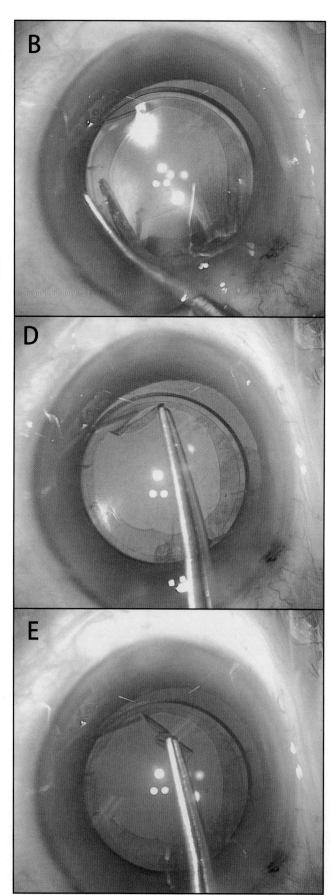

Figure 17-8. Case 3. Secondary enlargement of capsulorrhexis. (A) Trypan blue provides persistent capsule staining. (B) Uthoff-Gills scissors (Katena Eye Instruments, Denville, NJ) create an oblique anterior capsular cut to create a new flap. (C-E) The flap is advanced with the surgeon's right hand.

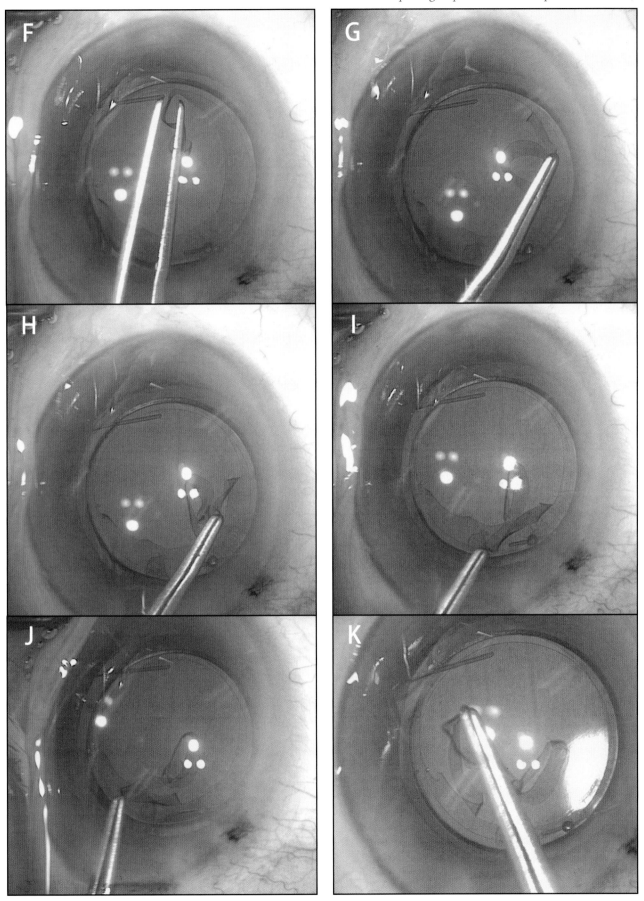

Figure 17-8 (continued). Case 3. Secondary enlargement of capsulorrhexis. (F-I) The surgeon changes to the left hand to advance the flap on the opposite side. (J-L) The right hand is used to complete the secondary enlargement.

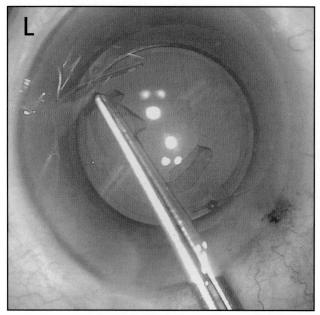

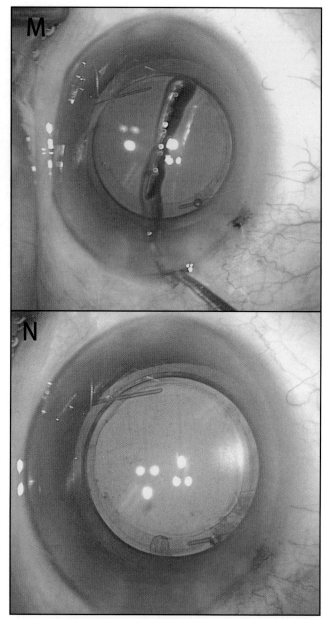

Figure 17-8 (continued). Case 3. Secondary enlargement of capsulorrhexis. (M) The ribbon of trimmed capsule is removed (N) leaving an enlarged capsulotomy diameter that still overlaps the circumferential optic edge.

capsule tends to move along with and in the same direction as the flap, the tear is difficult to control and will tend to veer radially.

Poor surgical technique whereby the capsular flap is allowed to become too long can also create pseudoelastic behavior. The farther the grasping point of the capsule forceps is from the tearing point, the more pliant the flap becomes and the more difficult it is to direct the tear. If the tear starts to spiral radially outward, the surgeon must regrasp the flap closer to the leading edge of the tear to improve control.

In higher-risk cases, the author considers the capsulorrhexis to be a "zonular stress test" because the first indication of how weak the zonules are becomes evident during this step. If the anterior capsule is not taut, the cystotome tip will tend to first dimple, wrinkle, and indent it, rather than immediately puncture it (Figure 17-9A-C; Figure 17-13). The appearance mimics that of using a dull cystotome. Next, as the surgeon tugs the capsular flap, the peripheral lens capsule is likely to stretch and move along with the flap toward the forceps (see Figure 17-12). With extreme zonular weakness, the entire lens may start to move with the capsule forceps. In addition to using capsule forceps to regrasp the flap more frequently, employing the tear out recovery technique described by Brian Little is invaluable in these situations and is described in the following section.[29]

If pseudoelasticity is severe, the surgeon can use iris hooks or specially designed capsule retractors to help anchor the bag during the capsulorrhexis step.[30,31] After completing several clock hours of the capsulorrhexis, one or

more capsule retractors can be used to stabilize the bag and provide helpful countertraction against the tugging flap. It is easy to exert too much tension on the capsule edge with the retractors, which will abruptly extend the tear peripherally. One should never insert a capsular tension ring (CTR) before completing the capsulorrhexis because the expansive force of the ring will extend the tear. If the pupil is of borderline size, enlarge its diameter with iris retractors. Optimal visualization of the peripheral capsular region is of far greater importance here than with a routine case.

Opinions differ regarding the target diameter of the capsulorrhexis in eyes with loose zonules. A larger-diameter capsulorrhexis will facilitate nuclear and cortical removal, but it is much harder to control and complete in eyes with capsular pseudoelasticity. In eyes with weakened zonules,

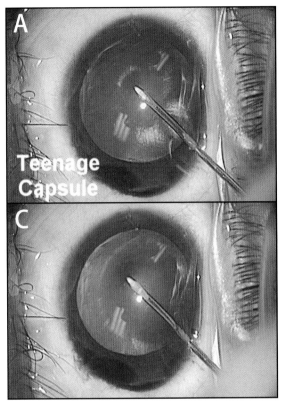

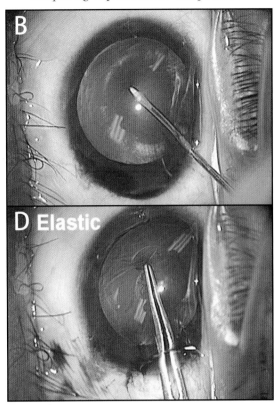

Figure 17-9. Case 4. Teenager with thin elastic capsule. (A-C) The sharp cystotome needle point is not able to incise the anterior capsule because it is so thin and elastic. By instead depressing the central anterior capsule, a halo light reflex is created. (D) The elastic peripheral capsule stretches during the capsulotomy, making it difficult to control the direction of the tear. The capsulotomy diameter is kept smaller, and the Little Maneuver is used in order to prevent a radial tear.

the more peripherally the tear advances, the more it wants to veer radially, and the more difficult it is to rescue the flap. By comparison, a smaller-diameter capsulorrhexis is much easier to control and increases the margin for error for recognizing and rescuing a peripherally escaping tear. Although a small-diameter capsulotomy may hinder subsequent surgical steps, it is far preferable to having a torn capsular edge, particularly when other risk factors are present. For this reason, and because a capsulorrhexis is a prerequisite for utilizing capsular retractors and a CTR, the author recommends aiming for a smaller diameter capsulorrhexis in the presence of significant zonular laxity. The surgeon should mentally visualize its diameter during nuclear emulsification, however, so as not to tear it with the chopper shaft or phaco tip. Bimanual instrumentation is superior for cortical clean-up in a floppy capsular bag and greatly improves subincisional access through a small capsulorrhexis. Finally, the surgeon should consider secondarily enlarging a small capsulorrhexis after the IOL and capsular tension ring are safely implanted, as discussed in the previous chapter.

RESCUE OF ERRANT CAPSULE TEAR

The Brian Little Tear Out Rescue Manuever is one of the most important capsulotomy skills to master, and is applicable to virtually every difficult situation[29] (Figure 17–14). The capsulotomy is normally created by pulling the free capsule flap ahead of its insertion point (Figure 17-7C-E). Control is maintained by continually regrasping the flap with forceps or re-engaging it with a sharp cystotome. When the surgeon starts to lose control, the tear can be seen to head radially outward rather than following the inward vector of the moving forceps tip (Figure 17-7F). Recognizing this, the surgeon must stop before the tear escapes too far peripherally and assess the cause. If the anterior chamber has shallowed, redeepening it with OVD and regrasping the flap closer to its base may help.

Often, lack of control is due to elevated intracapsular fluid pressure, capsular elasticity, or pseudoelasticity. One option is to abandon the flap and use capsule scissors to create a new flap that can be torn in the opposite direction. The problem is that to avoid a radial discontinuity, the

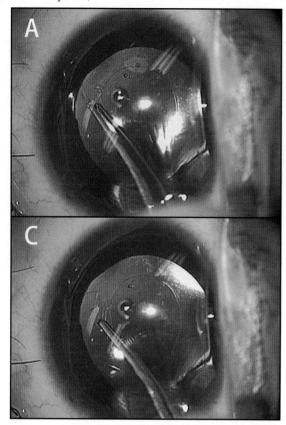
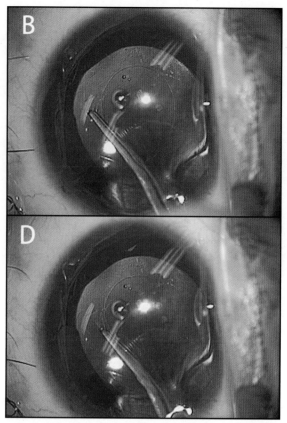

Figure 17-10. Case 4. (A) After IOL implantation, secondary enlargement of the capsulorrhexis is performed, but the tear is extending radially. (B-D) The Little Maneuver must be employed to control the flap, which stretches and wants to slingshot peripherally.

second tear must encompass and pass peripherally around the terminal point of the first tear before connecting. This is invariably difficult because the same conditions predisposing to radialization of the first tear still exist.

The Brian Little Tear Out Rescue Maneuver is an ingenious but counterintuitive method of redirecting an escaping anterior capsular tear. The first step is to unfold the flap backward and to place it on traction by pulling it away from the intended direction of the tear (see Figure 17-7G). By maintaining backward traction on the flap, one should be able to then redirect the tear back toward the center (see Figures 17-11H-I). Analogous to pulling on a bed sheet where one end is tucked in, this traction prevents the tear from moving in any direction other than that which the surgeon intends. Once the diverging tear has been successfully redirected, the flap can be folded forward and the traditional capsulotomy technique can be resumed (see Figures 17-7J-M).

TORN CAPSULORRHEXIS

The incidence of anterior capsule tears reported from 4 contemporary studies varies from 0.8% to 5%.[32-35] The highest rate was from a resident series.[33] In Dr. Robert Osher's series of more than 2600 consecutive eyes, the overall rate of anterior capsule tears was 0.8%, and the incidence of tears occurring during the capsulorrhexis step was 0.5%.[34] Forty-eight percent of these anterior capsular tears eventually extended into the posterior capsule and 19% of cases with a torn capsulorrhexis required an anterior vitrectomy. This study suggests that the risk of significant complications from a torn capsulorrhexis is very high, even in the most experienced hands.

If a peripheral radial anterior capsule tear occurs, one must consider any surgical comorbidities before deciding upon a surgical strategy. For a brunescent nucleus with weak zonules and a small pupil, converting to a large incision, manual extracapsular cataract procedure may be prudent. In this case, a can opener capsulotomy can be created,

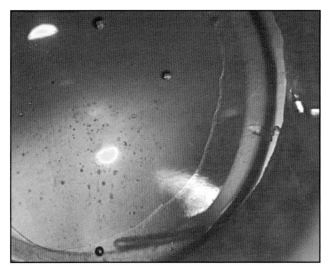

Figure 17-11. Close-up of jagged capsulorrhexis edge typical of a thin anterior capsule. The flap tends to veer radially in such a capsule.

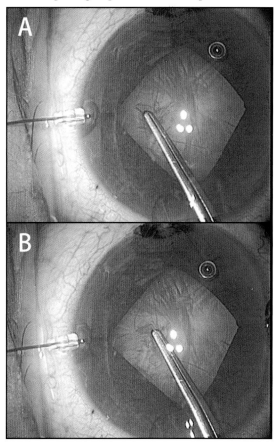

Figure 17-12. Pseudoelasticity. This patient with pseudoexfoliation has weak zonules which allows the peripheral capsule in this area to behave as though it were elastic. It moves excessively with manipulation of the capsule flap.

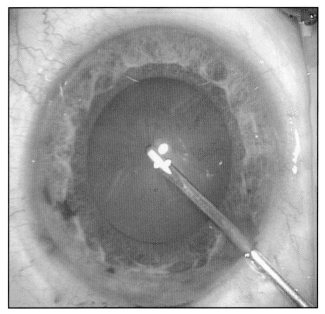

Figure 17-13. Pseudoexfoliation. Due to insufficient circumferential zonular tension, the anterior capsule is not taut and the cystotome needle tends to indent rather than incise the capsule, creating radiating capsular folds.

or at the very least, the continuous edge of the capsule should be incised in several places adjacent to the incision to avoid creating a capsular barrier to nucleus extraction. If one decides to phaco a brunescent nucleus because the zonules are normal, making 2 additional anterior capsule relaxing incisions 120 degrees away may reduce the chance for a wraparound posterior capsular tear by redistributing surgical forces to multiple points. If the nucleus is reasonably soft, one can opt to continue the continuous edge

capsulotomy from the opposite direction, prior to performing phaco in the presence of the single radial anterior capsular tear.

The surgical maneuver most likely to extend a single radial anterior capsular tear into the posterior capsule is intracapsular rotation of either the nucleus or the IOL. Rotating either structure with a single instrument requires that we first push it against the equator of the capsular bag to establish counter fixation prior to applying torque. In my opinion and experience, this is the moment at which a wraparound tear occurs. Therefore, emulsifying the nucleus without rotating it is one helpful strategy when proceeding with phaco in the presence of a capsulorrhexis tear (see Figure 18-11).

Gentle hydrodissection and hydrodelineation will not extend the anterior capsule tear, and in fact are critically important if one is to remove both the endonucleus and the epinucleus without rotation. With a smaller-sized endonucleus, hydrodissection may even be able to prolapse one pole of the nucleus out of the bag. If this can be

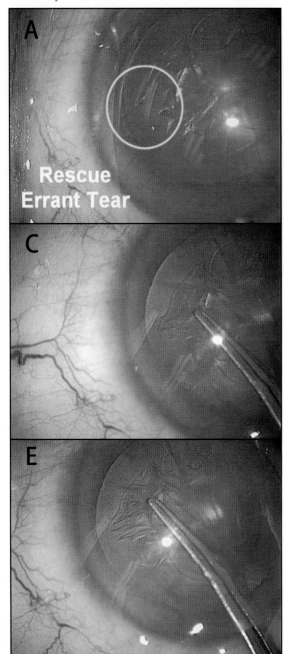

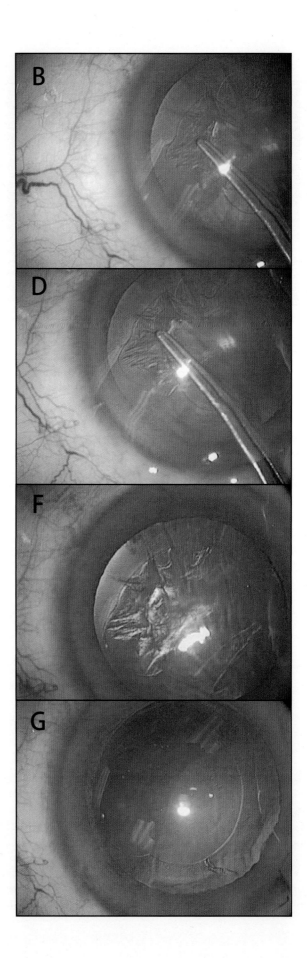

Figure 17-14. The Little Maneuver. (A) The capsulorrhexis tear is escaping peripherally due to focal zonular laxity. (B-E) The flap is pulled backward and placed on tension to improve directional control as the tear is advanced (F, G) and completed.

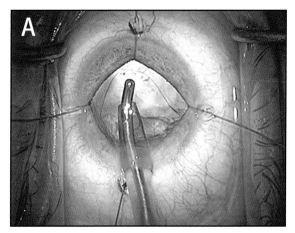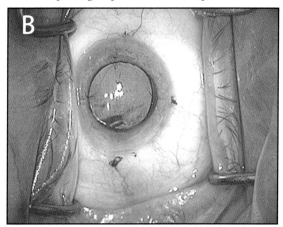

Figure 17-15. (A) A peripheral radial tear is visualized at the conclusion of cortical clean-up. (B) A single-piece acrylic IOL has been implanted with the haptics oriented 90 degrees away from the radial capsulorrhexis tear.

accomplished, flipping the nucleus into the supracapsular location will spare the capsular bag from the mechanical forces imparted by phaco. An alternative approach is to make the first 2 horizontal or vertical chops/fractures without rotating the nucleus (see Figures 18-11A-D). The first fragment that is created is lifted out of the capsular bag (see Figures 18-11G-H). Especially if the endonucleus is small enough, the remaining hemisections can be elevated out of the bag with the phaco tip or the horizontal chopper (see Figures 18-11I-N).

Following cortical clean-up, the bag should be filled with OVD. The capsulorrhexis will take on a tear drop shape because of the radial tear (Figure 17-15A). Injection of a single-piece hydrophobic acrylic lens can easily be performed while orienting the haptics 90 degrees away from the radial tear (Figure 17-15B). The haptics open slowly enough to rotate the IOL without applying any force against the capsular equator. However, if this IOL design is not available, a 3-piece IOL can also be safely placed inside the capsular bag with a single radial tear. The key is to avoid forcefully decentering the optic and haptic toward the quadrant where the capsulorrhexis is torn. One can accomplish this by first directing the lead haptic into the anterior chamber rather than into the capsular bag. This allows the surgeon to rotate the trailing haptic into the bag while all decentering forces are applied against the opposite anterior chamber angle. The second haptic is rotated into the bag by decentering the optic away from the capsulorrhexis tear. The haptics are then oriented approximately 90 degrees away from the location of the radial tear. The advantage of completing phaco in the presence of a single capsulorrhexis tear is that the intended IOL can still be placed inside the capsular bag with a low risk of postoperative decentration. IOL placement into the ciliary sulcus is an acceptable option, but increases the risk of a refractive surprise or postoperative decentration due to insufficient overall length.

REFERENCES

1. Arshinoff SA. Dispersive-cohesive viscoelastic soft shell technique. *J Cataract Refract Surg.* 1999;25:167-173.
2. Dick HB, Krummenauer F, Augustin AJ, Pakula T, Pfeiffer N. Healon 5 viscoadaptive formulation: comparison to Healon and Healon GV. *J Cataract Refract Surg.* 2001;27:320-326.
3. Arshinoff SA. Using BSS with viscoadaptives in the ultimate soft-shell technique. *J Cataract Refract Surg.* 2002;28:1509-1514.
4. Gimbel HV, Willerscheidt AB. What to do with limited view: the intumescent cataract. *J Cataract Refract Surg.* 1993;19:657-661.
5. Ermiss SS, Ozturk F, Inan UU. Comparing the efficacy and safety of phacoemulsification in white mature and other types of senile cataracts. *Br J Ophthalmol.* 2003;87:1356–1359.
6. Chen YJ, Wu PC. Automated irrigation/aspiration before phacoemulsification in eyes with white cataracts. *Ophthalmic Surg Lasers Imaging.* 2005;36:118-121.
7. Goldman JM, Karp CL. Adjunct devices for managing challenging cases in cataract surgery: capsular staining and ophthalmic viscosurgical devices. *Curr Opin Ophthalmol.* 2007;18:52-57. Review.
8. Kara-Junior N, de Santhiago MR, Kawakami A, Carricondo P, Hida WT. Mini-rhexis for white intumescent cataracts. *Clinics* (Sao Paulo). 2009;64:309-312.
9. Horiguchi M, Miyake K, Ohta I, Ito Y. Staining of the lens capsule for circular continuous capsulorrhexis in eyes with white cataract. *Arch Ophthalmol.* 1998;116:535-537.
10. Melles G, de Waard P, Pameyer J, Beekhuis W. Trypan blue capsule staining to visualize the capsulorrhexis in cataract surgery. *J Cataract Refract Surg.* 1999;25: 7-9.
11. Chang DF. Capsule staining and mature cataracts: a comparison of indocyanine green and trypan blue dyes. *Br J Ophthalmol.* 2000;84: video report.
12. Pandey SK, Werner L, Escobar-Gomez M, Roig-Melo EA, Apple DJ. Dye-enhanced cataract surgery. Part 1: anterior capsule staining for capsulorrhexis in advanced/white cataract. *J Cataract Refract Surg.* 2000;26:1052-1059.
13. Pandey SK, Werner L, Escobar-Gomez M, Roig-Melo EA, Apple DJ. Dye-enhanced cataract surgery. Part 2: learning critical steps of phacoemulsification. *J Cataract Refract Surg.* 2000;26:1060-1065.

14. Pandey SK, Werner L, Vroman DT, Apple DJ. Dye-enhanced anterior capsulorhexis: surgical techniques, guidelines, and recommendations for surgeons. *Comp Ophthalmol Update.* 2003;4:179-185.

15. Chang DF. Comments on: Dye-enhanced anterior capsulorhexis: surgical techniques, guidelines, and recommendations for surgeons. *Comp Ophthalmol Update.* 2003;4:187-188.

16. Jacob S, Agarwal A, Agarwal S, Chowdhary S, Chowdhary R, Bagmar AA. Trypan blue as an adjunct for safe phacoemulsification in eyes with white cataract. *J Cataract Refract Surg.* 2002;28:1819-1825.

17. Dada VK, Sharma N, Sudan R, Sethi H, Dada T, Pangtey MS. Anterior capsule staining for capsulorhexis in cases of white cataract: comparative clinical study. *J Cataract Refract Surg.* 2004;30:326-333.

18. Marques DMV, Marques FF, Osher RH. Three-step technique for staining the anterior lens capsule with indocyanine green or trypan blue. *J Cataract Refract Surg.* 2004;30:13-16.

19. Chung CF, Liang CC, Lai JSM, Lo ESF, Lam DSC. Safety of trypan blue 1% and indocyanine green 0.5% in assisting visualization of anterior capsule during phacoemulsification in mature cataract. *J Cataract Refract Surg.* 2005;31:938-942.

20. Jacobs DS, Cox TA, Wagoner MD, Ariyasu RG, Karp CL. Capsule staining as an adjunct to cataract surgery: a report from the American Academy of Ophthalmology. *Ophthalmology.* 2006;113:707-713.

21. Wong VW, Lai TY, Lee GK, Lam PT, Lam DS. A prospective study on trypan blue capsule staining under air vs under viscoelastic. *Eye* (Lond). 2006;20:820-825.

22. Brouzas D, Droutsas D, Charakidas A, Malias I, Georgiadou E, Apostolopoulos M, Moschos M. Severe toxic effect of methylene blue 1% on iris epithelium and corneal endothelium. *Cornea.* 2006;25:470-471.

23. Buzard K, Zhang JR, Thumann G, Stripecke R, Sunalp M. Two cases of toxic anterior segment syndrome from generic trypan blue. *J Cataract Refract Surg.* 2010;36:2195-2199.

24. Dick HB, Aliyeva SE, Hengerer F. Effect of trypan blue on the elasticity of the human anterior lens capsule. *J Cataract Refract Surg.* 2008;34:1367-1373.

25. Jardeleza MSR, Daly MK, Kaufman JD, Klapperich C, Legutko PA. Effect of trypan blue staining on the elastic modulus of anterior lens capsules of diabetic and nondiabetic patients. *J Cataract Refract Surg.* 2009;35:318-323.

26. Jaber R, Werner L, Fuller S, et al. Comparison of capsulorhexis resistance to tearing with and without trypan blue dye using a mechanized tensile strength model. *J Cataract Refract Surg.* 2012;38:507-512.

27. Saini JS, Jain AK, Sukhija F, et al. Anterior and posterior capsulorhexis in pediatric cataract surgery with or without trypan blue dye. Randomized prospective clinical study. *J Cataract Refract Surg.* 2003;29:1733-1737.

28. Chang DF. Phacoemulsification in high-risk cases. In: Wallace RB, ed. *Multifocal IOLs and Refractive Cataract Surgery.* Chapter 11. Thorofare, NJ: Slack Incorporated; 2001.

29. Little BC, Smith JH, Packer M. Little capsulorhexis tear-out rescue. *J Cataract Refract Surg.* 2006;32:1420-1422.

30. Lee V, Bloom P. Microhook capsule stabilization for phacoemulsification in eyes with pseudoexfoliation-syndrome-induced lens instability. *J Cataract Refract Surg.* 1999;25:1567-1570.

31. Mackool RJ. Capsule stabilization for phacoemulsification (letter). *J Cataract Refract Surg.* 2000;26:629.

32. Muhtaseb M, Kalhoro A, Ionides A. A system for preoperative stratification of cataract patients according to risk of intraoperative complications. *Br J Ophthalmol.* 2004;88:1242-1246.

33. Unal M, Yücel I, Sarici A, et al. Phacoemulsification with topical anesthesia: resident experience. *J Cataract Refract Surg.* 2006;32:1361-1365.

34. Marques FF, Marques DM, Osher RH, Osher JM. Fate of anterior capsule tears during cataract surgery. *J Cataract Refract Surg.* 2006;32:1638-1642.

35. Olali CA, Ahmed S, Gupta M. Surgical outcome following breach rhexis. *Eur J Ophthalmol.* 2007;17:565-570.

Please see companion narrated videos on the accompanying Web site at
www.Healio.com/phacochopvideos

18

Pearls for Hydrodissection and Hydrodelineation

David F. Chang, MD

The topic of hydrodissection receives relatively little attention compared to phacoemulsification and intraocular lens (IOL) insertion techniques and may therefore be the most underrated step of modern cataract surgery. A properly developed hydrodissection fluid wave should hug the internal capsular surface as it travels behind the nucleus (Figure 18-1A-C).[1,2] The subsequent hydrodelineation wave propagates along a more internal plane that cleaves the epinucleus apart from the endonucleus (Figure 18-1D).[2,3]

There are 3 important objectives for hydrodissection. First, because the phaco tip is confined to one location, nuclear rotation is integral to every phaco technique. Effective hydrodissection allows the entire nucleus to rotate without placing undue stress on the zonules. As a second benefit, the hydrodissection wave should loosen and facilitate removal of the epinuclear shell. Following hydrodelineation alone, a loosened endonucleus will rotate separately from the stationary epinucleus. However, it is hydrodissection that permits the epinucleus to be mobilized, spun, and flipped if its capsular attachments have been hydrostatically cleaved (Figure 18-2). Finally, an optimally positioned and executed hydrodissection wave should shear the cortical-capsular attachments, making cortical aspiration safer, faster, and more complete.[1-5] This, in turn, reduces the rate

of posterior capsular opacification, especially when combined with intracapsular nuclear rotation prior to phaco.[6-8]

There are several pearls that can help surgeons to consistently achieve these 3 important goals.

PEARL #1: DECOMPRESS THE ANTERIOR CHAMBER BEFORE STARTING

A common mistake is to initiate hydrodissection while the anterior chamber is over-inflated with an ophthalmic viscosurgical device (OVD). Hydrodissection is easier if the eye is somewhat soft and if the anterior chamber has been partially emptied. Of course, this condition is at odds with the preceding capsulorrhexis step during which the chamber has been pressurized with OVD.

Using OVD to deepen the chamber and flatten the anterior capsular convexity optimizes control of the capsulorrhexis tear. As discussed in Chapter 17, anterior chamber shallowing during the capsulotomy step increases the risk of the anterior capsule tearing peripherally. However, by

Chang DF.
*Phaco Chop and Advanced Phaco Techniques: Strategies for
Complicated Cataracts, Second Edition* (pp 195-207).
© 2013 SLACK Incorporated.

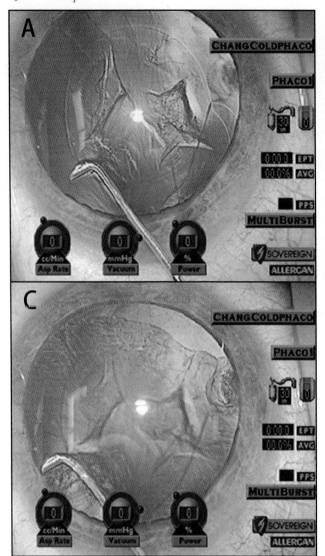
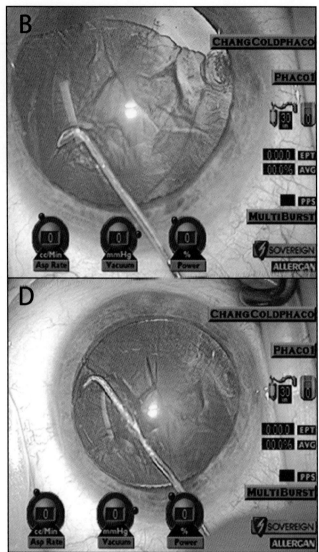

Figure 18-1. (A) Chang 23-gauge right angle hydrodissection cannula is placed just under the subincisional anterior capsule rim. (B, C) Hydrodissection wave with a scalloped leading edge advances toward contraincisional equator. (D) Rotating the tip slightly down into the nucleus creates a hydrodelineation wave upon injection.

exerting downward pressure against the nucleus, pressurizing the anterior chamber with OVD also increases the resistance that a posteriorly directed hydrodissection wave must overcome. Aggressive hydrodissection within an OVD-filled anterior chamber can result in excessive chamber deepening if the injected fluid cannot escape through the incision. This is particularly problematic with sodium hyaluronate 2.3% (Healon 5), which will not escape the chamber under pressure. It is therefore advisable to burp out some OVD immediately prior to initiating hydrodissection. This can be accomplished by gently pressing the tip or shaft of the hydrodissection cannula against the incision floor prior to the injection. Partially emptying the anterior chamber in this way will permit the nucleus to more readily separate and elevate away from the posterior capsule.

Pearl #2: Use Adequate Injection Force

For the wave to propagate posteriorly and shear the natural epinuclear-capsular adhesions, a sufficient hydrostatic force must be generated. However, fear of "blowing out" the capsule makes novice surgeons instinctively timid with the injection pressure. Because the volume of balanced salt solution (BSS) that can be injected into the anterior chamber is limited, the most effective fluid jet is one that is brief, sufficiently forceful, and radially directed. The resulting hydrostatic force is proportional to the rate of flow and the resistance of the cannula. Either a 30- or 27-gauge cannula (Figure 18-1A) provides enough resistance to generate the

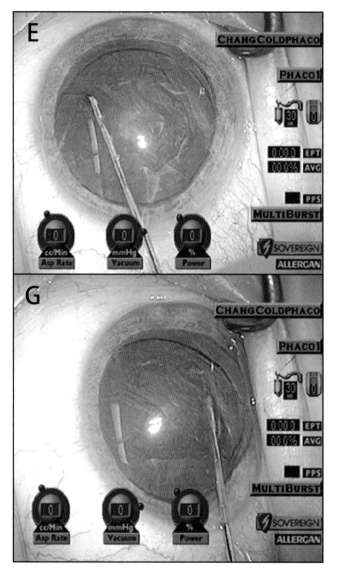

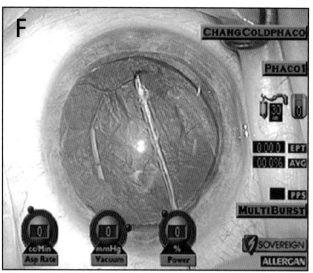

Figure 18-1 (continued). (E-G) Dull point of the cannula tip is used to engage the peripheral nucleus and rotate it in a clockwise direction.

necessary force with a small volume of fluid. Since tuberculin syringes hold insufficient volume, the preferred syringe size is 3 mL. In contrast to larger syringes, this size is small enough to provide good tactile feedback regarding the rate of flow as the plunger is advanced.

PEARL #3: AVOID CAPSULAR-LENTICULAR BLOCK

It is possible to rupture the posterior capsule during hydrodissection. Excessive injection force alone will not do this; the capsular-lenticular block is usually a prerequisite.[9-13] As a large, dense nucleus elevates, it may completely seal off the capsulorrhexis opening from below. If fluid cannot escape the capsular bag, continued infusion can over-inflate the bag enough to rupture the posterior capsule.[13] The surgeon may not be aware of this complication until the phaco tip is inserted. At this point, posterior nuclear displacement by the hydrostatic pressure will expand the posterior capsular rent, and the nucleus will descend into the vitreous cavity before or during the initial sculpting strokes. To avoid this complication, one should terminate the injection as soon as a brunescent nucleus "pops up" into the capsulorrhexis. Specifically, the surgeon should resist the temptation to continue injecting until the hydrodissection wave has completely crossed behind the nucleus. Instead, one should stop and reposit the nucleus posteriorly—thus breaking the capsular-lenticular block—before resuming hydrodissection or hydrodelineation.

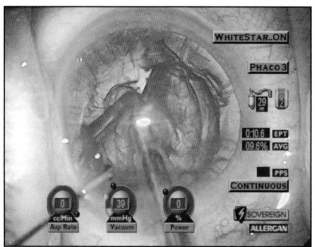

Figure 18-2. Well-performed hydrodissection loosens the epinucleus, facilitating mobilization with the phaco tip.

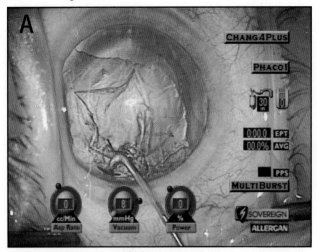
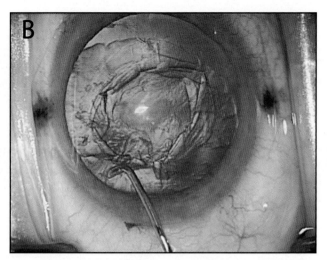

Figure 18-3. (A, B) Additional examples of the scalloped leading edge of the hydrodissection wave. Using a right-angled cannula preferentially loosens the subincisional cortex.

Pearl #4: Achieve Cortical Cleaving Hydrodissection

I. Howard Fine, MD emphasized the concept of cortical cleaving hydrodissection whereby the cortex is loosened by the fluid wave.[1] This is facilitated by tenting the anterior capsule slightly upward with the cannula tip in order to direct the fluid stream along the internal contour of the capsular bag (see Figure 18-1A). A wave that hugs the inner capsular surface will produce a slower advancing fluid front with scalloped edges (see Figures 18-1B, 18-1C, 18-3A, and 18-3B). These characteristics indicate the resistance that is encountered as the wave shears through the cortical-capsular adhesions, and confirm that all 3 hydrodissection goals will be achieved. Some surgeons advise leaving one's thumb off the plunger until the cannula tip is positioned properly. Otherwise, if even a tiny amount of fluid is trickling out, it may prevent the tip from properly tenting up the anterior capsule just prior to the definitive injection.

With hydrodissection, even if the wave propagates quickly, the surgeon will typically have a mental snapshot of its timing and direction. Provided that the lens is not mature, if the surgeon does not observe or perceive a fluid wave, it probably traveled along too internal an anatomic plane and may have resulted in hydrodelineation instead of hydrodissection (see Figure 18-1D). This error occurs more frequently in softer lenses where the epinucleus is proportionately larger. Without hydrodissection, hydrodelineation alone may permit the endonucleus to rotate within a stationery epinuclear shell, but it will not loosen the epinucleus and cortex. The adherent epinucleus will subsequently be difficult to aspirate, mobilize, or flip with the phaco tip.

Because either hydrodissection or hydrodelineation alone will permit rotation of a moderately dense endonucleus, proper hydrodissection may not be confirmed until the epinucleus and cortex are removed. In order to mobilize and flip the epinuclear shell, it is safer to aspirate the anterior shelf rather than the posterior portion in contact with the posterior capsule. If the anterior shelf breaks off as it is being aspirated, the surgeon can rotate the loosened epinucleus counterclockwise with a microfinger or horizontal chopper to position a fresh area of anterior shelf in the contraincisional quadrant. In contrast, an adherent epinucleus neither rotates nor flips, and the distally aspirated anterior shelf eventually breaks off. This leaves an adherent proximal epinuclear shell with nothing to safely grab on to, and turning the phaco tip toward the remaining shell increases the risk of aspirating the posterior capsule.

Finally, loosening the capsular attachments with hydrodissection facilitates automated cortical clean-up. For example, a mailing label easily separates in one piece from its waxed paper backing. However, once applied to a cardboard box, it becomes difficult to remove as a single piece. After one strip of the affixed label prematurely shreds and breaks off, one must again struggle to regrasp a new edge. The difference between these 2 situations is the strength of the adhesion. The tendency for hydrodissected cortex to separate easily in sheets, as opposed to small adherent strips, is particularly advantageous in the subincisional area.[4-6] The more adherent the cortex is to the posterior capsule, the greater the risk of aspirating or rupturing the posterior capsule becomes. Occasionally, the hydrodissected cortex becomes loose enough to be aspirated along with the epinucleus by the phaco tip (Figure 18-4).

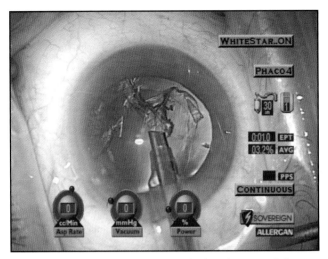

Figure 18-4. Cortical aspiration with the phaco tip following cortical-cleaving hydrodissection, as described by I. Howard Fine, MD.

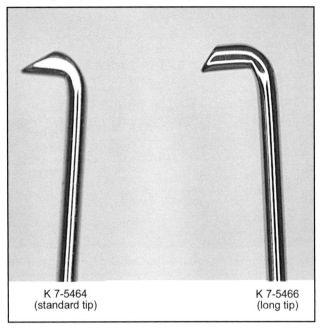

K 7-5464
(standard tip)

K 7-5466
(long tip)

Figure 18-5. Chang hydrodissection cannulae. Shorter tip model on left; longer tip model on right. (Reprinted with permission of Katena Products.)

PEARL #5: INITIATE THE WAVE PROXIMALLY

The hydrodissection wave often fails to completely traverse the posterior capsule. When a conventional straight cannula is used, a partially completed wave that started from the contraincisional fornix may not adequately loosen the subincisional cortex. The hydrodissection wave should ideally commence from the subincisional anterior capsular rim because of the importance of preferentially loosening subincisional cortex. For this reason, this author advocates using a right angle hydrodissection cannula tip. Like a right angle irrigation-aspiration (I/A) tip, this configuration can access the proximal 180 degrees of anterior capsular rim (see Figure 18-3A and 18-3B). In contrast, a straight cannula can only access the distal 120 degrees of capsular rim, and a J-shaped cannula is limited to the subincisional quadrant of capsular rim.

PEARL #6: ROTATE THE NUCLEUS WITH THE CANNULA

Another helpful hint is to sever the last remaining capsular attachments by using the cannula tip to rotate the nucleus within the bag prior to phaco.[7] The right angle hydrodissection cannula tip works well at engaging the peripheral anterior nuclear surface and rotating it with circular raking motions (see Figure 18-1E-G). By not having to remove the tip, the surgeon can readily repeat the hydrodissection step if necessary.

TECHNIQUE USING A RIGHT-ANGLED HYDRODISSECTION CANNULA

The Chang hydrodissection cannula (Katena Products, Denville, NJ; Mastel Precision, Rapid City, SD; and Rhein Medical) is a reusable, 27-gauge cannula with a short, 1-mm right-angled tip (Figure 18-5). The short 90-degree tip has been flattened to create a slightly fan-shaped fluid stream that allows it to more snugly nestle beneath the proximal anterior capsular rim. A disposable version is manufactured by Oasis Medical (Glendora, CA). Hydrodissection success is determined more by technique than by instrumentation. Nevertheless, the small right angle design of this cannula provides several ergonomic advantages such as the following:

1. By angling the shaft within the tunneled incision, one can position the 1-mm cannula tip just underneath the proximal capsulorrhexis edge-either slightly to the left or right of the incision (see Figure 18-1A). Initiating hydrodissection from this position preferentially loosens the subincisional cortex. A right-angled I/A tip configuration provides better access to aspirate subincisional cortex for the same reason.

2. The 1-mm long bent tip is small enough to flip around while still inside the anterior chamber. This allows one to sequentially hydrodissect or hydrodelineate both lateral quadrants without having to reinsert the instrument.

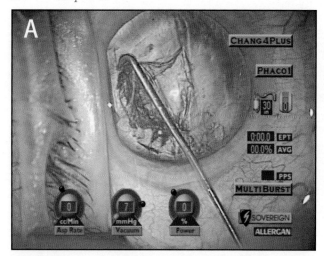

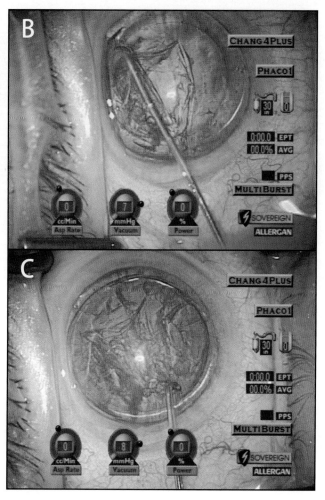

Figure 18-6. (A, B) Hydrodelineation with resulting golden ring. Note the more internal path of the fluid wave relative to hydrodissection. (C) Hydrodelineation with resulting golden ring.

3. Because of the tip's 90-degree bend, rotating it along the axis of the shaft can angle the tip so that it points either slightly above or below the plane of the capsulorrhexis. By initially angling it slightly upward, the undersurface of the anterior capsule is tented. This forces the ensuing hydrodissection wave to hug the inside contour of the capsule. By next angling it slightly downward, the tip rotates into a more internally directed cleavage plane for hydrodelineation (Figure 18-6A-C).

4. Used like a dull pick, the short right-angled tip can spin the nucleus by engaging its anterior surface peripherally and exerting a rotational motion (see Figure 18-1E-G). This repetitive raking motion manually shears the remaining capsular adhesions and confirms successful nuclear rotation. As shown in a study by Vasavada, nuclear rotation (prephaco) also mechanically loosens the lens epithelial cells enough to reduce posterior capsular opacification when compared to omitting this step.[7] The Chang cannula has a dull point at the tip to further facilitate this maneuver. If the nucleus will not rotate, the cannula is repositioned for additional hydrodissection attempts.

5. The right angle design keeps the shaft out of the way as fluid is injected behind the nucleus. This can facilitate efforts to prolapse one pole of the endonucleus through the capsulorrhexis and out of the capsular bag. This maneuver can be used in supracapsular flip techniques or for manual small incision extracapsular cataract extraction (ECCE).[14]

OTHER HYDRODISSECTION PITFALLS

Inability to Rotate the Nucleus

Inability to rotate the nucleus and epinucleus forces the phaco tip to be aimed in a direction other than toward the contraincisional quadrant. Particularly with epinucleus, turning the phaco tip bevel laterally or posteriorly increases the risk of aspirating the posterior capsule. Causes include ineffective hydrodissection, a very soft nucleus, and significant zonular laxity. As with a pillow, a soft nucleus absorbs the rotational instrument forces and is less likely to revolve as a unit. Weak zonules may not provide the necessary capsular counter fixation for the nucleus to separate and rotate easily.

In order to rotate the nucleus with a single instrument, one needs a stationary platform—the capsular bag—against which to push the nucleus to generate enough torque. With severe zonular laxity, this platform is too unstable; overly

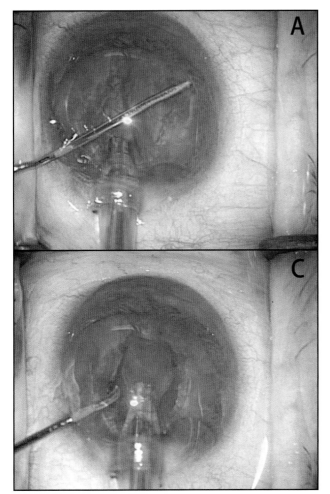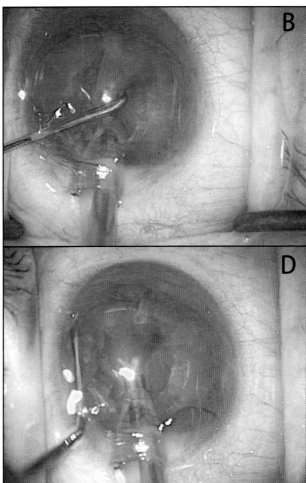

Figure 18-7. (A) Horizontal chop of a soft nucleus that will not rotate. Without rotation following the initial chop, the horizontal chopper hooks the equator several clock hours to the right. (B) Second chop toward the phaco tip creates the first mobile pie-shaped fragment. (C) First fragment is aspirated out of the bag. (D) Without rotation, the next chop is initiated by hooking the nuclear equator several clock hours to the left.

forceful attempts at rotation may tear the zonules. Using 2 Sinskey-type hooks for bimanual counter-rotation will often succeed in rotating the lens while minimizing pressure against the weakened zonules. This is because each hook uses the other as a platform to push off against, and spares the loosened capsular bag from having to sustain these torsional forces.

If hydrodissection fails and the nucleus will not spin, phaco chop can create several nuclear fragments without any sculpting or rotation. This is because the chopper is more versatile and maneuverable as compared to the phaco tip. After the nucleus is bisected with the first chop, the second chop is performed after repositioning the chopper several clock hours to one side and reimpaling with the phaco tip. The second chop will create an initial pie-shaped piece, which can then be aspirated or tumbled out (Figure 18-7). This greater maneuverability of the chopper overcomes the limitations of the divide-and-conquer method for a nucleus that will not rotate. Hydrodissection

of the remaining nucleus can be reattempted after one or more fragments have been removed. It can also be repeated after the endonucleus has been removed in an attempt to mobilize the epinucleus.

There are 2 situations in which the author intentionally avoids nuclear rotation. The first is with posterior polar cataracts, for the reasons discussed in the following section. The second is the presence of a single radial anterior capsular tear. Achieving nuclear rotation requires exerting sufficient torsional pressure against the counter-fixating capsular bag. This is probably the most forceful maneuver experienced by the capsular-zonular complex and the maneuver most likely to extend a radial capsulorrhexis tear into the posterior capsule. In this situation, the author tries to perform the initial chops and nuclear disassembly without nuclear rotation. As soon as the nuclear fragments are small enough, they can be aspirated and elevated out of the capsular bag for subchopping within the anterior chamber.

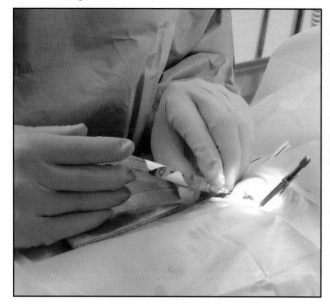

Figure 18-8. Hand positions for injecting through a hydrodissection or other cannula. The dominant right hand thumb is pushing the plunger. The left hand index finger contacts and steadies the cannula.

Projectile Cannula

With any small gauge cannula tip, forceful fluid injection can dislodge the cannula hub and suddenly produce an intraocular projectile. Although the scrub nurse and surgeon should check that the Luer lock is properly fastened prior to use, many surgeons have experienced this complication.[15] A recommended habit is to routinely place the tip of the index finger from the nondominant hand against the cannula hub prior to injection. For a surgeon holding a syringe with the right hand thumb against the plunger, this means steadying cannula with the tip of the left index finger (Figure 18-8). This not only stabilizes the instrument but provides instantaneous tactile feedback should the cannula accidentally separate from the syringe. The surgeon will immediately and instinctively cease injecting at this point. This sensory feedback loop is much faster than visualizing an intraocular projectile as the first sign of separation. In my experience, it has repeatedly been able to prevent this dangerous complication.

Posterior Polar Cataracts

Because of a possible central defect or weakness, posterior capsule rupture is more likely with posterior polar cataracts (Figure 18-9 to 18-11).[16-21] Several surgical steps can tear the weakened central posterior capsule, including hydrodissection, nuclear rotation, and phaco maneuvers. Because these patients are frequently younger, decreased scleral rigidity can exaggerate chamber depth fluctuation

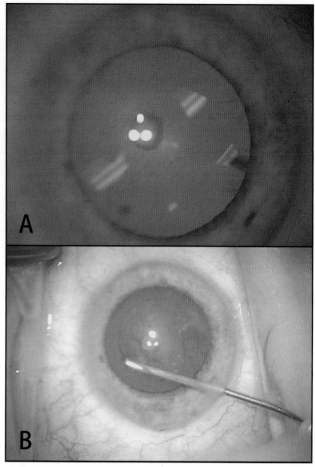

Figure 18-9. (A) Posterior polar cataract. (B) Capsulorrhexis sized 5.0 mm in diameter.

and lead to anterior chamber collapse as the phaco or I/A tip is withdrawn. Even forward bulging of the posterior capsule associated with chamber collapse can lead to a tear. There has been some suggestion that the risk of capsular rupture may increase with increasing diameter of the posterior polar opacity.[22]

Care should be taken to make the capsulorrhexis diameter smaller than the IOL optic to permit sulcus placement with optic capture in the event of posterior capsular rupture (see Figure 18-9B). Hydrodissection should be avoided with posterior polar cataracts because of the risk of tearing the posterior capsule with hydrostatic pressure.[21] Hydrodelineation can be used to mobilize the endonucleus because the fluid plane is internal and should not impart hydrostatic force against the posterior capsule (see Figure 18-10E).[21,23] Intentionally omitting hydrodissection will make it difficult to rotate the nucleus and to remove the adherent epinucleus, however. Having an immobile and adherent epinucleus increases the risk of aspirating or tearing the posterior capsule with the phaco or I/A tip.

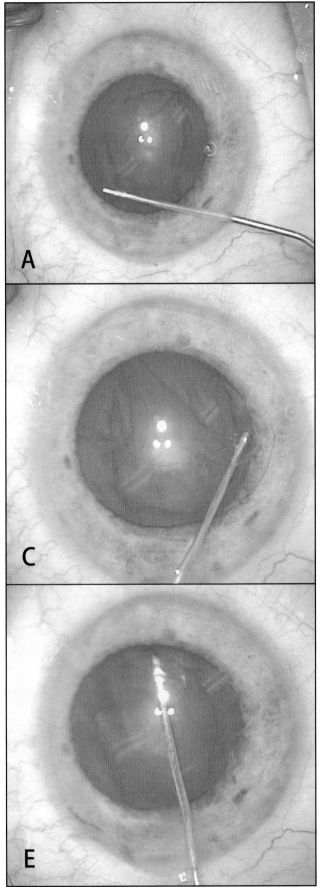

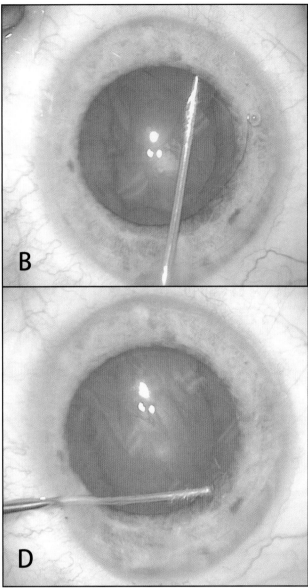

Figure 18-10. (A) Viscodissection using sodium chondroitin sulfate (Viscoat) through (B, C) right sideport incision, and (D) left sideport incisions. (E) The right-angled cannula is used to perform hydrodelineation, but not hydrodissection. This is the same case as in Figure 18-9.

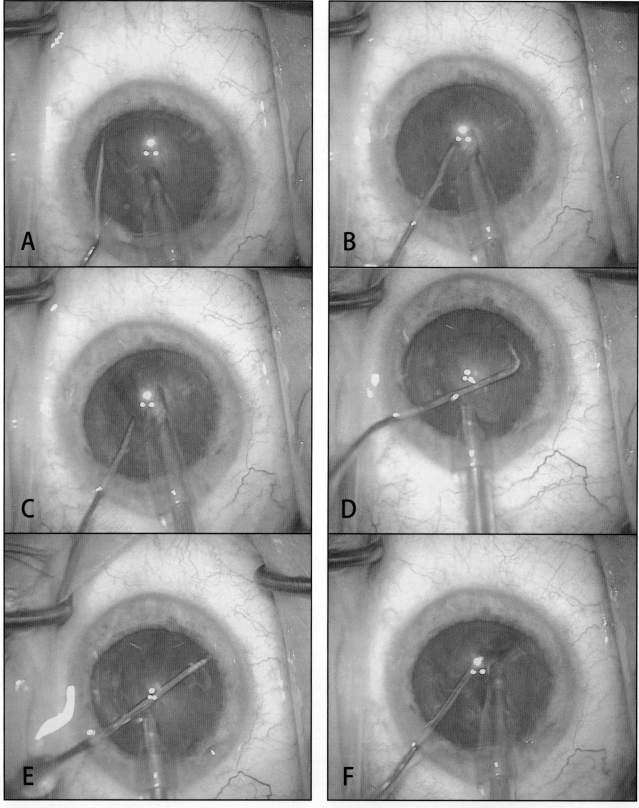

Figure 18-11. Horizontal chop without rotation of the nucleus. (A-C) Initial chop is angled slightly from the left. (D-F) Second chop is made by hooking the nuclear equator slightly to the right. This is the same case as in Figures 18-9 and 18-10.

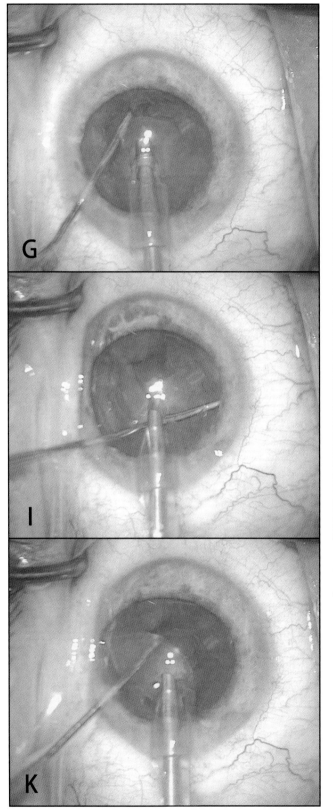

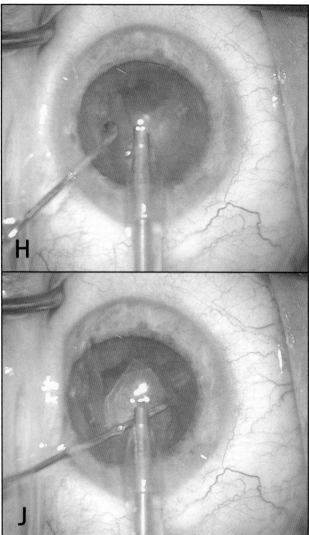

Figure 18-11 (continued). Horizontal chop without rotation of the nucleus. (G, H) First pie-shaped fragment is removed. (I-K) Right hand fragment is flipped into the anterior chamber. This is the same case as in Figures 18-9 and 18-10.

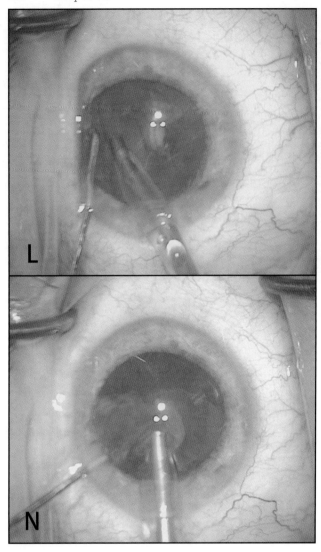

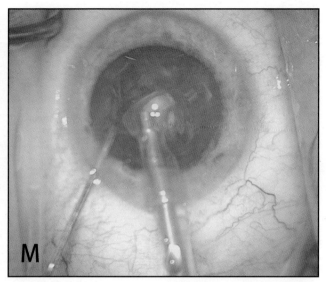

Figure 18-11 (continued). Horizontal chop without rotation of the nucleus. (L, M) Left hand fragment is aspirated by angling the phaco tip. (N) Epinucleus is flipped. This is the same case as in Figures 18-9 and 18-10.

Viscodissection for Posterior Polar Cataracts

Richard J. Mackool, MD has advocated the technique of viscodissection, in which a dispersive OVD is used in place of BSS to hydrodissect the nucleus.[24,25] The rationale is that injecting a dispersive OVD behind the nucleus should cushion the posterior capsule from forceful maneuvers and instrument contact. Achieving true posterior capsular viscodissection is difficult, but the author has found equatorial viscodissection to be very useful for posterior polar cataracts.[26]

Using a dispersive OVD for partial viscodissection of the nucleus will loosen and facilitate subsequent removal of the epinuclear shell with the phaco or I/A tip. The OVD cannula is introduced through multiple incisions with the goal of separating the epinucleus from the anterior and equatorial capsule in different quadrants (Figure 18-10A-D). Unlike with BSS, it is easier to confine the passage of dispersive

OVD to the capsular equator and to prevent it from crossing behind the nucleus. One must be careful to continually burp dispersive OVD out of the incision to avoid overly distending the anterior chamber.

As with a radial anterior capsule tear, avoiding nuclear rotation is desirable if there is a weakened posterior capsule. This is because nuclear rotation generally imparts more force against the zonules and posterior capsule than any other single surgical maneuver. The phaco chop method outlined earlier for a nonrotating nucleus is ideal for these cases (see Figure 18-11). The fact that these nuclei are typically soft makes stationary division by the chopper easier. Finally, because of decreased scleral rigidity in younger patients, one should consider filling the anterior chamber with viscoelastic before withdrawing the phaco or I/A tip from the eye. This will prevent the chamber from abruptly emptying and the hyaloid face and posterior capsule from vaulting forward as the incision is unplugged.

CONCLUSION

Because surgeons are limited to a single incision in phacoemulsification, cortical cleaving hydrodissection facilitates removal of the nucleus, epinucleus, and cortex. One cannot as safely remove subincisional nucleus and epinucleus if they cannot be rotated. Overly adherent subincisional cortex increases the risk of snagging or tearing the posterior capsule during cortical aspiration. Successful hydrodissection improves surgical efficiency, reduces the risk of capsular rupture, and—by cleaving the cortical attachments—reduces the risk of retained cortex and posterior capsular opacification.[4-8] Surgeons can reliably achieve these benefits on a consistent basis by optimizing the hydrodissection technique and instrumentation.

REFERENCES

1. Fine IH. Cortical cleaving hydrodissection. *J Cataract Refract Surg.* 1992;18:508-512.

2. Gimbel HV. Hydrodissection and hydrodelineation. *Int Ophthalmol Clin.* 1994;34:73-90.

3. Koch DD, Liu JF. Multilamellar hydrodissection in phacoemulsification and planned extracapsular surgery. *J Cataract Refract Surg.* 1990;16:559-562.

4. Vasavada AR, Singh R, Apple DJ, et al. Effect of hydrodissection on intraoperative performance: Randomized study. *J Cataract Refract Surg.* 2002;28:1623-1628.

5. Vasavada AR, Goyal D, Shastri L, Singh R. Corticocapsular adhesions and their effect during cataract surgery. *J Cataract Refract Surg.* 2003;29:309-314.

6. Peng Q, Apple DJ, Visessook N, et al. Surgical prevention of posterior capsule opacification. Part 2: Enhancement of cortical clean up by focusing on hydrodissection. *J Cataract Refract Surg.* 2000;26:188-197.

7. Vasavada AR, Raj SM, Johar K, Nanavaty MA. Effect of hydrodissection combined with rotation on lens epithelial cells: surgical approach for the prevention of posterior capsule opacification. *J Cataract Refract Surg.* 2006;32:145–150.

8. Vasavada AR, Dholakia SA, Raj SM, Singh R. Effect of cortical cleaving hydrodissection on posterior capsule opacification in age-related nuclear cataract. *J Cataract Refract Surg.* 2006;32:1196-1200.

9. Hurvitz LM. Posterior capsular rupture at hydrodissection (letter). *J Cataract Refract Surg.* 1991;17:866.

10. Kershner RM. Capsular rupture at hydrodissection (letter). *J Cataract Refract Surg.* 1992;18:423.

11. Yeoh R. The 'pupil snap' sign of posterior capsule rupture with hydrodissection in phacoemulsification (letter). *Br J Ophthalmol.* 1996;80:486.

12. Ota I, Miyake S, Miyake K. Dislocation of the lens nucleus into the vitreous cavity after standard hydrodissection. *Am J Ophthalmol.* 1996;121:706-708.

13. Miyake, K. et al. New classification of capsular block syndrome. *J Cataract Refract Surg.* 1998;24:1230-1234.

14. Blumenthal M, Ashkenazi I, Assia E, Cahane M. Small-incision manual extracapsular cataract extraction using selective hydrodissection. *Ophthalmic Surg.* 1992;23:699-701.

15. Pandey P, Kirkby G. Cannula detachment during cataract surgery: results of a survey. *Can J Ophthalmol.* 2012;47:280-283.

16. Osher RH, Yu BC-Y, Koch DD. Posterior polar cataracts: a predisposition to intraoperative posterior capsular rupture. *J Cataract Refract Surg.* 1990;16:157-162.

17. Vasavada AR, Singh R. Phacoemulsification in eyes with posterior polar cataract. *J Cataract Refract Surg.* 1999;25:238-245.

18. Allen D, Wood C. Minimizing risk to the capsule during surgery for posterior polar cataract. *J Cataract Refract Surg.* 2002;28:742-744.

19. Fine IH, Packer M, Hoffman RS. Management of posterior polar cataract. *J Cataract Refract Surg.* 2003;29:16-19.

20. Hayashi K, Hayashi H, Nakao F, Hayashi F. Outcomes of surgery for posterior polar cataract. *J Cataract Refract Surg.* 2003;29:45-49.

21. Vasavada AR, Raj SM, Vasavada V, Shrivastav S. Surgical approaches to posterior polar cataract: a review. *Eye* (Lond). 2012;26:761-770.

22. Kumar S, Ram J, Sukhija J, Severia S. Phacoemulsification in posterior polar cataract: does size of lens opacity affect surgical outcome? *Clin Experiment Ophthalmol.* 2010;38:857-861.

23. Vasavada AR, Raj SM. Inside-out delineation. *J Cataract Refract Surg.* 2004;30:1167-1169.

24. Mackool RJ, Nicolich S, Mackool R Jr. Effect of viscodissection on posterior capsule rupture during phacoemulsification. *J Cataract Refract Surg.* 2007;33:553.

25. Vasavada V, Vasavada VA, Werner L, Mamalis N, Vasavada AR, Crandall AS. Corticocapsular cleavage during phacoemulsification: viscodissection versus hydrodissection. Miyake-Apple view analysis. *J Cataract Refract Surg.* 2008;34:1173-1180.

26. Taskapili M, Gulkilik G, Kocabora MS, Ozsutcu M. Phacoemulsification with viscodissection in posterior polar cataract: minimizing risk of posterior capsule tear. *Ann Ophthalmol* (Skokie). 2007;39:145-149.

19

Strategies for the Rock Hard Nucleus

David F. Chang, MD

Virtually every step of cataract surgery is more difficult in the setting of a mature, brunescent nucleus. Successful management requires that surgeons first understand and then employ specific strategies to overcome these intimidating obstacles.

VISUALIZATION

A poor red reflex impedes visualization of the capsulorrhexis and makes the surgeon more likely to tear its edge with the chopper or phaco tip. Fortunately, trypan blue dye persists long enough to make the edge of the capsulorrhexis visible during nuclear emulsification.[1,2] Some operating microscopes (eg, OPMI Lumera, Carl Zeiss Meditec Inc, Dublin, CA) have dual control over separate oblique and coaxial illumination sources. This allows the surgeon to turn off the oblique illuminating beam and to use only the stereo coaxial beam in order to dramatically enhance the red reflex for the capsulorrhexis step (see Figure 21-8A-C). This illumination technique may render capsular staining unnecessary in many cases with dense nuclei. With ultra-brunescent lenses, however, trypan blue staining is often necessary or advisable to allow adequate anterior capsule

visualization (Figure 19-1). Awareness and visualization of the capsulorrhexis edge during nuclear emulsification is important to avoid tearing it during sculpting or chopping (see Figures 19-1D and 19-1E).

CAPSULAR BLOCK

During hydrodissection, an elevating bulky and brunescent nucleus is more likely to seal the capsulorrhexis from below, causing a capsular-lenticular block.[3-5] Because it cannot escape the capsular bag, injecting any additional hydrodissection fluid at this point will distend and eventually rupture the posterior capsule. The surgeon may not recognize any problem until the nucleus suddenly descends through the torn posterior capsule following the first sculpting stroke. This is because a posterior capsular defect will not widen until mechanical or hydrostatic irrigation pressure against the nucleus propels it posteriorly.

To avoid capsular-lenticular block, one should terminate hydrodissection as soon as the solid nucleus elevates against the capsulorrhexis. One must avoid the temptation to continue injecting until the migrating posterior fluid wave completely crosses behind the nucleus. Instead, tap

Chang DF.
Phaco Chop and Advanced Phaco Techniques: Strategies for Complicated Cataracts, Second Edition (pp 209-220).
© 2013 SLACK Incorporated.

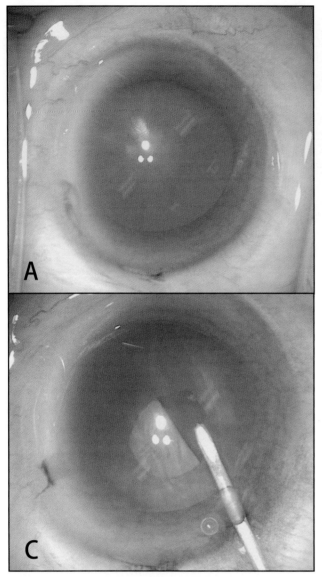

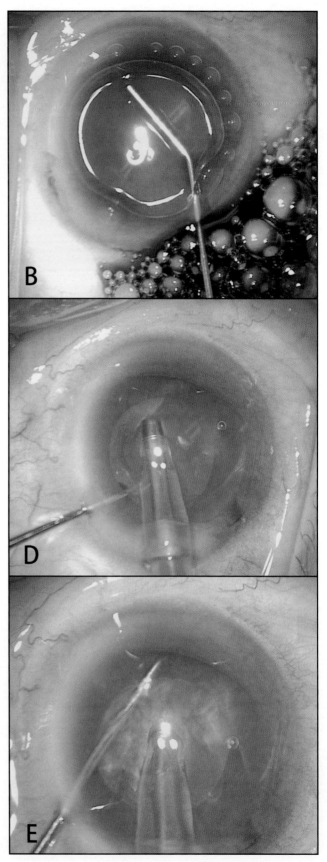

Figure 19-1. Case 1. (A) Mature ultra-brunescent nucleus. (B) Trypan blue is injected beneath an air bubble. (C) The blue staining is intense enough to stand apart from the brown nucleus. Persistent capsular staining helps in avoiding the anterior capsule edge with (D) the phaco tip or (E) the chopper.

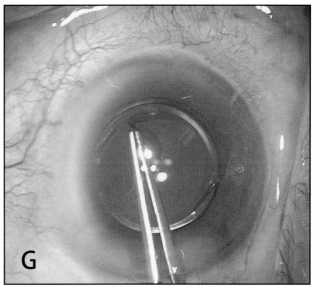

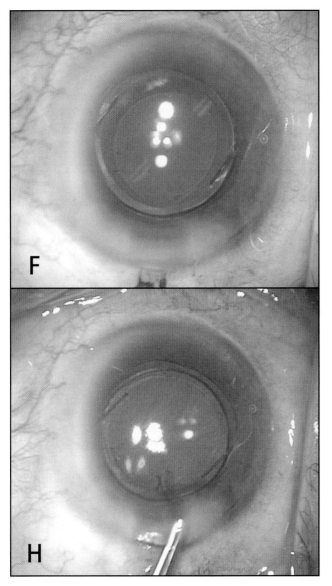

Figure 19-1 (continued). Case 1. (F-H) The blue capsular stain persists even after the intraocular lens (IOL) has been implanted and facilitates secondary capsulorrhexis enlargement.

is the combination of longer phaco time and greater phaco needle stroke length that generates excessive heat compared to routine cases.

Combining chopping with a lower phaco duty cycle can significantly reduce the production of energy and heat during nuclear emulsification. Using torsional phaco alone with brunescent nuclei may result in a clogged tip; combining some longitudinal phaco tip motion to dislodge and advance the thicker emulsate is recommended. Finally, one should aspirate any retentive OVD just above the anterior nuclear surface prior to initiating phaco to lessen the chance of tip clogging from a sludge-like mixture of OVD and nucleus.

ENDOTHELIAL CELL LOSS

There are 3 clinical settings in which the risk of endothelial cell loss is much greater than normal. The first is with a very shallow anterior chamber, where the closer proximity of the phaco tip to the cornea increases the likelihood of endothelial cell loss. The second is in the setting of weakened zonules, where trampolining of a lax posterior capsule occurs as more and more of the nucleus is removed. As the last nuclear fragments are emulsified, this forces the surgeon to elevate the phaco tip closer to the endothelium in order to increase the margin of posterior capsular safety.

Finally, as evidenced by increased corneal edema on the first postoperative day, the odds of endothelial cell loss are significantly increased with a brunescent nucleus.[7,8] The increased density and volume of nuclear material necessitates greater ultrasound power and time to emulsify it.

the center of the elevated nucleus to dislodge it posteriorly before resuming hydrodissection from the opposite quadrant. A right-angled hydrodissection cannula facilitates the latter step.

WOUND BURN

Incisional burns are also much more likely to occur with brunescent nuclei. If the overlying OVD is not initially aspirated away, it can mix together with the brunescent nuclear emulsate to clog the phaco tip.[6] Absent any exiting fluid, there can be no gravity-fed irrigation inflow and a burn immediately develops once ultrasound commences. Particularly with a clear corneal incision, moderate whitening and heat shrinkage can result from the higher levels of continuous phaco power typically employed for 4+ nuclei. It

There is poor followability and much greater chatter occurring at the phaco tip because of the increased stroke length associated with higher phaco power and because rigid nuclear fragments do not mold as well to the phaco tip. This produces excessive particulate turbulence within the anterior chamber and this microscopic nuclear "shrapnel" emanating from the phaco tip mechanically bombards the endothelium. This is more likely responsible for the greater endothelial cell trauma and loss than the phaco energy itself.

PEARLS FOR REDUCING ENDOTHELIAL TRAUMA

Maximally Retentive Ophthalmic Viscosurgical Device

With the prolonged operative times associated with brunescent nuclei, ophthalmic viscosurgical device (OVD) washout is a far greater problem than with most typical cases (Figure 19-2). Dispersive OVDs, such as sodium chondroitin sulfate (Viscoat) and sodium hyaluronate 3% (Healon EndoCoat) or viscoadaptive and highly retentive OVDs such as sodium hyaluronate 2.3% (Healon 5) or DisCoVisc, if properly utilized, are able to coat and protect the endothelium for longer periods than their cohesive counterparts.[9-12] All OVDs eventually wash away, and one should stop to replenish the protective endothelial layer partway through the nuclear removal step when dealing with a brunescent lens (see Figure 19-2R). Repeatedly recoating the endothelium with dispersive OVD during phaco should be considered in other higher risk cases, such as those with a crowded anterior chamber or with Fuchs dystrophy.

Maximizing Anterior Chamber Depth

Sufficient chamber depth for the capsulorrhexis step can usually be achieved by using a enough OVD. However, this will wash out as soon as nuclear emulsification is initiated. To minimize the risk of having microscopic particles bombarding the endothelium, one must be conscious of keeping the phaco tip as deep as possible while the fragments are being emulsified. This author also aims and rotates the bevel more posteriorly when endothelial protection is paramount. Placing the curved chopper tip a few millimeters directly opposite the phaco tip opening allows the surgeon to aim the tip downward during fragment removal with negligible risk of aspirating the posterior capsule during any momentary postocclusion surge.

Occasionally, eyes at the far extreme of the shallow chamber spectrum are encountered. In these cases, viscoelastic injection may be unable to adequately deepen the chamber without first causing iris prolapse or a dangerously firm globe. In these situations, performing a vitreous tap prior to viscoelastic injection can expand the chamber to a safer depth.[13] This technique is discussed in Chapter 26.

Phaco Chop

By replacing sculpting with manual fracture of the nucleus, phaco chop leads to an overall reduction in total ultrasound power and time.[14-17] The effect of this on endothelial cell loss probably varies with the nuclear density, with less of a difference appreciated with soft to medium nuclei.[17,18] However, with denser nuclei, the reduction in ultrasound power achieved by phaco chop results in decreased endothelial cell loss.[19]

Power Modulations

The ability to reduce the duty cycle produces a major reduction in cumulative ultrasound time. These changes significantly reduce heat production and total ultrasound energy delivered by the phaco tip, and practically eliminate the risk of wound burn.[20-22] As nicely captured in Dr. Teruyuki Miyoshi's American Society of Cataract and Refractive Surgery (ASCRS) award-winning videos using ultra high speed digital photography, alternating each ultrasound pulse with rest periods of "OFF" time (OFF-T) diminishes the repelling force of the vibrating phaco tip. This, in turn, reduces the chatter and turbulence of small lens particles at the phaco tip that cause collateral endothelial damage.

Alcon's OZil replaces traditional axial phaco needle movement with the torsional oscillation of a bent Kelman tip. Several studies have documented a decrease in cumulative ultrasound energy, endothelial cell loss, and wound distortion with this modality.[23-28] Miyoshi's videos were able to confirm the significant reduction in longitudinal repelling forces at the phaco tip, which dramatically improves followability and reduces fragment chatter. The Ellips (Signature; Abbott Medical Optics [AMO], Santa Ana, CA) blends some longitudinal movement with a transverse elliptical tip path. Retaining some longitudinal motion is done to improve the tip's ability to cut dense nuclear material. The enhanced followability which characterizes the torsional and transversal modes is most dramatic and obvious when used on dense nuclei.

POSTERIOR CAPSULE RUPTURE

Posterior capsule rupture is more likely with 4+ nuclei for several reasons.[29] There is proportionally more endonucleus and less epinucleus with brunescent cataracts, which can double the volume of solid material requiring emulsification. This also forces the phaco tip to work much

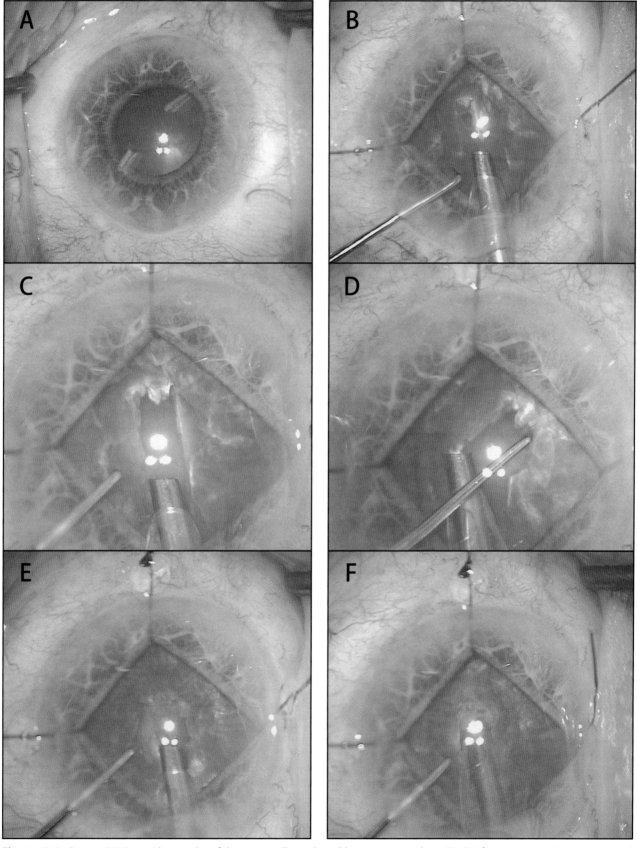

Figure 19-2. Case 2. (A) Eye with pseudoexfoliation, small pupil, and brunescent nucleus. (B, C) After inserting iris retractors and completing the capsulorrhexis, the anterior epinucleus is aspirated prior to sculpting a half trench. (D, E) The nucleus is rotated 180 degrees, and (F) the phaco tip impales the nucleus in burst mode at the base of the half trench.

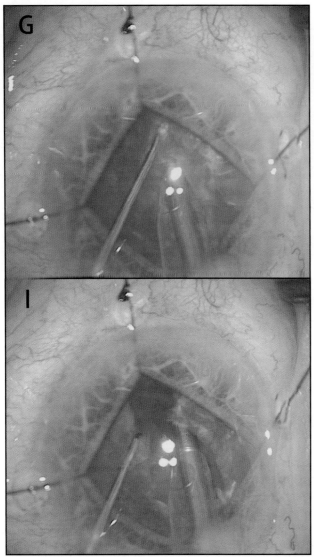

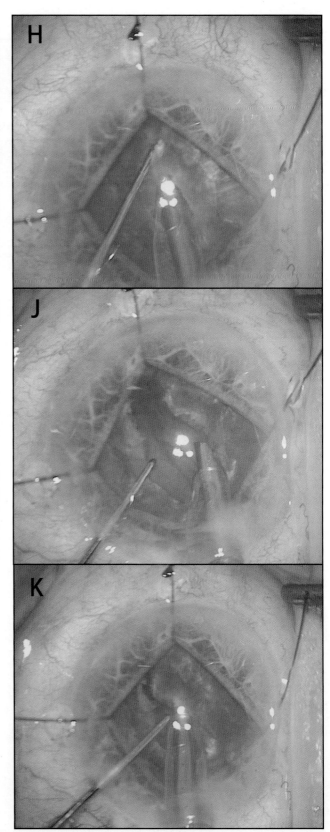

Figure 19-2 (continued). Case 2. (G-I) The Chang vertical chopper is used to initiate the first chop. (J) The initial crack propagates along the deeply sculpted half trench on the proximal side. The phaco tip (K) impales one heminucleus in order to (L-N) initiate a second (O-Q) and a third vertical chop.

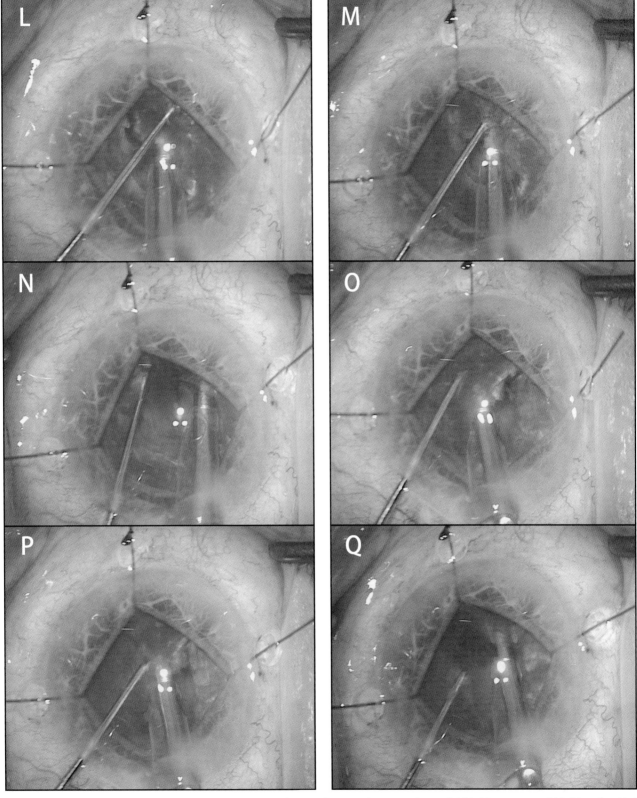

Figure 19-2 (continued). Case 2. The phaco tip (K) impales one heminucleus in order to (L-N) initiate a second (O-Q) and a third vertical chop.

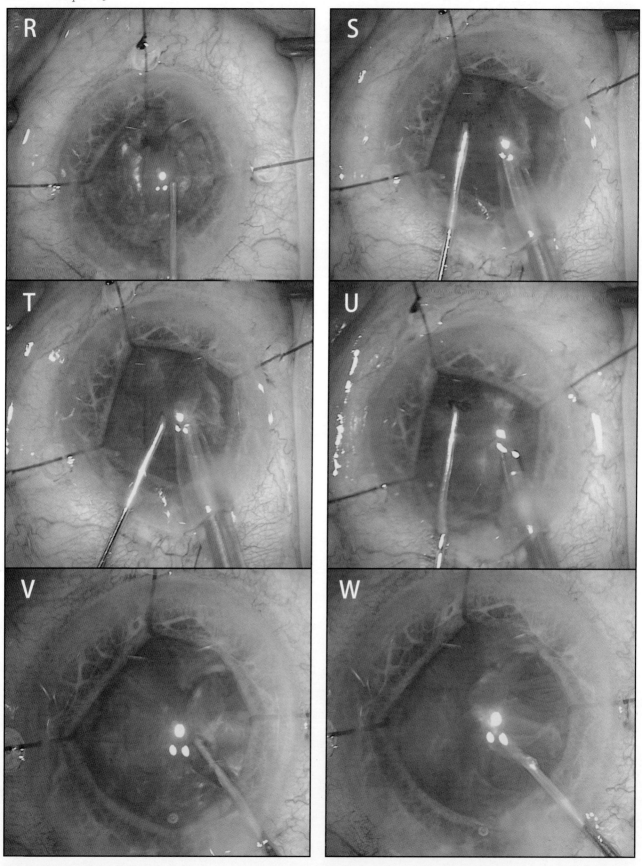

Figure 19-2 (continued). Case 2. (R) Phaco is interrupted to recoat the endothelium with dispersive OVD. (S, T) Pie-shaped brunescent fragments are subchopped with the horizontal chopper. (U) A thin, leathery posterior plate abuts the posterior capsule. (V) The OVD cannula is inserted through a fissure in the plate to inject dispersive OVD beneath the nuclear plate (W) and to distance it from the posterior capsule.

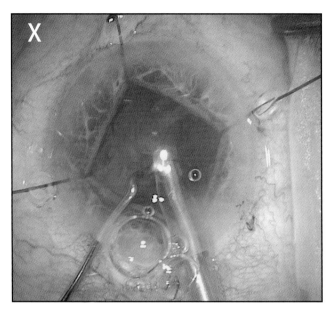 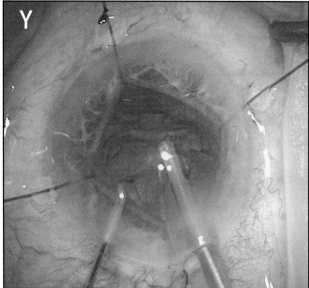

Figure 19-2 (continued). Case 2. (X) This elevation of the nuclear plate allows the phaco tip to get beneath it. (Y) The thin epinucleus is aspirated.

closer to the peripheral and posterior capsule, particularly when sculpting a deep central trough. Unlike a softer nucleus, which absorbs instrument pressure like a pillow, a dense nucleus is as rigid as a wooden board. As a result, it more directly transmits all of the instrument forces directly to the posterior or peripheral capsule and zonules.

Ultra-brunescent nuclei are often associated with weak zonules. This comorbidity may be associated with advanced age, or perhaps the greater mass of the lens imparts more force against the zonules with each ocular saccade, producing a cumulative zonular weakening over time. Weak zonules are particularly problematic if there is little or no epinucleus present. Normally, the soft epinuclear shell restrains a lax posterior capsule from trampolining toward the phaco tip as the last nuclear fragment is removed. Without the epinucleus, the exposed posterior capsule is more likely to billow toward the phaco tip with even the slightest degree of postocclusion surge. The sharp edges of the brunescent fragments and the greater capsular laxity caused by weak zonules further increase the risk of capsular puncture. If one reacts defensively by emulsifying the last fragment closer to the cornea, then one further increases endothelial cell loss.

Chopping is a superior phaco technique for the brunescent nucleus because it reduces stress on the zonules and decreases the overall procedural phaco power and time.[14-17,30-32] In the absence of any epinuclear shell, horizontal phaco chop is contraindicated. Vertical chop is also better able to transect the leathery posterior plate.[30-32] Sculpting a half trench or a deep pit in the center of the nucleus allows the surgeon to penetrate the bulky nucleus more deeply and peripherally with the phaco tip than if the nucleus was impaled without any debulking (see Figure 19-2B-F). To

better impale the nucleus, one should maximally retract the irrigation sleeve and bury the tip to the hilt. A very sharp vertical chopper will best incise into the dense nuclear face without displacing it (see Figure 19-2G-I). As discussed in Chapter 4, one can first place the vertical Chang chopper peripherally beneath the blue-stained anterior capsule, and then chop in a diagonal direction toward the buried phaco tip (see Figure 19-1E). This adds a slight horizontal vector force that compresses the fragment against the phaco tip during the vertical chop.[30]

While advantageous under ordinary circumstances, burst mode and high vacuum combine to provide a maximal grip with the densest nuclear material. Inadequate holding power makes it more likely that the vertical chopper will dislodge pieces from the phaco tip, and makes it more difficult to elevate large fragments out of the bag. Particularly with a brunescent lens, continuous mode cavitation cores out the firm material surrounding the phaco tip. This facilitates sculpting, but by eroding the seal, continuous mode phaco may not achieve the complete tip occlusion necessary to achieve high vacuum levels.

With a brunescent 4+ nucleus, regardless of whether the initial fragmentation is accomplished by divide-and-conquer, stop and chop, or pure chopping, the resulting fragments are much larger and denser than those encountered with typical nuclei. One can employ horizontal chopping to subdivide these large fragments into smaller, bite-sized pieces[30] (see Figure 19-2S and 19-2T). This reduces the tendency of oversized fragments to deflect away from the vibrating phaco tip toward the endothelium.

Capsule retractors can stabilize a wobbly nucleus with weak zonules during phaco (see Figure 23-4). Their insertion is dependent upon effective staining and capsulorrhexis

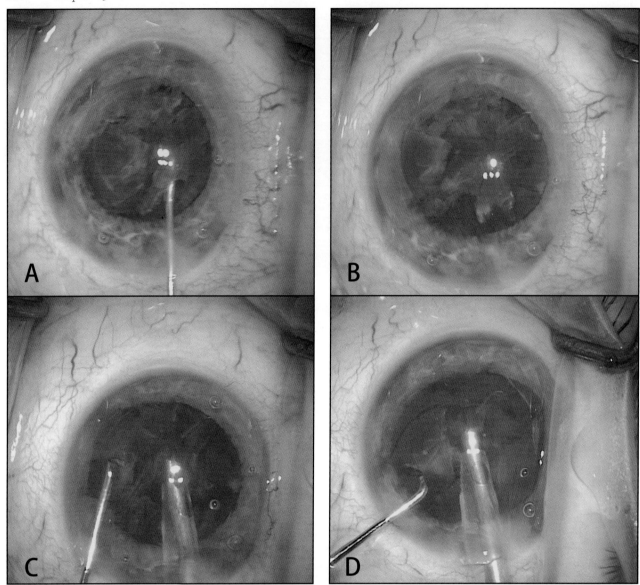

Figure 19-3. Case 3. "Visco-vault." (A, B) Dispersive OVD is injected behind the leathery 4+ posterior nuclear plate to elevate it away from the posterior capsule. (C) This enables the phaco tip to get behind the nuclear plate. (D) As the last brunescent nuclear fragments are removed, the dispersive OVD blocks the lax posterior capsule from trampolining toward the phaco tip. This permits the final brunescent fragment to be safely emulsified at the iris plane, instead of near the endothelium to avoid a trampolining posterior capsule.

visualization. As a single device, capsule retractors are preferable to a capsule tension ring (CTR) for stabilizing the lens during phaco. CTRs also impede cortical clean-up and do not provide the anterior-posterior support or torsional stability for the bag that the capsule retractors do. However, CTRs are certainly invaluable for stabilizing a moderately weakened capsular bag for IOL implantation and longer-term centration.

Roger F. Steinert, MD coined the term *viscoelastic vault* to describe a technique for deploying a dispersive OVD as an artificial epinucleus for the brunescent nucleus. In cases of weakened zonules or in cases where the epinucleus is scant or absent, one should temporarily stop phaco before removing the last remaining fragments. A generous amount of dispersive OVD is injected in front of and behind the fragments in order to partially fill the capsular bag (Figure 19-3). Because a dispersive OVD better resists aspiration by the phaco tip, it will better restrain the lax and exposed posterior capsule from trampolining toward the phaco tip. This OVD layer also cushions the capsule from being poked by the sharper contours of the brunescent fragments and distends it for cortical clean-up in the presence of weakened zonules. With less concern about proximity to the posterior capsule, the surgeon is less likely to phaco the last fragment too close to the endothelium (see Figure 19-3D).

This technique is also useful when a posterior connecting plate of nucleus is encountered. Although sequential deep fractures of the nucleus may be successfully initiated, they may not intersect at the posterior pole of the endonucleus. This may result in stubborn bridges of posterior endonucleus that connect the partially separated brunescent fragments at their deepest apical point. The safest strategy is to inject a dispersive OVD underneath the posterior pole of the endonucleus until it arches and vaults away from the posterior capsule (see Figures 19-3A and 19-3B). Inserting the OVD cannula tip through chopped fissures in the nucleus may be necessary (see Figure 19-2V). Once the thin connecting posterior plate has been elevated away from the posterior capsule, it can be ultrasonically severed with the phaco tip (see Figures 19-2W and 19-2X).

CONTINGENCY PLAN

The combination of an ultra-brunescent nucleus and weak zonules dramatically increases the risk of endothelial cell loss, posterior capsular rupture, and dropped lens material. It is during the capsulorrhexis or initial stages of nuclear emulsification that the extent of zonular abnormality may first become apparent to the surgeon. Despite the helpful devices and strategies reviewed in this chapter, each surgeon must assess his or her own personal limit in terms of how brunescent a lens they can safely emulsify.

Given the advantages of phacoemulsification, it is difficult for surgeons to attain and maintain proficiency with manual extracapsular cataract extraction (ECCE). However, with the most advanced and brunescent lenses, converting to manual ECCE and the inconvenience of a larger incision is far more preferable to corneal decompensation, capsular rupture, or a dropped nucleus. Performing a regional anesthetic block in anticipation of this possibility should be considered. Even when proceeding with phaco, the surgeon must have a contingency plan for unexpected problems such as weak zonules or poor visibility. One should consider separately packaging a sterilized contingency kit of instruments that will be readily available in the event that the surgeon is required to convert to a standard ECCE (see Figure 27-13).

REFERENCES

1. Chung CF, Liang CC, Lai JSM, Lo ESF, Lam DSC. Safety of trypan blue 1% and indocyanine green 0.5% in assisting visualization of anterior capsule during phacoemulsification in mature cataract. *J Cataract Refract Surg.* 2005;31:938–942.
2. Jacobs DS, Cox TA, Wagoner MD, Ariyasu RG, Karp CL. Capsule staining as an adjunct to cataract surgery: a report from the American Academy of Ophthalmology. *Ophthalmology.* 2006;113:707–713.
3. Yeoh R. The 'pupil snap' sign of posterior capsule rupture with hydrodissection in phacoemulsification (letter). *Br J Ophthalmol.* 1996:80:486.
4. Ota I, Miyake S, Miyake K. Dislocation of the lens nucleus into the vitreous cavity after standard hydrodissection. *Am J Ophthalmol.* 1996;121:706-708.
5. Miyake K, Ota I, Ichihashi S, Miyake S, Tanaka Y, Terasaki H. New classification of capsular block syndrome. *J Cataract Refract Surg.* 1998;24:1230–1234.
6. Ernest P, Rhem M, McDermott M, Lavery K, Sensoli A. Phacoemulsification conditions resulting in thermal wound injury. *J Cataract Refract Surg.* 2001;27:1829–1839.
7. Hayashi K, Hayashi H, Nakao F, Hayashi F. Risk factors for corneal endothelial injury during phacoemulsification. *J Cataract Refract Surg.* 1996;22:1079–1084.
8. Singh R, Vasavada AR, Janaswamy G. Phacoemulsification in brunescent and black cataracts. *J Cataract Refract Surg.* 2001;27:1762–1769.
9. Kim EK, Cristol SM, Kang SJ, Edelhauser HF, Kim HL, Lee JB. Viscoelastic protection from endothelial damage by air bubbles. *J Cataract Refract Surg.* 2002;28:1047–1053.
10. Ravalico G, Tognetto D, Baccara F, Lovisato A. Corneal endothelial protection by different viscoelastics during phacoemulsification. *J Cataract Refract Surg.* 1997;23:433–439.
11. Storr-Paulsen A, Nørregaard JC, Farik G, Tårnhøj J. The influence of viscoelastic substances on the corneal endothelial cell population during cataract surgery: a prospective study of cohesive and dispersive viscoelastics. *Acta Ophthalmol Scand.* 2007;85:183–187.
12. Koch DD, Liu JF, Glasser DB, et al. A comparison of corneal endothelial changes after use of Healon or Viscoat during phacoemulsification. *Am J Ophthalmol.* 1993;115:188–201.
13. Chang DF. Pars plana vitreous tap for phaco in the crowded eye. *J Cataract Refract Surg.* 2001;27:1911–1914.
14. DeBry P, Olson RJ, Crandall AS. Comparison of energy required for phaco-chop and divide and conquer phacoemulsification. *J Cataract Refract Surg.* 1998;24:689–692.
15. Ram J, Wesendahl TA, Auffarth GU, Apple DJ. Evaluation of in situ fracture versus phaco chop techniques. *J Cataract Refract Surg.* 1998;24:1464–1468.
16. Wong T, Hingorani M, Lee V. Phacoemulsification time and power requirements in phaco chop and divide and conquer nucleofractis techniques. *J Cataract Refract Surg.* 2000;26:1374–1378.
17. Vajpayee RB, Kumar A, Dada T, Titiyal JS, Sharma N, Dada VK. Phaco-chop versus stop-and-chop nucleotomy for phacoemulsification. *J Cataract Refract Surg.* 2000;26:1638–1641.
18. Storr-Paulsen A, Norregaard JC, Ahmed S, Storr-Paulsen T, Pedersen TH. Endothelial cell damage after cataract surgery: divide-and-conquer versus phaco-chop technique. *J Cataract Refract Surg.* 2008;34:996–1000.

19. Pirazzoli G, D'Eliseo D, Ziosi M, Acciarri R. Effects of phaco-emulsification time on the corneal endothelium using phaco-fracture and phaco chop techniques. *J Cataract Refract Surg.* 1996;22:967–969.

20. Soscia W, Howard J, Olson R. Bimanual phacoemulsification through two stab incisions: a wound temperature study. *J Cataract Refract Surg.* 2002;28:1039–1043.

21. Soscia W, Howard J, Olson R. Microphacoemulsification with WhiteStar: A wound temperature study. *J Cataract Refract Surg.* 2002;28:1044–1046.

22. Donnenfeld E, Olson R, Solomon R, et al. Efficacy and wound-temperature gradient of White Star phacoemulsification through a 1.2-mm incision. *J Cataract Refract Surg.* 2003;29(6):1097–1100.

23. Liu Y, Zeng M, Liu X, et al. Torsional mode versus conventional ultrasound mode phacoemulsification: randomized comparative clinical study. *J Cataract Refract Surg.* 2007;33(2):287–292.

24. Berdahl JP, Jun B, DeStafeno JJ, Kim T. Comparison of a torsional handpiece through microincision versus standard clear corneal cataract wounds. *J Cataract Refract Surg.* 2008;34:2091–2095.

25. Rękas M, Montés-Micó R, Krix-Jachym K, Kluś A, Stankiewicz A, Ferrer-Blasco T. Comparison of torsional and longitudinal modes using phacoemulsification parameters. *J Cataract Refract Surg.* 2009;35:1719–1724.

26. Vasavada AR, Raj SM, Patel U, Vasavada V, Vasavada VA. Comparison of torsional and microburst longitudinal phaco-emulsification: a prospective, randomized, masked clinical trial. *Ophthalmic Surg Lasers Imaging.* 2010;41:109–114.

27. Vasavada AR, Vasavada V, Vasavada VA, Praveen MR, Johar SR, Gajjar D, Arora AI. Comparison of the effect of torsional and microburst longitudinal ultrasound on clear corneal incisions during phacoemulsification. *J Cataract Refract Surg.* 2012;38:833–839.

28. Rosado-Adames N, Afshari NA. The changing fate of the corneal endothelium in cataract surgery. *Curr Opin Ophthalmol.* 2012;23:3–6. Review.

29. Artzén D, Lundström M, Behndig A, Stenevi U, Lydahl E, Montan P. Capsule complication during cataract surgery: case-control study of preoperative and intraoperative risk factors: Swedish Capsule Rupture Study Group report 2. *J Cataract Refract Surg.* 2009;35:1688–1693.

30. Chang D. Converting to phaco chop: Why? Which technique? How? *Ophthalmic Practice.* 1999;17(4):202–210.

31. Vasavada AR, Desai JP. Stop, chop, chop and stuff. *J Cataract Refract Surg.* 1996;22:526–529.

32. Vasavada A, Singh R. Step-by-step chop in situ and separation of very dense cataracts. *J Cataract Refract Surg.* 1998;24:156–159.

Please see companion narrated videos on the accompanying Web site at
www.Healio.com/phacochopvideos

Advanced Phaco Techniques for Brunescent Nuclei
Cross-Action Chop Circumferential Disassembly

Lisa B. Arbisser, MD

Brunescent nuclear sclerosis challenges phacoemulsification surgeons with its leathery interdigitated posterior fibers and the rubbery density unique to this cataract type. Patients often experience symmetric progression and do not notice the slow deterioration of contrast sensitivity and acuity. Unless a discrete opacity develops, patients tolerate advanced disease before seeking surgery. These eyes have minimal cortical cushioning and a fragile zonular apparatus, which increase interventional risk. The goal of immediate visual rehabilitation and clear corneas on postoperative day 1 can be attained in almost 100% of cases with modern phacoemulsification technology and meticulous attention to detail. Even the most brunescent black or tan lens can be safely and predictably conquered without planned extracapsular techniques, sharp choppers, leaving the safe central zone within the capsulorrhexis, or sculpting of any kind. This chapter will detail the technique that is used to facilitate attaining this goal in even the most challenging eyes. It is called cross-action vertical chop with circumferential disassembly.[1,2]

PREREQUISITES

Brunescent cases require a little extra time in the schedule. As long as the patient can fixate on the indirect light during the preoperative exam, standard topical anesthesia is adequate. Employ modern phacoemulsification machines that permit a noncontinuous delivery of ultrasound.

This technique requires a minimum 5-mm pupil dilation to permit an adequate continuous curvilinear capsulorrhexis (CCC; Figures 20-1 and 20-2). Staining the anterior capsule helps because nuclear brunescence dulls the red reflex. Vertical chop with circumferential disassembly allows the CCC to be tailored to the optic size rather than to the size of the nucleus.[3,4]

The primary incision should be snug (appropriate to the phaco tip), and the paracentesis should not exceed 0.5 mm to achieve a closed chamber with minimal leak.

The author strongly prefers the Rosen splitter (Katena Products, Denville, NJ) for chopping. It fits easily through the small paracentesis, is blunt at the tip and outer edge, and has a hatchet-like inner aspect.

Chang DF.
Phaco Chop and Advanced Phaco Techniques: Strategies for Complicated Cataracts, Second Edition (pp 221-228).

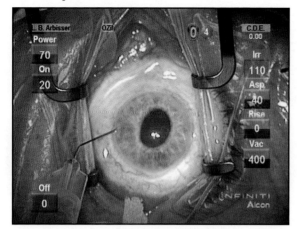

Figure 20-1. Inadequate pupil in ischemic eye.

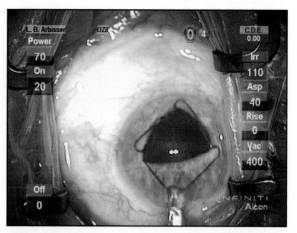

Figure 20-2. Malyugin ring for optimal exposure.

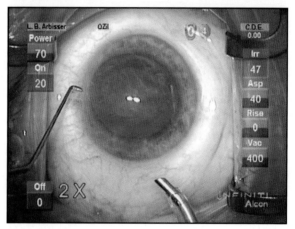

Figure 20-3. Note settings, retracted sleeve, and Rosen splitter.

Thorough hydrodissection to establish nuclear rotation without stressing the zonular network is essential. The very brunescent lens contains little space for fluid. Sensitive and sparing force should be used in creating the fluid wave around the lens while slightly depressing the center of the lens to burp the bag. Multidirectional hydrodissection with "J" cannulas may be helpful to complete the release of any cortical adhesion. Nuclear rotation is best attempted with a 2-handed technique or with the chamber refilled with dispersive viscoelastic ophthalmic viscosurgical device (OVD). Carefully attend to vector force to avoid zonular stress.

Endothelial protection, ideally a soft-shell technique utilizing dispersive OVD, significantly reduces the likelihood of postoperative corneal edema.

Our goal in all ocular surgery is to keep the eye as normotensive as possible, preventing over-deepening or collapse of the anterior chamber. Keeping all tissues in their normal anatomic relationship minimizes complications.

CROSS-ACTION VERTICAL CHOP

Specific parameters mentioned in this chapter refer to the author's current Infinity phacoemulsification technology (Alcon Laboratories, Fort Worth, TX); however, all modern phacoemulsification platforms on the market work well.[5]

The author prefers the bent Kelman-style 0.9-mm mini-flared 30-degree Aspiration Bypass System phaco tip. The bend in the tip makes it easier to imbed into the nucleus without lifting the incision and provides useful angles when debulking an endonucleus. The smaller gauge is ideal for maneuverability and reduced surge. The 30-degree tip allows for excellent occlusion, which is more important to this technique than cutting ability.

The author retracts the sleeve as far as possible without allowing irrigation into the incision tunnel to avoid chamber collapse. The retracted sleeve exposes about 2 mm of phaco needle; this permits adequate entry into the nucleus to gain purchase on the material facilitating vertical chop. The exposed needle acts like a dipstick, creating a visual clue to confirm its safe depth in the nucleus when imbedded to the edge of the sleeve (Figure 20-3).

The author prefers to enter the chamber on foot pedal position 0 (FP0) by first filling the anterior chamber with dispersive OVD. This controlled entry assures excellent endothelial protection, prevents flinching by the topical patient, and allows Descemet's membrane to be visualized and protected. Enter the chamber with the bottle initially low in a myopic or post-vitrectomy eye to prevent reverse pupillary block and over-deepening of the anterior chamber. The bottle is elevated to the normal height once a stable and relatively physiologic chamber depth is achieved. If needed, the iris is lifted off the anterior capsule with the second hand instrument, preventing or resolving reverse pupil block.

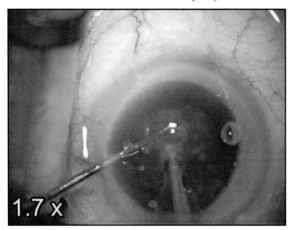

Figure 20-4. Bury phaco tip to sleeve.

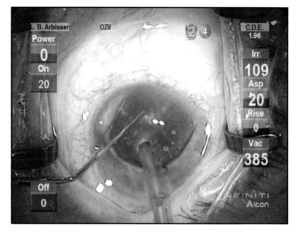

Figure 20-5. Beginning position of splitter for first chop.

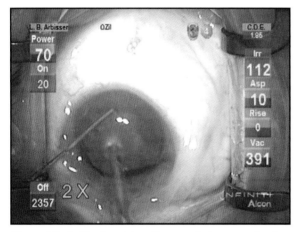

Figure 20-6. Dig in with splitter and draw proximal to meet phaco tip.

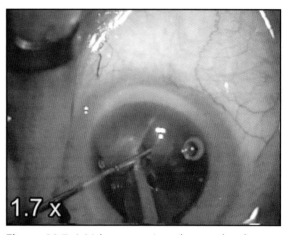

Figure 20-7. Initial cross action chop to barely open clamshell.

The author always begins in FP2 (aspiration) to establish flow, preventing incision burn while removing superficial cortex to clear the view. Fluidics are adjusted to create a stable chamber while providing efficiency. The author generally works at fixed settings of 400 mm Hg vacuum, 40 cc/min flow rate, and positions the bottle at 110 cm. A 0 rise time is preferred so that the pump does not change speed upon occlusion. For the chopping (disassembly) portion of any case the author uses burst mode with longitudinal ultrasound only (not torsional). The fixed panel set power is tailored to the density of nucleus from 15% for Grade 1 nuclei to 70% to 80% power for the truly brunescent lens. The burst is set at 20 ms on burst width so that the burst interval is linear but the burst width is fixed. The tip is directed into the lens just proximal of the CCC center (Figure 20-4). Burst mode allows the surgeon to see the ease of travel into the "meat" of the lens, confirming appropriate power delivered. Individual bursts are used until the phaco needle is buried just beyond half depth near the nucleus' center. With vacuum engaged and a Rosen splitter as the nondominant hand (let us assume the left hand)

instrument through the paracentesis about 90 degrees away from the main incision, the splitter is used to slice into the nucleus starting just inside the distal edge of the CCC rim (Figure 20-5). It is drawn proximal, toward the phaco tip just to the right side of center until it makes contact with the phaco tip (Figure 20-6). This initiates a fault formation in the nucleus as the 2 instruments are moved apart in a cross-wise fashion with the splitter moving to the right and the phaco tip moving to the left opposite direction (Figure 20-7). Unlike classic vertical chop where the splitter moves to the left and the phaco tip to the right, this technique does not require vacuum maintenance because there is no lifting motion to effect the chop or fault line propagation. Rather, the 2 instruments work more like a prechopper, helping the 2 sides of the lens to part. There are several major advantages to this cross-action chop maneuver over the classic direct action chop. The 2 instruments remain in the same Z plane rather than having one push down and the other lift, which discourages dangerous tilting of a stiff and dense nucleus. Second, because vacuum is not critical to the maneuver's success, the foot position can go to 1 or 0 once

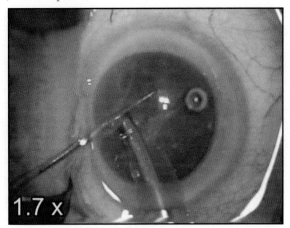

Figure 20-8. Rotate for subsequent chops.

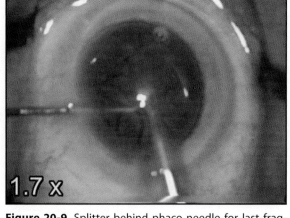

Figure 20-9. Splitter behind phaco needle for last fragments.

the fault line is initiated. This obviates the risk of a soft lens nucleus' aspiration at the apogee of the split, avoiding the risk of posterior capsule aspiration and rupture. Lastly, the technique is easier for inexperienced surgeons to reproduce once the concept is understood because the perfect coordination of foot pedal with hand motion is not critical as in direct action classical phaco chop. Like all vertical phaco chop, the 2 instruments are always kept within the safe zone inside the CCC, the same drastic reduction in phaco energy compared to sculpting techniques is enjoyed, and there is no drag on proximal zonules.

For the average nucleus, this first fault line advances through the posterior plate, allowing the formation of 2 hemispheres. The nucleus is then rotated clockwise, and this splitting maneuver is repeated as often as necessary to allow the phaco-assisted aspiration of all of the pie sections at the iris plane or slightly up into the anterior chamber (Figure 20-8). A small air bubble often remains stuck in the viscoelastic layer under the endothelium; this signals a lack of turbulence near these delicate cells. A combination of standard direct action chop and cross-action chop can be used as deemed convenient until complete. Avoid removing the largest piece last. The shallower the chamber and the denser the nucleus, the smaller the pie wedges are appropriately divided in order to avoid challenging the endothelium with a large fragment in the anterior chamber. Except in the truly brunescent nucleus, where it is most efficient to remain in burst mode until the last thin pieces of epinucleus, the author prefers to use torsional (intelligent phaco OZil; Alcon Surgical) for section removal. The author's quadrant removal setting is continuous torsional starting at 25% with linear up to 100%. The author will toggle between the 2 modes if sections come early, or do all chopping first and then remove segments with one mode change.

During removal of the last pieces the author positions the Rosen splitter with its blunt tip under the phaco needle to protect the posterior capsule in the event of surge

(Figure 20-9). For soft nuclei, hydrodelineation to create a golden ring allows the endonucleus to be easily divided with cross-action chop and the 2 hemispheres are removed without further division. In rubbery nuclei (often encountered in diabetics or the elderly with minimal anterior sclerosis but denser posterior nuclear plates), a maneuver called *back cracking* can be very helpful as an adjunct to standard or cross-action chop. As long as there is any one full-thickness crack anywhere in the nucleus, the Rosen splitter (which is smooth on its outer edge and tip) can be maneuvered under the nucleus along the posterior capsule within the crack between the posterior capsule and nucleus. The splitter is then lifted upward while the phaco tip is merely held, without engaging lens material, above the nucleus next to the splitter to stabilize the nucleus. Upward motion of the splitter then creates a crack, which presents the section for removal from its central apex rather than, as usual, from the nucleus periphery. This obviates the necessity to follow a receding nuclear edge out close to the peripheral capsule and eliminates the need to thin the material with sculpting. Once all dense nuclear material is evacuated, any remaining epinucleus is usually engaged and aspirated without altering fluidics.

Brunescent Lens Phaco: Circumferential Disassembly

The author modifies this basic technique for the densely brunescent lens. The posterior plates of these lenses feature rubbery interdigitated fibers. This causes unacceptable stress on the bag when the surgeon attempts to create 2 hemispheres with the first chop. The author never sculpts or craters but instead developed a technique called *circumferential disassembly*. This entails making the first chop in the usual fashion but with the goal of creating a

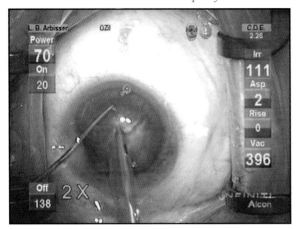

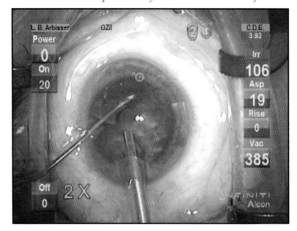

Figure 20-10. (A) Second anterior radial chop. (B) Endonuclear plane exposed.

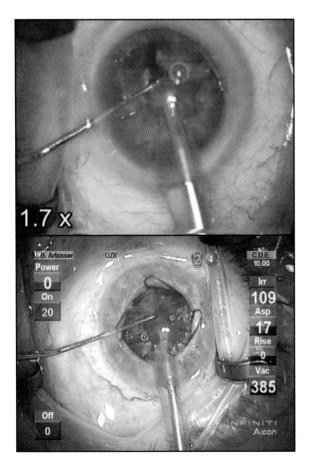

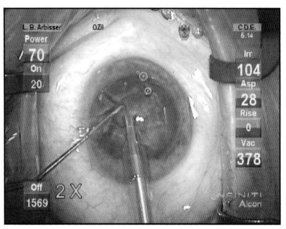

Figure 20-11. (A) Debulking small segments. (B) Poised to split dense lens into small parts so no bulk enters anterior chamber. (C) Endonucleus debulked without sculpting.

superior superficial chop, slowly prying apart the 2 hemispheres to about the middle of the depth of the nucleus only and not through the posterior plate. The plan is to gain access to the endonucleus but not to split the lens all the way down to the epinucleus. The lens is then turned slightly and the surgeon makes multiple very small radial pie wedges, which are complete on the anterior surface of the lens but not posteriorly (Figure 20-10A). This permits the nucleus to be flayed open enough to engage the endonucleus within the nuclear and epinuclear framework, analogous to removing

the clam from its shell (Figure 20-10B). These lamellae are not totally fused but adhere firmly in the brunescent lens. The natural planes that permit hydrodelineation of the immature cataract, creating a golden ring, are occult. Surgeons, of course, cannot hydrodelineate the brunescent lens, but can still mechanically find this division and debulk the nucleus in a circumferential manner, peeling out dense fibers while simultaneously creating our usual radial disassembly (Figures 20-11A and 20-11B). The lens is rotated many times, constantly thinning the remaining shell in a symmetrical fashion, without stress on zonules (as excellent hydrodissection has already been established; Figure 20-12). The outer shell of nucleus keeps the bag well expanded while multiple sections of endonucleus are evacuated—all in the safe zone within the CCC and deep in the chamber, away from the endothelium. The Rosen splitter, with its hatchet-shaped inner aspect, can be used with a sweeping motion from peripheral to central to help lyse the tough interdigitated strands as a small piece of endonucleus is lollipopped with the phaco tip and drawn centrally, freeing each segment from its apical attachment for

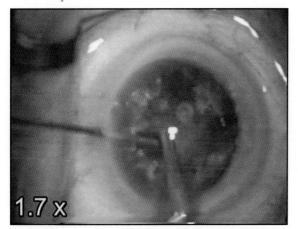

Figure 20-12. Thinning to the point of red reflex.

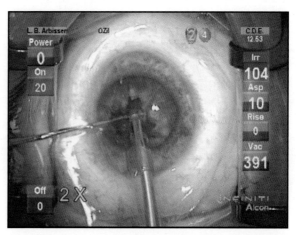

Figure 20-13. Sweeping with splitter to lyse central fibers and free section for aspiration.

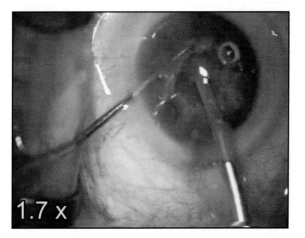

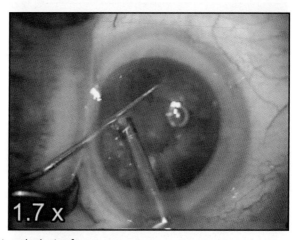

Figure 20-14. (A) Finding dense endonucleus to debulk. (B) Rotating clockwise for next segment.

phaco-assisted aspiration (Figure 20-13). The author finds burst mode with longitudinal phaco to be most efficient with brunescent lenses because even with newer mixed modes (IP OZil), a very brunescent lens is more apt to clog the tip when any torsional component is added. Burst mode allows the judicious use of power to latch onto a small piece, permitting its disassembly from the whole by the application of mechanical force with the splitter (Figure 20-14). Ultrasound is only used again to assist aspiration in its removal. A cumulative dispersed energy (CDE) of 40 s is rarely exceeded, even for the blackest nucleus. Virtually all of the ultrasound energy is delivered within the posterior chamber. Once the endonucleus is debulked evenly without any remaining thick sections and the outer shell is divided into small radial pies anteriorly, the dispersive OVD can be replaced through the paracentesis if it has dissipated (Figure 20-15). The remaining nucleofied epinuclear shell is lifted into the anterior chamber and fed into the phaco tip with the Rosen splitter after re-establishing flow to avoid incision burn. Sometimes this is best done by allowing it to fold inward and nibbling the anterior peripheral edges (Figure 20-16). Otherwise, it is best to lift it centrally; one

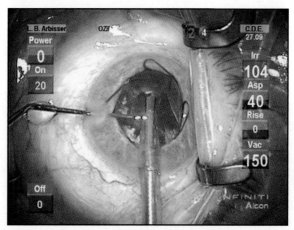

Figure 20-15. Reinjection of OVD before final removal in anterior chamber.

burst can loosen any remaining structural attachment of the sections to each other. At this point, the fluidics can be somewhat stepped down (for this author it goes from 400 to 320 mm HG vacuum and from 40 to 32 cc/min flow rate; Figure 20-17). Removal is completed with care to keep

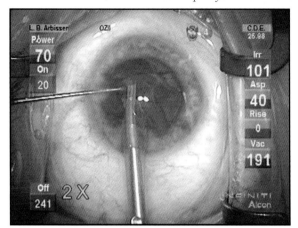

Figure 20-16. Tumbling epinucleus.

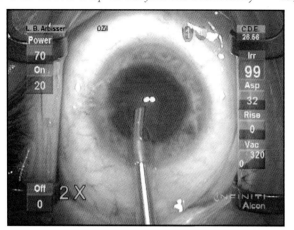

Figure 20-17. Note stepdown of fluidics for endonucleus, clear cornea, and final CDE.

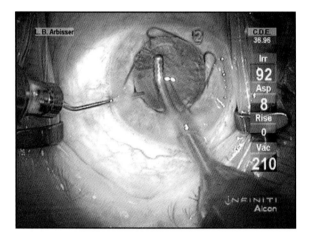

Figure 20-18. Peripheral cortex removed with high vacuum.

the second hand instrument below the phaco tip to protect the posterior capsule when actually applying phaco bursts. This maneuver protects against any surge encountered. Take care not to withdraw the sleeve into the incision tunnel, allowing the chamber to shallow. Circumferential disassembly has the major advantage of "keeping the shoe tree in the shoe"; it maintains the expanded bag during all of the action until the last of the epinucleus is gone. Most brunescent lenses have friable zonular attachment and no cushion of posterior cortex to protect the capsule. The rigid posterior plate (thinned but in place until the end) provides this protection. This circumferential strategy is extremely safe to zonules, the posterior capsule, and endothelium. If an eye has normal zonules to begin with, both the author's complication rate and first-day postoperative visual acuity are no different for the brunescent lens than for the average lens. As the author does in every case prior to removing the phaco tip from the eye, she trades the Rosen splitter for a syringe with balanced salt solution on a 27-gauge cannula and irrigates through the paracentesis while removing the phaco tip from the main incision to prevent anterior

chamber collapse while awaiting the irrigation and aspiration handpiece.

CORTEX REMOVAL

The brunescent mature cataract often presents its own challenging cortical removal issues because the central cortex is often nonexistent; however, there is often copious cortical remnant peripherally.[6] For standard irrigation and aspiration (I/A) where the anterior leaf of cortex protrudes central to the CCC, the author's settings are 600 mm Hg linear vacuum and 40 cc/min fixed aspiration (Figure 20-18). An alternate I/A setting, which is used to vacuum anterior capsule flaps in all cases, is useful in this scenario. The upper level vacuum setting is limited to 50 mm Hg linear with aspiration set at 10 cc/min fixed. This allows safe "fishing" under the CCC in the fornix to sequentially clean each clock hour, emptying the bag entirely for the best short-term and long-term outcome (Figure 20-19A). Be certain when closing the incision to irrigate and burp the wound to flush any residual chip that could have become lodged in OVD. This is important for every case, but retained chips are more common after brunescent cataract.

IMMEDIATE POSTOP

Glaucoma patients or those at risk for pressure rise—including all brunescent lens patients—receive 1 oral acetazolamide sequel upon discharge if they have no sulfa allergy. They are otherwise routine patients and are instructed to use a fluoroquinolone, nonsteroidal anti-inflammatory drug (NSAID), and a steroid every 3 hours while awake until he or she return for the 1-day postoperative visit.

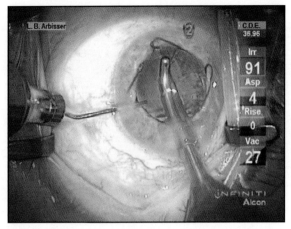 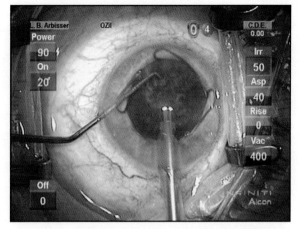

Figure 20-19. (A) Significant cortex hides at equator removed with low vacuum. (B) Black nucleus uses highest ultrasound setting.

CONCLUSION

We stand on the shoulders of the giants who initiated our path with awesome technology and insight. Cataract surgery today remains wonderfully rewarding. No 2 cases are exactly alike, so I am never bored. I particularly enjoy the challenge of patients with dense brunescence, whose "oohs and aahs" at the forgotten colors of the world are the icing on the cake of restoring their vision (Figures 20-19B and 20-20).

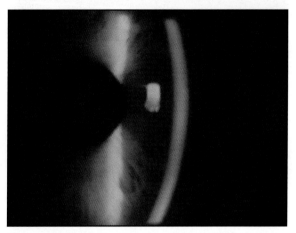

Figure 20-20. A 6+ brunescent cataract with clear cornea on day 1 postop.

REFERENCES

1. Arbisser LB. *Phacoemulsification Technique With Vertical Chop Clam Shell Circumferential Disassembly for Brunescent Cataract.* Philadelphia: Lippincott Williams & Wilkins; 2005.
2. Arbisser LB. Osher's Video Journal of Cataract and Refractive Surgery: Circumferential Disassembly of the Brunescent Cataract. 2006;1(XXll):Issue 1.
3. Singh R, Vasavada AR, Janaswamy G. Phacoemulsification of brunescent and black cataracts. *J Cataract Refract Surg.* 2001;27(11):1762-1769.
4. Vasavada AR. Multilevel chop technique. *J Cataract Refract Surg.* 2011;37:2092–2094.
5. Fine IH, Packer M, Hoffman RS. Use of power modulations in phacoemulsification: choo-choo chop and flip phacoemulsification. *J Cataract Refract Surg.* 2001;27:188–197.
6. Artzén D, Lundström M, Behndig A, et al. Capsule complication during cataract surgery: Case-control study of preoperative and intraoperative risk factors: Swedish Capsule Rupture Study Group report 2. *J Cataract Refract Surg.* 2009;35:1688–1693.

21

Strategies for Small Pupils

David F. Chang, MD

Small pupils pose 2 sets of problems that increase the risk for posterior capsule rupture during phaco. First, working space in the pupillary plane is limited. This restricts the diameter of the capsulorrhexis and increases the chance of traumatizing the pupillary or capsular edge with the phaco tip, irrigation/aspiration (I/A) tip, or second instrument. If the surgeon unknowingly lacerates the capsulorrhexis edge with the phaco tip, subsequent nuclear rotation can extend the tear into the posterior capsule.

The second problem is impaired visualization of the lens and capsular bag. The iris hides the peripheral lens, and the intensity of the red reflex is significantly reduced with each millimeter less of pupil diameter. A poor red reflex makes it difficult to see the anterior capsule edge both during and after completion of the capsulorrhexis. The iris may also obscure optimal positioning of the hydrodissection cannula just beneath the capsulorrhexis rim, leading to flawed or failed hydrodissection. During phaco, a poor red reflex makes it difficult to judge the depth at which the phaco tip is cutting. This is a problem for divide-and-conquer techniques where a long, deep central trench is needed to crack the nucleus in half. Visually confirming full posterior separation of the heminuclei becomes difficult as well.

Finally, a small diameter pupil and capsulorrhexis hinder instrument access to the capsular bag periphery. Along with impaired visualization, this complicates removing the peripheral nucleus, epinucleus, and cortex, and implanting the IOL. Removing subincisional cortex is particularly difficult in eyes with a small diameter pupil and capsulorrhexis. Intraoperative floppy iris syndrome (IFIS) involves special considerations that are covered in greater detail in the following chapter.

STRATEGIES

Use of a pledget or instrument wipe soaked in solution of dilating medications can improve pharmacologic mydriasis of marginal pupils (Figure 21-1). Direct intracameral injection of alpha agonists such as phenylephrine or epinephrine (off label) is a safe and simple pharmacologic strategy to try and may be particularly effective for IFIS.[1-6]

In the United States, 1:1000 epinephrine has been commercially available from several manufacturers. The 30 mL bottle contains the preservative chlorobutanol and should not be used in the eye. Preservative-free 1:1000 epinephrine is packaged in single use 1 mL vials (1 mg/mL) and comes in 2 forms—with and without 0.1% bisulfite as a stabilizing agent. Bisulfite improves the stability of the solution by delaying oxidation of the active substance, but is toxic to the corneal endothelium due to its high buffer capacity. In addition, epinephrine taken directly from the vial has a low pH of approximately 3.0. Therefore, direct intracameral injection of undiluted 1:1000 epinephrine should be avoided. Instead, a 1:4000 epinephrine solution can be easily constituted by adding 0.2 mL of commercially available 1:1000 epinephrine to 0.6 mL of plain balanced salt solution

Chang DF.
Phaco Chop and Advanced Phaco Techniques: Strategies for Complicated Cataracts, Second Edition (pp 229-243).
© 2013 SLACK Incorporated.

(BSS) or BSS Plus in a 3-mL disposable syringe. This dilution raises the pH to a physiologic level and appears to sufficiently dilute the bisulfite stabilizing agent.[1,5]

Although bisulfite-free 1:1000 epinephrine is theoretically preferred for intracameral injection, there has been a nationwide shortage in the United States at the time of this writing. The 1:4 dilution of bisulfite-containing epinephrine has been safely used by the author, and was endorsed in a 2013 ASCRS clinical alert whenever bisulfite-free epinephrine is unavailable. Adding bisulfite-containing epinephrine to a 500 mL BSS irrigation bottle (off label) will not cause corneal endothelial toxicity because of the significant dilution. However, shortages of even bisulfite-containing 1:1000 epinephrine are now being reported in the United States. The author has noted an increased incidence of IFIS despite the absence of systemic alpha antagonists whenever epinephrine is omitted from the BSS irrigation bottle.

Several publications report the safety and efficacy of unpreserved 1.5% intracameral phenylephrine for both IFIS prevention and routine surgical mydriasis.[2,3,5,6] One of these studies found no significant reduction in endothelial cell counts compared to non-treated eyes.[6] Preservative-free phenylephrine 2.5% is only commercially available outside the United States. Because these preparations still contain bisulfite, a 1:4 dilution with BSS, BSS Plus, or preservative-free lidocaine is also recommended.

Lacking a commercial source in the United States, many surgeons (including the author) obtain bisulfite-free intracameral phenylephrine 1.5% prepared by compounding pharmacies. To avoid potential toxicity from preservative-containing phenylephrine, ophthalmologists should specify that only the unpreserved (raw) drug should be used as a compounding source. Prudent precautions for any drug compounded for intracameral injection include appropriate testing for pH, osmolality, and sterility. Ophthalmologists should check to see if the compounding pharmacy is accredited by the Pharmacy Compounding Accreditation Board (PCAB).

There are several excellent options that can be utilized to surgically expand the pupil intraoperatively.[7] Beside improving the red reflex and increasing the surgical working space, a parallel objective is to preserve a functional pupil size.[8] The minimum pupil diameter required for a safe surgery will depend on the surgeon's skill level and the presence of other risk factors such as pseudoexfoliation or a brunescent nucleus. Posterior synechiae should be lysed with a metal spatula or ophthalmic viscosurgical device (OVD) injection (Figure 21-2). In some cases, a ribbon-like pigmented membrane underlying and constraining the pupillary margin can be stripped away with capsule forceps (see Figure 21-2C-E).

The bimanual pupil stretching technique of Luther L. Fry, MD is simple in requiring only 2 Lester or collar-button

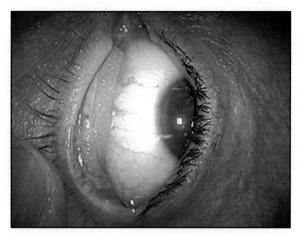

Figure 21-1. Pledget soaked in dilating solution placed in inferior fornix.

style hooks[9] (Figure 21-3). Mechanically stretching the pupil creates tiny, partial thickness tears in the iris sphincter that will preserve a functional pupil size.[10-12] This is particularly effective if the pupillary margin is stiff and fibrotic, such as in patients who chronically used pilocarpine. The Beehler pupil dilator (Microtech Inc, Garnet Valley, PA) achieves this objective with a single instrument.[7,13] If the pupil margin is more elastic and tends to simply stretch without tearing, intraocular MST microscissors can be used to make multiple partial thickness cuts in the iris sphincter prior to stretching.[7,14] Care must be taken to avoid transecting the 1-mm wide sphincter muscle, which would cause permanent mydriasis. Pupil stretching is ineffective and should be avoided in eyes with IFIS.[15]

Although preferences for OVDs vary widely, sodium hyaluronate 2.3% (Healon 5) is a maximally cohesive single agent that is particularly well suited for viscomydriasis and for blocking the iris from prolapsing in IFIS (see Figure 22-3). Particularly if mydriasis is insufficient after injecting an intracameral alpha agonist, Healon 5 can be used to mechanically expand the pupil further[16] (see Figure 22-3A-C). Viscomydriasis facilitates the capsulorrhexis and combines with the epinephrine-induced iris rigidity to block iris prolapse. However, low flow and vacuum parameters (eg, < 175 to 200 mm Hg; < 26 mL/min) should be used to avoid immediately aspirating Healon 5 out of the eye. One should therefore not rely on this strategy if high vacuum and aspiration flow settings are desired for denser nuclei. In this situation dispersive OVDs, such as DisCoVisc, sodium chondroitin sulfate (Viscoat), or sodium hyaluronate 3% (Healon EndoCoat) may persist longer within the anterior chamber. Finally, combining Healon 5 with Viscoat has been advocated as a combination strategy whereby the Viscoat will better resist aspiration and delay the evacuation of Healon 5.

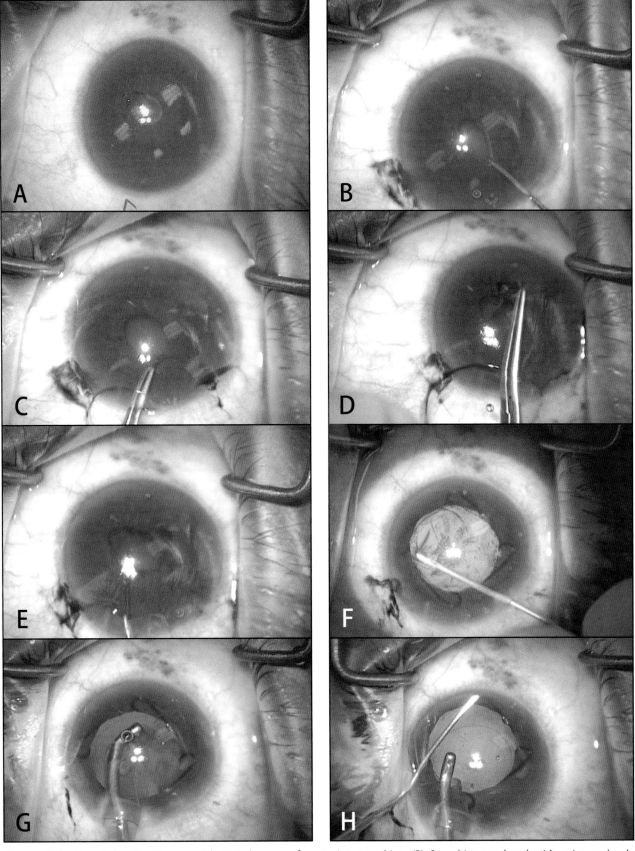

Figure 21-2. Case 1. (A) Uveitic eye with 360 degrees of posterior synechiae. (B) Synechiae are lysed with a Lester hook. (C-E) Pigmented, fibrotic pupillary membrane is grasped with capsule forceps and peeled away. (F) Initial capsulotomy diameter is limited by Malyugin ring exposure. (G) During or following cortical aspiration, (H) the Malyugin ring can be moved like a picture frame to better expose the periphery without stretching the pupil any further.

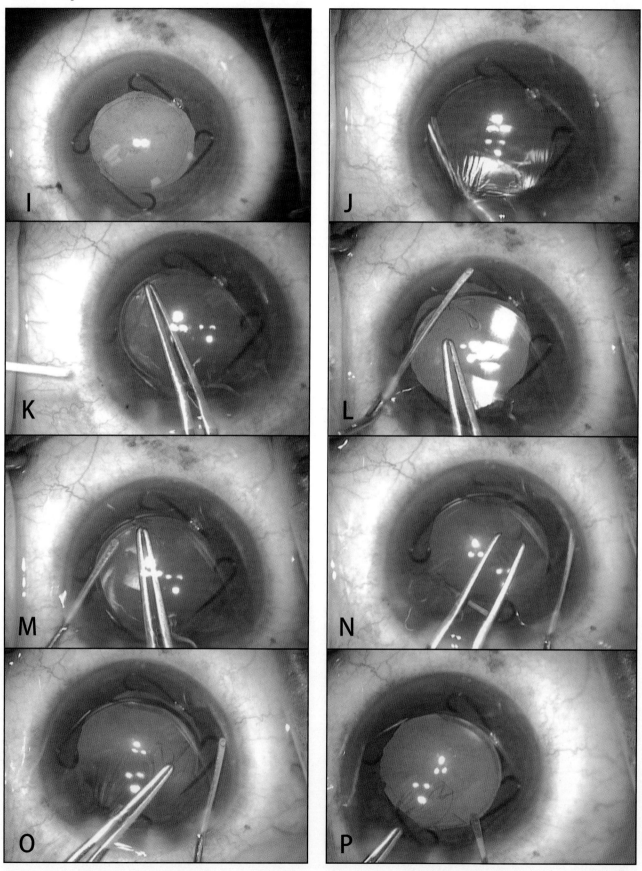

Figure 21-2 (continued). Case 1. (I) Vitreous cells are visible after cataract extraction. Likewise, moving the ring sequentially exposes the peripheral optic area so that the capsulotomy can be secondarily enlarged. (J-Q) The capsulorrhexis is widened out to the very edge of the optic in order to prevent posterior synechiae formation to the capsular rim.

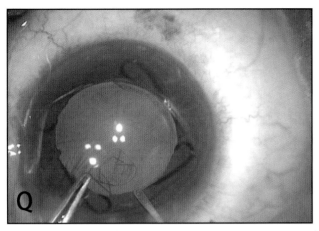

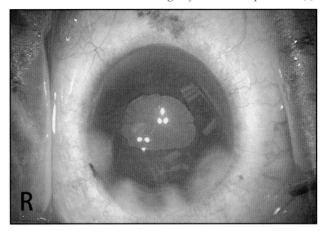

Figure 21-2 (continued). Case 1. (R) After Malyugin ring removal, the fibrotic pupil immediately returns to physiologic size because the sphincter has not been excessively stretched.

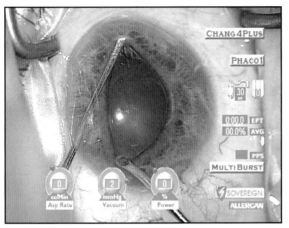

Figure 21-3. Bimanual stretch technique for pupil enlargement. Note that the pupil must be stretched much wider than the desired diameter in order to cause microscopic relaxing sphincter tears.

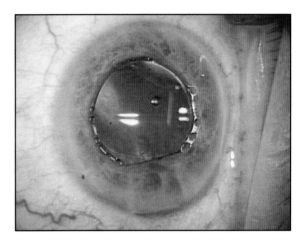

Figure 21-4. Morcher pupil expansion ring in eye with IFIS.

Pupil Expansion Rings

Pupil expansion rings are disposable devices that mechanically expand and maintain the intraoperative pupil diameter. Disposable polymethylmetacrylate (PMMA) rings, such as the Morcher 5S pupil ring (Figure 21-4; FCI Ophthalmics, Marshfield Hills, MA) and the Milvella Perfect Pupil (Figure 21-5; Milvella, Savage, MN), have grooved contours that are threaded alongside the pupillary margin with dedicated metal injectors.[17,18] Eagle Vision's Graether disposable silicone pupil expansion ring is inserted with a single use plastic injector (Eagle Vision, Memphis, TN).[19] All of these rings are relatively difficult to position if the pupil is less than 4 mm wide or if the anterior chamber is shallow. They will fail to engage the iris if the pupil diameter is larger than 7 mm.

Most surgeons find the Malyugin ring (MicroSurgical Technology, Redmond, WA) to be the easiest and fastest pupil expansion device to insert and remove[20] (see Figure 21-2 and Figure 21-6). This is a 5-0 polypropylene

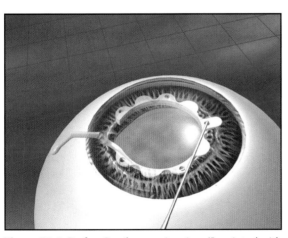

Figure 21-5. Perfect Pupil expansion ring. (Reprinted with permission of BD Ophthalmic.)

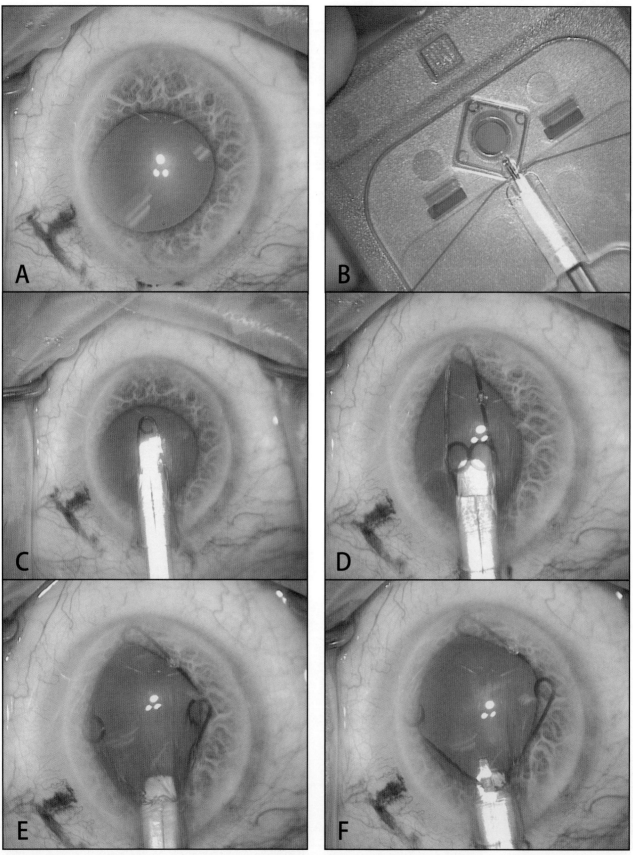

Figure 21-6. Case 2. Malyugin ring. (A) Pupil dilates poorly. (B) Disposable Malyugin ring injector system. (C) The injector tip should be positioned close to the nasal iris margin so that the leading coil can easily engage the pupil. (D, E) As the lead and lateral coils engage the pupil margin, the injector tip is slowly moved toward the incision. (F) The injector hook is disengaged.

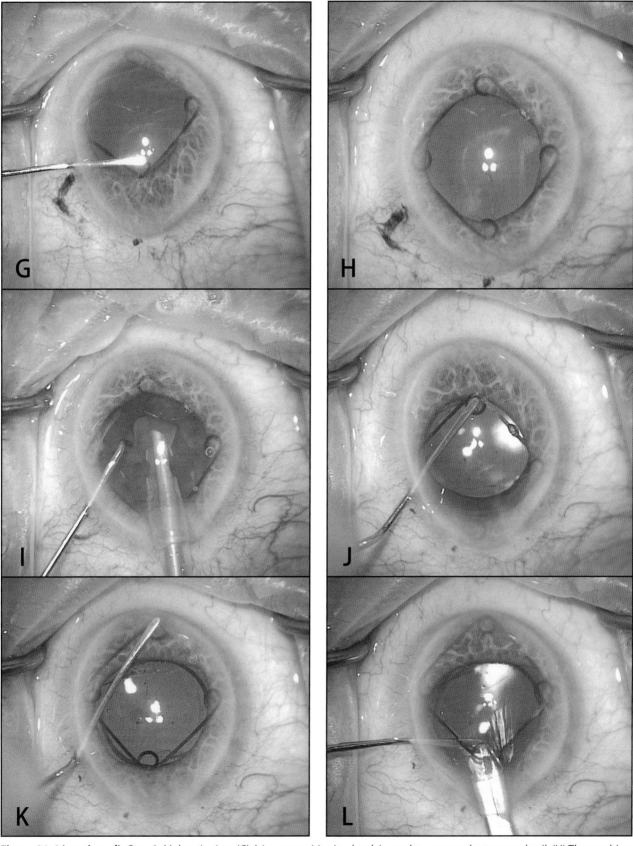

Figure 21-6 (continued). Case 2. Malyugin ring. (G) A Lester positioning hook is used to engage the temporal coil. (H) The resulting pupil diameter is 6 mm and rounded due to 8 points of contact. (I) The low profile of the ring does not impede instrument movement or access. (J) For removal, the distal coil is first disengaged. (K) Sliding the ring slightly nasally frees the proximal coil. (L) The Lester hook elevates the proximal coil to facilitate capture with the hooked injector tip.

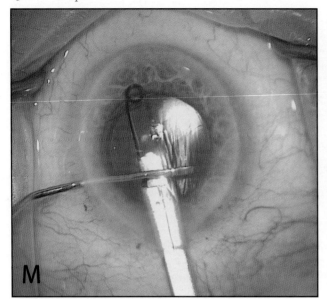

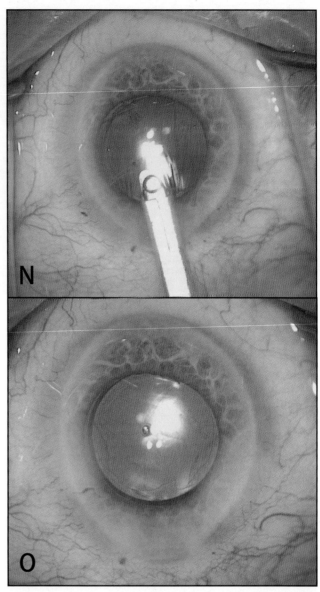

Figure 21-6 (continued). Case 2: Malyugin ring. (M, N) The ring is collapsed into the injector as the hook is withdrawn. (O) The pupil returns to its preoperative diameter without any sphincter tear.

Table 21-1.

OVERCOMING HISTORICAL OBJECTIONS TO IRIS RETRACTORS

OBJECTION	REBUTTAL
Too costly	Reusable iris hooks are very cost effective.
Time consuming to place	Stiffer 4–0 polypropylene hooks are much easier to handle and manipulate compared to 6-0 nylon.
Iris sphincter will be torn and damaged	With IFIS, the sphincter is elastic rather than fibrotic. Maximal stretching can therefore occur without excessive trauma to the sphincter muscle. Otherwise, aim smaller with the expectation of progressive widening during phaco.
Iris is tented up in front of the phaco tip	The diamond configuration avoids this problem and the associated iris chafing.
Insufficient surgical exposure	The diamond configuration and the ability to maximally stretch an IFIS pupil provide superb visualization and exposure.

single use device that is introduced with a disposable injector (see Figure 21-6B-F). The way in which the iris drapes over the sides of the device creates a round 6- or 7-mm pupil diameter, depending on which of the 2 available sizes is used (see Figure 21-6H). The disposable injector tip fits through a 2.5-mm incision and is used to both place and extract the ring. Compared to bulkier and more rigid plastic expansion rings, the thin profile of the Malyugin ring reduces the risk of accidental corneal or incisional trauma and does not impede instrument access to the cataract (see Figure 21-6I). The avoidance of multiple paracentesis sites is advantageous in the presence of a bleb, a pterygium, and multiple radial keratotomy (RK) scars and avoids the problem of iris hooks being pushed against the lid speculum with a tight palpebral fissure. Finally, the smooth coils are very gentle on the pupil margin, and generally minimize iris sphincter damage (see Figures 21-2R and 21-6O). A similar iris expander device has been introduced by Oasis Medical.

IRIS RETRACTORS

The author prefers reusable 4–0 polypropylene retractors (available from Katena Products, Denville, NJ, and FCI Ophthalmics) to disposable 6–0 nylon retractors, which are available through Alcon[21] (Figure 21-7). Measuring 0.15 mm in diameter, the 4–0 retractors are the same size and stiffness as the polypropylene haptic of an IOL (see Figure 21-7D). This greater rigidity, when compared to 6–0 nylon retractors, makes 4–0 retractors more durable and easier to manipulate. Furthermore, the 4-0 polypropylene hooks can be repeatedly autoclaved in the manufacturer supplied storage case, which makes them more cost

effective than disposable hooks or pupil expansion rings (see Figure 21-7I).

Before initiating the capsulorrhexis, 1-mm limbal paracenteses are created in each quadrant, including a separate stab incision just posterior to the temporal clear corneal incision (see Figure 21-7A-C). In this way, the phaco tip passes through a separate incision directly alongside and above the track for the subincisional retractor (see Figure 21-7F). As originally advocated by Oetting and Omphroy, placing the hooks in this diamond configuration has several advantages (see Figure 21-7E).[22,23] The subincisional hook retracts the iris downward and out of the path of the phaco tip. This not only provides excellent access to subincisional cortex, but also avoids tenting the iris up in front of the phaco tip, which is what occurs when the retractors are placed in a square configuration (see Figures 21-7F and 21-7G). This configuration also maximizes temporal exposure directly in front of the phaco tip as well as nasal exposure for placement of the chopper tip (see Figure 21-7G). Following IOL implantation, the iris retractors are removed, rinsed in balanced salt solution, and gently dabbed with an instrument wipe to remove any viscoelastic residue. They are then stored in the autoclavable storage container (see Figure 21-7I).

Iris retractors both enlarge and maintain an adequate pupillary size throughout the course of surgery. They provide sufficient tension to the iris stroma so that no prolapse can occur with IFIS. If the pupil is fibrotic, such as with chronic pilocarpine use or longstanding posterior synechiae, overstretching the iris can cause bleeding, tear the sphincter, and result in permanent mydriasis. It is therefore advisable to start with a smaller target diameter than needed with the expectation that the pupil opening will widen further during phaco (Figure 21-8B). The likely

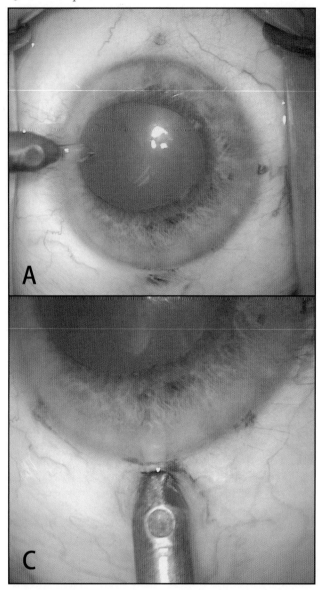

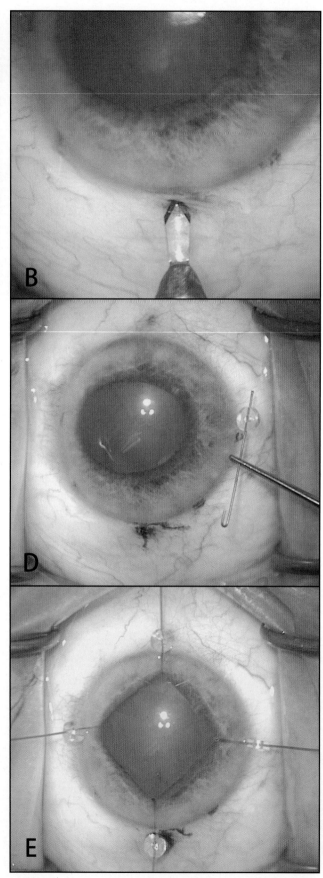

Figure 21-7. Case 3. Prolene iris retractors. Although the pupil dilates reasonably well in this patient taking tamsulosin, the opposite eye displayed IFIS during cataract surgery despite the use of intracameral epinephrine. It was decided to place iris retractors prior to the capsulorrhexis. (A) A diamond blade makes a 1-mm paracentesis. (B, C) A separate limbal stab incision is made just behind the temporal clear corneal incision and angled toward the pupil margin. (D) The reusable 4–0 polypropylene iris retractors (Katena Products, Inc; FCI Ophthalmics) are stiffer and easier to manipulate than 6–0 nylon retractors. (E) Unlike with pseudoexfoliation, posterior synechiae, or chronically miotic pupils, the IFIS pupil stretches without tearing and can be maximally dilated.

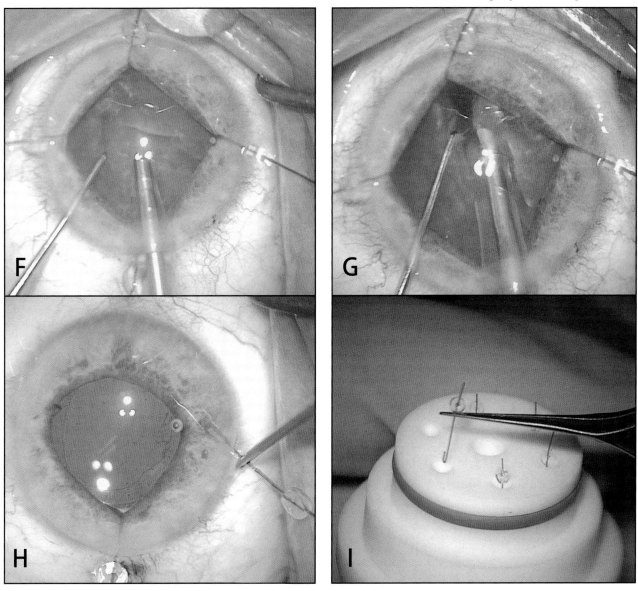

Figure 21-7 (continued). Case 3. Prolene iris retractors. Although the pupil dilates reasonably well in this patient taking tamsulosin, the opposite eye displayed IFIS during cataract surgery despite the use of intracameral epinephrine. It was decided to place iris retractors prior to the capsulorrhexis. (F) When placed in a diamond configuration, the subincisional retractor pulls the iris down and away from the phaco tip. The phaco tip slides above the subincisional retractor lying within a separate tunnel (G) while the nasal retractor maximizes surgical exposure for the chopper. (H) Because the IFIS pupil stretches without tearing, it immediately constricts as the retractors are removed. With toric IOLs, placement of iris retractors near the toric axis provides excellent visibility of the alignment marks. (I) The reusable retractors are rinsed, cleaned, and returned to the autoclavable sterilizing case.

reason for this is that the hydrostatic irrigation force propels the iris posteriorly against the 4-point restraints of the anchored retractors. This effectively acts to mechanically stretch the pupil margin, resulting in microscopic sphincter muscle tears. The exception is the IFIS pupil, which tends to be elastic and stretches maximally without tearing (see Figure 21-7E-H). Maximal widening with iris retractors can be employed with IFIS eyes.

Iris retractors are advantageous when a toric IOL is used, because 2 of the retractors can often be aligned with the astigmatic axis. This not only externally marks the axis, but allows the surgeon to visually confirm the location of the peripheral optic astigmatic markings (see Figure 21-7H). A particular advantage of using iris retractors for small pupils associated with pseudoexfoliation is that they can be readily repositioned around the capsulorrhexis edge to serve as capsule retractors if necessary (see Figure 21-8).

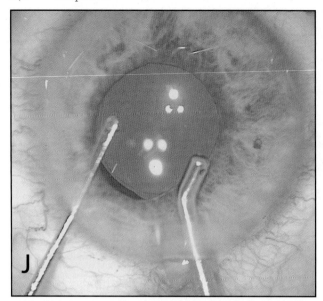

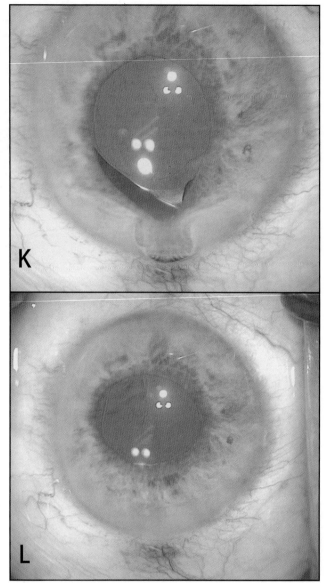

Figure 21-7 (continued). Case 3. Prolene iris retractors. Although the pupil dilates reasonably well in this patient taking tamsulosin, his opposite eye displayed IFIS during cataract surgery despite the use of intracameral epinephrine. It was decided to place iris retractors prior to the capsulorrhexis. (J, K) Iris prolapse and miosis occur during OVD aspiration following removal of iris retractors. (L) Despite maximal pupil stretching, the IFIS pupil immediately returns to a small diameter.

PHACO TECHNIQUE

Compared to divide-and-conquer, chopping offers several advantages for small pupil cases.[24,25] With either horizontal or vertical chop, the phaco tip generally remains in the central 2-mm zone of the pupil, where it is far less likely to aspirate or lacerate the iris or the anterior capsule. This also eliminates the necessity of sculpting behind the iris. Because chopping is a kinesthetic technique that, unlike sculpting, does not require visualization of the depth of the phaco tip, there is less dependence on a bright red reflex. One needs only to see the horizontal chopper pass beneath the anterior capsule before hooking the nucleus. Because peripheral placement of the horizontal chopper is not visualized with ordinary pupil sizes, a smaller pupil does not further complicate this maneuver (Figure 21-9).

During cortical clean-up, one can employ a Lester hook to focally retract the iris where peripheral access and visibility are impaired. Inserting the IOL through a small capsulorrhexis can also be challenging. Because the entire IOL must pass through the opening in the cartridge tip, as long as the tip fits inside the capsulorrhexis, the IOL can be delivered into the bag without stretching or tearing the anterior capsular edge. Once the IOL has been implanted, the small diameter capsulorrhexis can be secondarily enlarged, as discussed in Chapter 16. Retracting the iris with a Lester hook can also facilitate this step as well (see Figure 16-6D-J).

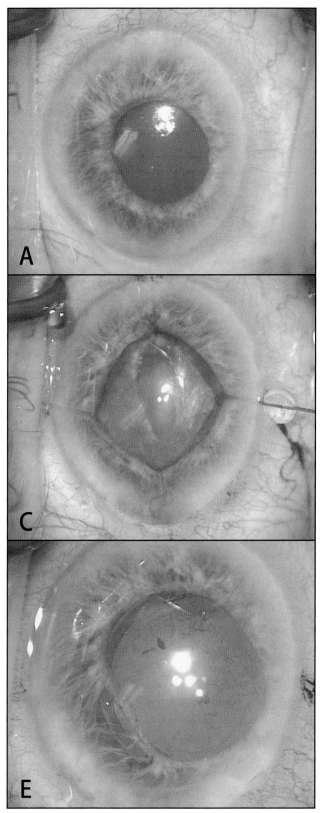

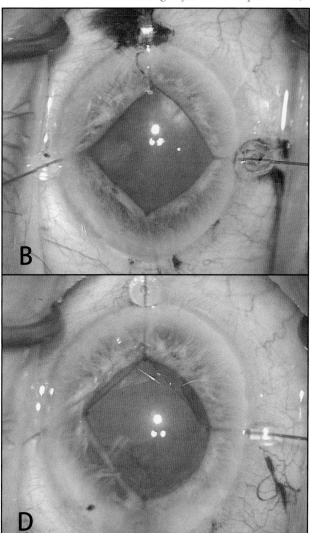

Figure 21-8. Case 4. (A) Small pupil in a tamsulosin patient with pseudoexfoliation and a brunescent lens. (B) Four Prolene iris retractors are placed prior to the capsulotomy and trypan blue dye staining. (C) Because diffuse and significant zonular weakness is noted during the capsulorrhexis step, the iris retractors are advanced around the edge of the capsulotomy to support the bag during lens removal. (D) Following nuclear removal, the retractors can remain in place during the cortical clean-up because they do not trap the cortex (unlike a CTR). (E) The retractors are removed after a STAAR AQ-2010 V 3-piece foldable IOL has been placed in the ciliary sulcus. Some stromal iris trauma has occurred following iris prolapse to the left-hand sideport incision during phaco.

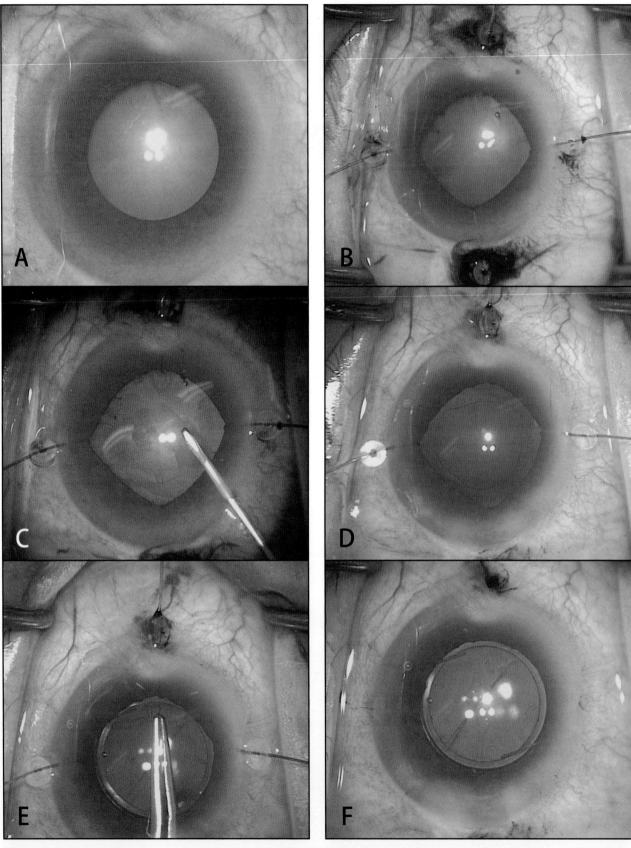

Figure 21-9. Case 5. Prolene iris retractors. (A, B) In a non-IFIS eye, the pupil must not be over-stretched. (C) With a small pupil, the red reflex is enhanced with the Zeiss Lumera microscope by using only the stereo coaxial illumination beam. (D) Following phaco, the pupil is slightly enlarged because of stretching of the sphincter as the iris is hydrostatically displaced posteriorly. (E) The smaller capsulorrhexis is secondarily enlarged prior to removing the hooks. (F) Sphincter tears and permanent mydriasis are avoided by not maximally stretching the pupil.

References

1. Shugar JK. Intracameral Epinephrine for Prophylaxis of IFIS [letter]. *J Cataract Refract Surg.* 2006;32:1074-1075.

2. Gurbaxani A, Packard R. Intracameral phenylephrine to prevent floppy iris syndrome during cataract surgery in patients on tamsulosin. *Eye.* 2007;21:331-332.

3. Manvikar S, Allen D. Cataract surgery management in patients taking tamsulosin. *J Cataract Refract Surg.* 2006;32:1611-1614.

4. Myers WG, Shugar JK. Optimizing the intracameral dilation regimen for cataract surgery: Prospective randomized comparison of 2 solutions. *J Cataract Refract Surg.* 2009;35:273-276.

5. Myers WG, Edelhauser HF. Shortage of bisulfite-free preservative-free epinephrine for intracameral use. *J Cataract Refract Surg.* 2011;37:611.

6. Lorente R, DeRojs V, Vazquez DE, Targa P, Moreno C, Varella J, Landaluce ML, Mendez J, Lorente B. Intracameral phenylephrine 1.5% for prophylaxis against intraoperative floppy iris syndrome: prospective, randomized fellow eye study. *Ophthalmology.* 2012;119:2053-2058.

7. Bartlett JD, Miller KM. Phacoemulsification techniques for patients with small pupils. *Comp Ophthalmol Update.* 2003;4:171-176.

8. Masket S. Relationship between postoperative pupil size and disability glare. *J Cataract Refract Surg.* 1992;18:506-507.

9. Fry LL. Miscellaneous Surgical Procedures I Have Found Helpful. Film Festival, Symposium on Cataract, IOL and Refractive Surgery. Seattle. May 1993.

10. Miller KM, Keener GT Jr. Stretch pupillopolasty for small pupil phacoemulsification. *Am J Ophthalmol.* 1994;117:107-108.

11. Shepherd DM. The pupil stretch technique for miotic pupils in cataract surgery. *Ophthalmic Surg.* 1993; 24; 851-852.

12. Dinsmore JC. Modified stretch technique for small pupil phacoemulsification with topical anesthesia. *J Cataract Refract Surg.* 1996;22:27-30.

13. Barboni P, Zanini M, Rossi A, Savini G. Monomanual pupil stretcher. *Ophthalmic Surg Lasers.* 1998;29:772-773.

14. Fine IH. Pupilloplasty for small pupil phacoemulsification. *J Cataract Refract Surg.* 1994;20:192-196.

15. Chang DF, Braga Mele R, Mamalis N, et al. ASCRS Cataract Clinical Committee. ASCRS white paper: intraoperative floppy iris syndrome—a clinical review. *J Cataract Refract Surg.* 2008;34:2153-2162.

16. Arshinoff SA. Modified SST-USST for tamsulosin-associated intraocular floppy iris syndrome. *J Cataract Refract Surg.* 2006;32:559-561.

17. Akman A, Yilmaz G, Oto S, Akova Y. Comparison of various pupil dilatation methods for phacoemulsification in eyes with a small pupil secondary to pseudoexfoliation. *Ophthalmology.* 2004;111:1693-1698.

18. Kershner RM. Management of the small pupil for clear corneal cataract surgery. *J Cataract Refract Surg.* 2002;28:1826-1831.

19. Graether JM. Graether pupil expander for managing the small pupil during surgery. *J Cataract Refract Surg.* 1996;22:530-535.

20. Chang DF. Use of Malyugin pupil expansion device for intraoperative floppy iris syndrome: Results in 30 consecutive cases. *J Cataract Refract Surg.* 2008;34:835-841.

21. Nichamin LD. Enlarging the pupil for cataract extraction using flexible nylon iris retractors. *J Cataract Refract Surg.* 1993;19:793–796.

22. Oetting TA, Omphroy LC. Modified technique using flexible iris retractors in clear corneal cataract surgery. *J Cataract Refract Surg.* 2002;28:596–598.

23. Dupps WJ, Oetting TA. Diamond iris retractor configuration for small-pupil extracapsular or intracapsular cataract surgery. *J Cataract Refract Surg.* 2004;30:2473–2475.

24. Chang D. Converting to Phaco Chop: Why? Which Technique? How? *Ophthalmic Practice.* 1999;17(4):202-210.

25. Vasavada A, Singh R. Phacoemulsification in eyes with a small pupil. *J Cataract Refract Surg.* 2000;26:1210-1218.

Please see companion narrated videos on the accompanying Web site at
www.Healio.com/phacochopvideos

22

Intraoperative Floppy Iris Syndrome

David F. Chang, MD

Intraoperative floppy iris syndrome (IFIS) in association with current or prior tamsulosin (Flomax) use was first described in 2005.[1] Beside a tendency for poor preoperative pupil dilation, severe IFIS exhibits a triad of intraoperative signs—iris billowing and floppiness, iris prolapse to the main and sideport incisions, and progressive intraoperative miosis (Figure 22-1). Numerous studies have confirmed our initial suspicion that when such iris behavior is unexpected, the rate of cataract surgical complications is increased.[2-7] Based on parallel large retrospective and prospective clinical studies that John Campbell and the author had conducted, we identified a strong association of IFIS with either current or prior use of tamsulosin.[1] This systemic alpha-1 antagonist is the most commonly prescribed medication for the symptomatic relief of benign prostatic hyperplasia (BPH). The association of IFIS with other systemic alpha-1 antagonists such as doxazosin, terazosin, and alfuzosin has since been documented as well.[4]

CLINICAL FEATURES

Although our original paper described a triad of signs with what we would now call severe IFIS, there is a wide range of clinical severity seen in clinical practice. In a prospective study of 167 eyes in patients taking tamsulosin, we classified IFIS as being mild (good dilation; some iris billowing without prolapse or constriction), moderate (iris billowing with some constriction of a moderately dilated pupil), or severe (classic triad and poor preoperative dilation).[2] Using this scale, the distribution of IFIS severity was 10% no IFIS, 17% mild IFIS, 30% moderate IFIS, and 43% severe IFIS. The tendency for iris prolapse often first appears during hydrodissection. Iris billowing may be seen when irrigation from the phaco tip is introduced, followed shortly thereafter by iris prolapse to both the incision and sideport paracentesis. Progressive intraoperative pupil constriction may occur with our without accompanying iris prolapse. The combination of progressive miosis and iris floppiness increases the likelihood of aspirating the iris with the phaco tip.

When surgeons have not recognized or anticipated IFIS, the rate of reported intraoperative complications increases. Multiple retrospective studies have published higher rates of capsular rupture and vitreous loss.[1,4-7] Complications of iris prolapse or aspiration include iridodialysis, iris sphincter damage, hyphema, and significant iris stromal or transillumination defects. Such iris trauma can cause permanent

Chang DF.
Phaco Chop and Advanced Phaco Techniques: Strategies for
Complicated Cataracts, Second Edition (pp 245-252).

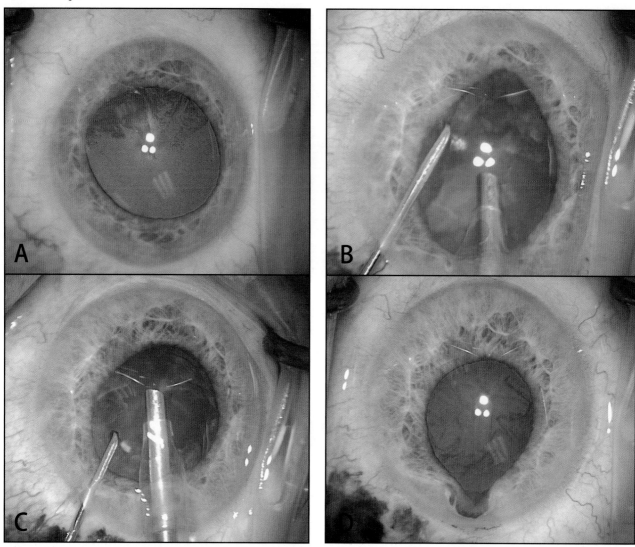

Figure 22-1. (A) Patient on tamsulosin showing preoperative dilation, (B) intraoperative iris billowing, (C) intraoperative miosis with iris prolapse to the phaco and sideport incisions, and (D) iris prolapse following instrument removal.

pupil deformity with glare or photophobia. In 2009, a retrospective Canadian study of nearly 100,000 male patients who underwent cataract surgery documented a doubling of the rate of serious postoperative complications including retinal detachment, retained nuclear fragments, and severe inflammation in tamsulosin patients.[7]

One important caution with IFIS is that partial thickness sphincterotomies and manual pupil stretching are ineffective and can exacerbate iris billowing and prolapse.[1,4] A medical history of systemic alpha-1 antagonist use should alert the cataract surgeon to anticipate IFIS and to consider alternative small pupil management strategies. Our multicenter prospective study of 169 consecutive cataract surgeries in tamsulosin patients attained excellent outcomes with low surgical complications by employing 4 specific operative techniques either alone or in combination.[2] Using sodium hyaluronate 2.3% (Healon 5) viscomydriasis, iris retractors, preoperative topical atropine administration, or pupil expansion rings, the incidence of posterior capsule rupture and vitreous loss was less than 1% in this clinical trial. However, because these were highly experienced cataract surgeons, this study may not be representative of the general surgical experience with IFIS. In a 2008 American Society of Cataract and Refractive Surgery (ASCRS) membership survey, 95% of the respondents reported that tamsulosin increased the difficulty of cataract surgery and 77% believed that it also increased the risk of complications.[3] Specifically, during the prior 2 years, IFIS had increased the rate of posterior capsular rupture for 52% of respondents and the rate of significant iris trauma for 23% of respondents.

PHARMACOLOGY AND MECHANISM OF INTRAOPERATIVE FLOPPY IRIS SYNDROME

Alpha-1 antagonists relax smooth muscle in the bladder, neck, and prostate. This facilitates more complete bladder emptying and thereby reduces the lower urinary tract symptoms of benign prostatic hyperplasia (BPH). There are at least 3 common human alpha-1 receptor subtypes: alpha-1A, alpha-1B, and alpha-1D. Doxazosin (Cardura), terazosin (Hytrin), and alfuzosin (Uroxatral) are considered nonselective alpha-1 antagonists. Tamsulosin, however, is very selective for the alpha-1A receptor subtype, which predominates in the prostate as well as in the iris dilator smooth muscle. Because, theoretically, it should not block the vascular smooth muscle alpha-1D receptors, tamsulosin has a lower risk of causing postural hypotension. Although BPH is by far the most common indication, both men and women may take alpha-1 antagonists for other conditions. Tamsulosin is often briefly prescribed as an adjunctive medication to facilitate renal stone passage following shock wave lithotripsy. It may also be prescribed for urinary retention in women, and IFIS has been well documented in female patients taking tamsulosin. Finally, alpha-1 antagonists, such as doxazosin, terazosin, and prazosin, have long been prescribed for systemic hypertension. Ophthalmologists should also become familiar with 2 newer drugs prescribed for BPH symptoms. Silodosin (Rapaflo) is a systemic alpha blocker that was FDA approved for BPH in 2008. Like tamsulosin, it is also selective for the alpha-1A subtype, and is similar to tamsulosin in its strong propensity to cause IFIS. Jalyn is the brand name for the combination of dutasteride and tamsulosin, and was FDA approved in 2010. The combination of these 2 agents was shown in a large prospective clinical trial to be more effective at reducing the progression of BPH compared to either drug alone.

All alpha-1 antagonists may inhibit pupil dilation and cause IFIS. A number of retrospective and prospective studies, however, have shown that the frequency and severity of IFIS is much higher with tamsulosin as compared with nonselective alpha-1 antagonists.[3-10] For example, the large retrospective Canadian study discussed previously reported that tamsulosin significantly increased the rate of postoperative complications, but that nonselective alpha antagonists did not.[7] A second Canadian retrospective study found that 86% of patients taking tamsulosin developed IFIS compared to only 15% of patients taking alfuzosin.[6] A prospective masked trial from Italy comparing phaco in patients taking tamsulosin versus nonselective alpha blockers and a large 2011 meta-analysis of the literature reached this same conclusion: that IFIS is more common and severe with tamsulosin.[9,10] These and other studies were further supported by the 2008 ASCRS survey finding that 90% of respondents with sufficient experience believed that IFIS was more common with tamsulosin than with nonselective alpha-1 antagonists.[3] IFIS may also occur in patients without any history of alpha antagonist use. In addition to confirming that IFIS was strongly correlated with alpha-1 antagonists, one prospective study found that IFIS was also associated with systemic hypertension in the absence of alpha blockers.

In the original publication, Campbell and the author hypothesized that IFIS was a manifestation of decreased iris dilator muscle tone and loss of intraoperative structural rigidity.[1] Two separate slit lamp OCT studies have reported significant thinning of the mid iris stromal thickness in tamsulosin patients when compared to control eyes.[11] Another surprising but widespread finding is that IFIS can occur more than one year after tamsulosin has been discontinued.[1-4] Ninety-five percent of ASCRS survey respondents have experienced IFIS in patients with only a prior history of alpha-1 antagonist use.[3] Tamsulosin can even be recovered from aqueous samples taken 1 to 4 weeks after discontinuing the drug, suggesting that is has a very prolonged receptor binding time. One morphologic study of iridectomy samples from eyes demonstrating IFIS showed vacuolar degeneration of iris smooth muscle cells.[12] A subsequent large histopathologic study of autopsy eyes from patients taking tamsulosin (26 eyes) also showed atrophy of the iris dilator muscle, which was consistent with a permanent drug effect on iris morphology.[13] In 2012, Goseki and coauthors published an in vitro and histologic rabbit studies showing that, in addition to smooth muscle alpha-1 receptors, tamsulosin also binds strongly to pigment granules in the iris.[14] Pigment epithelial cells share nuclei with the adjacent smooth muscle cells, and this unique morphology may explain the histopathologic finding of dilator muscle atrophy in tamsulosin treated rabbits. Clearly, cataract surgical patients should be questioned about any prior alpha-1 antagonist use for this reason.

Summary

The mechanism of IFIS is not fully understood. There are several anecdotal reports of IFIS occurring within days of initiating tamsulosin treatment, meaning that chronic drug use is not necessary to cause this syndrome. However, the stronger association with tamsulosin compared to nonselective alpha-1 antagonists and the occurrence of IFIS without any prior alpha blocker use suggests a more complex mechanism than that simply mediated by blockade of the alpha-1A receptor. IFIS appears to result from a combination of pharmacologic inhibition of iris smooth muscle contraction and longer term smooth muscle degeneration relating to drug accumulation in adjacent iris pigment epithelial cells.[14] These permanent structural changes would explain the occurrence of IFIS long after

Table 22-1.
EXPERIENCE WITH IFIS PREOPERATIVE STRATEGIES (2008 ASCRS SURVEY)

DO YOU:	STOP TAMSULOSIN PRIOR TO CATARACT SURGERY?	USE PREOPERATIVE TOPICAL ATROPINE FOR TAMSULOSIN PATIENTS?
Never	64.2% (642)	56.9% (545)
Occasionally (< 20%)	11.4% (109)	12.3% (118)
Sometimes (20% to 50%)	5.0% (48)	4.8% (46)
Usually (> 50%)	8.6% (82)	7.4% (71)
Routinely	10.9% (104)	18.5% (177)

tamsulosin cessation. A stronger binding affinity to iris pigment granules and alpha-1A receptors might explain the greater propensity for tamsulosin to cause IFIS compared to nonselective alpha antagonists. Finally, the strong affinity for some systemic medications, such as psychotropic drugs, to bind to iris pigment granules might explain the occasional occurrence of IFIS in patients who have never taken alpha antagonists.

CLINICAL AND SURGICAL MANAGEMENT OF INTRAOPERATIVE FLOPPY IRIS SYNDROME

Preoperative Management

The possibility of IFIS increases the importance of taking the patient's medication history prior to cataract surgery. A history of systemic alpha antagonists may not be elicited without direct questioning about current or prior use of prostate medication.[3]

As discussed earlier, stopping tamsulosin preoperatively is of unpredictable and questionable value. With so many reported cases of IFIS occurring up to several years after the drug had been stopped, it is clear that ophthalmologists cannot rely solely upon drug cessation to prevent this condition. In the multicenter prospective trial mentioned earlier, tamsulosin was discontinued prior to surgery in 19% of patients, but did not result in any significant reduction in IFIS severity in this subgroup of eyes.[2] In the 2008 ASCRS IFIS survey, 64% of respondents said that they never stop tamsulosin prior to surgery compared to 11% who routinely do.[3]

Preoperative atropine drops (eg, 1% t.i.d. for 1 to 2 days preoperatively) can enhance cycloplegia as a means of preventing intraoperative miosis.[15] However, the multicenter prospective tamsulosin study demonstrated that atropine, as a single strategy, is often ineffective for more severe cases of IFIS.[2] In the ASCRS IFIS survey, 57% of respondents said that they never use topical atropine prior to surgery, compared to 19% who routinely do.[3]

Surgical Management

The inter-individual variability in the severity of IFIS makes it difficult to determine whether one surgical strategy is superior to another. The severity of IFIS is likely to be greater in patients taking tamsulosin. Poor preoperative pupil dilation and billowing of the iris immediately following instillation of intracameral lidocaine are also predictive of greater IFIS severity.[2,4,9] In contrast, if the pupil dilates well preoperatively, mild to moderate IFIS is more likely but the surgeon should still be prepared for iris prolapse and miosis. Patients taking nonselective alpha-1 antagonists or who have already discontinued these medications for several months are most likely to display mild to moderate IFIS.

Ideally, surgeons should be adept at using several different strategies that may be used alone or in combination to manage the iris in IFIS. Tables 22-1 and 22-2 show the preferences and experiences of the 2008 ASCRS survey respondents for IFIS surgical strategies.[3] In general, one should make a constructed shelved clear corneal incision, perform hydrodissection very gently, and consider reducing the irrigation and aspiration flow parameters if possible. Partial thickness sphincterotomies and mechanical pupil stretching are ineffective for IFIS and may worsen the iris prolapse and miosis.[1,4]

Intracameral injection of alpha agonists such as phenylephrine or epinephrine, as first reported by Richard Packard and Joel Shugar, respectively, is both a safe and inexpensive strategy for IFIS. By presumably saturating the alpha-1A receptors, these agonists can further dilate the pupil (Figure 22-2). It may take a minute before the pupil

Table 22-2.
EXPERIENCE WITH IFIS SURGICAL STRATEGIES (2008 ASCRS SURVEY)

YOUR SATISFAC-TION FOR MANAG-ING IFIS:	WITH VISCO-ADAPTIVE OVD (HEALON 5)?	WITH IRIS RETRACTORS?	WITH PUPIL EXPANSION RINGS?	WITH INTRACAM-ERAL EPINEPHRINE OR PHENYLEPHRINE?
Never have used	46.2% (442)	17.2% (165)	69.9% (669)	28.9% (277)
Tried, but not satisfied	17.7% (169)	13.7% (131)	11.7% (112)	18.2% (174)
Use, but not always	21.6% (207)	46.3% (443)	14.6% (140)	14.8% (142)
Use routinely	14.5% (139)	22.8% (218)	3.8% (36)	38.0 % (364)

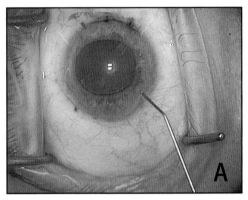 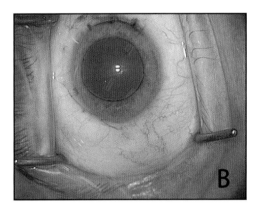

Figure 22-2. (A) Tamsulosin patient with pupil diameter before, and (B) after intracameral injection of 1:4000 unpreserved epinephrine mixture.

slowly dilates further, but even if it does not, the alpha agonist will often increase iris dilator muscle tone, which reduces billowing and the tendency for prolapse or sudden miosis. Because of the variable severity of IFIS, intracameral alpha agonists work well in some eyes but may have no detectable effect in others.[16-19,4] The preparation of intracameral epinephrine and phenylephrine is discussed in Chapter 21.

As first suggested by Robert H. Osher, MD and Douglas D. Koch, MD, sodium hyaluronate 2.3% (Healon 5) is a maximally cohesive ophthalmic viscosurgical device (OVD) that is particularly well suited for viscomydriasis and for blocking iris prolapse in IFIS (Figure 22-3). If mydriasis is still suboptimal after injecting epinephrine, Healon 5 can then be used to further mechanically expand the pupil (see Figure 22-3B and 22-3C). Viscomydriasis facilitates the capsulorrhexis and combines with the epinephrine-induced iris rigidity to block iris prolapse. However, to avoid immediately aspirating Healon 5, one must employ low flow and vacuum parameters (eg, < 175 to 200 mm Hg; < 26 mL/min). This strategy is therefore less suitable if high vacuum settings are desired for denser nuclei. At higher aspiration flow rates, others have suggested that more dispersive OVDs, such as DisCoVisc or sodium chondroitin sulfate (Viscoat),

may persist for longer periods within the eye. Finally, combining Healon 5 with Viscoat has been advocated as a combination strategy whereby the Viscoat will better resist aspiration and delay the evacuation of Healon 5.[20]

Mechanical pupil expansion with iris retractors or devices, such as the Malyugin ring, assures a reliably wide pupil diameter that cannot abruptly constrict during surgery (Figure 22-4).[21] The use of these mechanical devices was discussed in Chapter 21. Mechanical devices also permit surgeons to use their preferred OVD, phaco technique, and fluidic parameters. It is easier and safer to insert these devices prior to the creation of the capsulorrhexis. If the pupil dilates poorly preoperatively (eg, 3 to 5 mm diameter), or billows during injection of intracameral lidocaine, one should consider proceeding directly to mechanical devices because of the likelihood of severe IFIS. If the pupil dilates well preoperatively but begins to constrict or prolapse after hydrodissection or during phaco, combining intracameral epinephrine and Healon 5 can be an excellent rescue technique that may avoid the need to insert mechanical devices. If iris retractors are used, one should retract the pupil margin with a second instrument to avoid hooking the capsulorrhexis margin with the retractors.

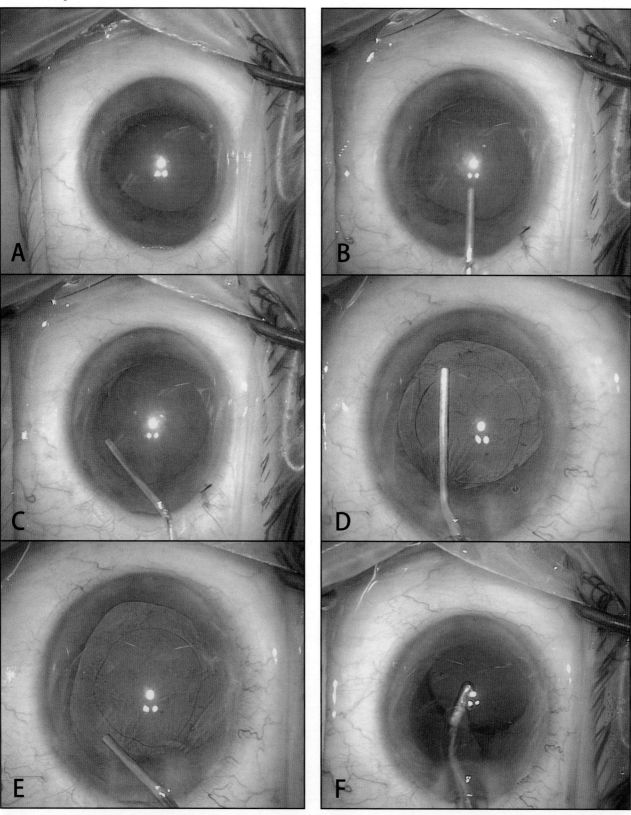

Figure 22-3. (A) Pupil in patient taking tamsulosin is not well dilated even after intracameral epinephrine administration. (B, C) Healon 5 widens the pupil diameter prior to the capsulorrhexis step. (D, E) Reinjection of Healon 5 produces viscomydriasis prior to IOL insertion. (F) Healon 5 is aspirated from behind the IOL.

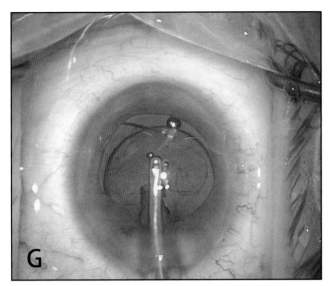

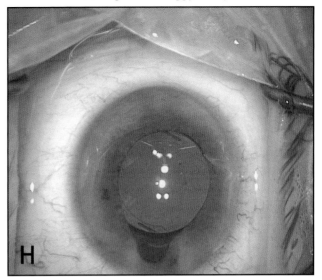

Figure 22-3 (continued). (G) As more Healon 5 is removed, the pupil constricts, and (H) prolapses following I/A tip removal.

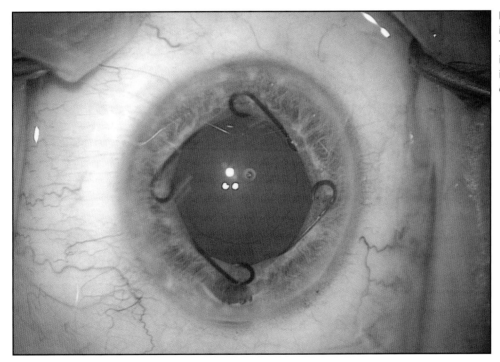

Figure 22-4. Malyugin ring in eye with IFIS (MicroSurgical Technology). The floppy iris is still able to prolapse to the incision, but the pupil cannot constrict.

Eliciting a history of current or prior alpha-1 antagonist use should alert surgeons to anticipate IFIS and to employ these strategies either alone or in combination with each other. Because of the variability in IFIS severity, many surgeons use a staged-management approach.[4,18] Pharmacologic measures alone may be sufficient for mild to moderate IFIS cases. Even if they fail to enlarge the pupil, intracameral alpha agonists can reduce or prevent iris billowing and prolapse by increasing iris dilator muscle tone. If the pupil diameter is still inadequate, viscomydriasis with Healon 5 can further expand it for the capsulorrhexis step. Finally, mechanical expansion devices assure the best surgical exposure for severe IFIS, and should be considered when other risk factors, such as weak zonules or a brunescent nucleus, are present.

REFERENCES

1. Chang DF, Campbell JR. Intraoperative floppy iris syndrome associated with tamsulosin (Flomax). *J Cataract Refract Surg.* 2005;31:664-673.

2. Chang DF, Osher RH, Wang L, Koch DD. Prospective multicenter evaluation of cataract surgery in patients taking tamsulosin (Flomax). *Ophthalmology.* 2007;114:957-964.

3. Chang DF, Braga-Mele R, Mamalis N, et al. for the ASCRS Cataract Clinical Committee. Clinical experience with intraoperative floppy-iris syndrome. Results of the 2008 ASCRS member survey. *J Cataract Refract Surg.* 2008;34:1201-1209.

4. Chang DF, Braga Mele R, Mamalis N, et al. for the ASCRS Cataract Clinical Committee. ASCRS White Paper: Intraoperative Floppy Iris Syndrome–A Clinical Review. *J Cataract Refract Surg.* 2008;34:2153-2162.

5. Chadha V, Borooah S, Tey A, et al. Floppy iris behaviour during cataract surgery: associations and variations. *Br J Ophthalmol.* 2007;91:40-42.

6. Blouin M, Blouin J, Perreault S, et al. Intraoperative floppy iris syndrome associated with alpha-1 adrenoreceptors. Comparison of tamsulosin and alfuzosin. *J Cataract Refract Surg.* 2007;33:1227-1234.

7. Bell CM, Hatch WV, Fischer HD, et al. Association between tamsulosin and serious ophthalmic adverse events in older men following cataract surgery. *JAMA.* 2009;301:1991-1996.

8. Palea S, Chang DF, Rekik M, et al. Comparative effect of alfuzosin and tamsulosin on the contractile response of isolated rabbit prostatic and iris dilator smooth muscles. Possible model for intraoperative floppy iris syndrome. *J Cataract Refract Surg.* 2008;34: 489-496.

9. Chatziralli IP, Sergentanis TN. Risk factors for intraoperative floppy iris syndrome: a meta-analysis. *Ophthalmology.* 2011;118:730-735.

10. Casuccio A, Cillino G, Pavone C, et al. Pharmacologic pupil dilation as a predictive test for the risk of intraoperative floppy-iris syndrome. *J Cataract Refract Surg.* 2011;37:1447-1454.

11. Prata TS, Palmiero PM, Angelilli A, et al. Iris morphologic changes related to alpha(1)-adrenergic receptor antagonists implications for intraoperative floppy iris syndrome. *Ophthalmology.* 2009;116:877-881.

12. Goseki T, Shimizu K, Ishikawa H, et al. Possible mechanism of intraoperative floppy iris syndrome: a clinicopathological study. *Br J Ophthalmol.* 2008;92:1156-1158.

13. Santaella RM, Destafeno JJ, Stinnett SS, et al. The effect of alpha1-adrenergic receptor antagonist tamsulosin (Flomax) on iris dilator smooth muscle anatomy. *Ophthalmology.* 2010;117:1743-1749.

14. Goseki T, Ishikawa H, Ogasawara S, et al. Effects of tamsulosin and silodisin on isolated albina and pigmented rabbit iris dilators–Possible mechanism of IFIS. *J Cataract Refract Surg.* 2012;38:1643-1649.

15. Masket S, Belani S. Combined preoperative topical atropine sulfate 1% and intracameral nonpreserved epinephrine hydrochloride 1:4000 [corrected] for management of intraoperative floppy-iris syndrome. *J Cataract Refract Surg.* 2007;33:580-582.

16. Shugar, JK. Intracameral Epinephrine for Prophylaxis of IFIS [letter]. *J Cataract Refract Surg.* 2006;32:1074-1075.

17. Gurbaxani A, Packard R. Intracameral phenylephrine to prevent floppy iris syndrome during cataract surgery in patients on tamsulosin. *Eye.* 2007;21:331-332.

18. Manvikar S, Allen D. Cataract surgery management in patients taking tamsulosin. *J Cataract Refract Surg.* 2006;32:1611-1614.

19. Lorente R, DeRojs V, Vazquez DE, Targa P, Moreno C, Varella J, Landaluce ML, Mendez J, Lorente B. Intracameral phenylephrine 1.5% for prophylaxis against intraoperative floppy iris syndrome: prospective, randomized fellow eye study. *Ophthalmology.* 2012;119:2053-2058.

20. Arshinoff SA. Modified SST-USST for tamsulosin-associated intraocular floppy iris syndrome. *J Cataract Refract Surg.* 2006;32:559-561.

21. Chang DF. Use of Malyugin pupil expansion device for intraoperative floppy iris syndrome: results in 30 consecutive cases. *J Cataract Refract Surg.* 2008;34:835-841.

Please see companion narrated videos on the accompanying Web site at
www.Healio.com/phacochopvideos

23

Strategies for Weak Zonules

David F. Chang, MD

Weak zonules complicate every step of the cataract procedure and challenge surgeons to diagnose and manage intraoperative zonulopathy[1-9] (Figure 23-1). Even if the capsular bag is successfully preserved, the surgeon must also consider and optimize long-term IOL fixation and centration in light of concurrent and potentially progressive zonular abnormality.[10] The most common predisposing risk factors for zonular weakness include pseudoexfoliation, advanced age, prior trauma, retinopathy of prematurity, and prior intraocular surgery (eg, prior vitrectomy or trabeculectomy). Less common risk factors would be conditions such as Marfans, retinitis pigmentosa, and myotonic dystrophy.

PREOPERATIVE SIGNS OF ZONULOPATHY

The presence of a traumatic angle recession, mydriasis, iridodialysis, and vitreous herniation is invariably associated with traumatic zonulopathy. Suspicion should also be high with a history of traumatic hyphema. In the absence of preoperative phacodonesis or visible zonular dialysis, however, the extent of zonular weakness is usually not known until the initiation of surgery. Robert H. Osher, MD has identified subtle signs of zonular weakness that include a wider iridolenticular gap (space between the iris and the anterior lens surface), a decentered nucleus, focal iridodonesis, and visibility of the peripheral lens equator upon lateral gaze.[11]

With pseudoexfoliation, the zonulopathy is progressive and the whitish deposits are found not only on the zonules but also on the posterior iris surface and pupillary margin. Therefore, smaller pupils are often associated with more advanced zonulopathy. Likewise, a brunescent nucleus is frequently accompanied by weak zonules. The most ominous sign with pseudoexfoliation, however, is a shallow anterior chamber despite a normal axial length; this invariably indicates extremely weak zonules.[4,9] One should consider a retrobulbar or peribulbar anesthetic block in cases carrying the higher risk of capsular rupture. Because of the progressive nature of the associated zonulopathy, it can be argued that cataract surgery in pseudoexfoliation eyes should be performed at the earlier end of the elective surgical window.

Chang DF.
Phaco Chop and Advanced Phaco Techniques: Strategies for Complicated Cataracts, Second Edition (pp 253-266).
© 2013 SLACK Incorporated.

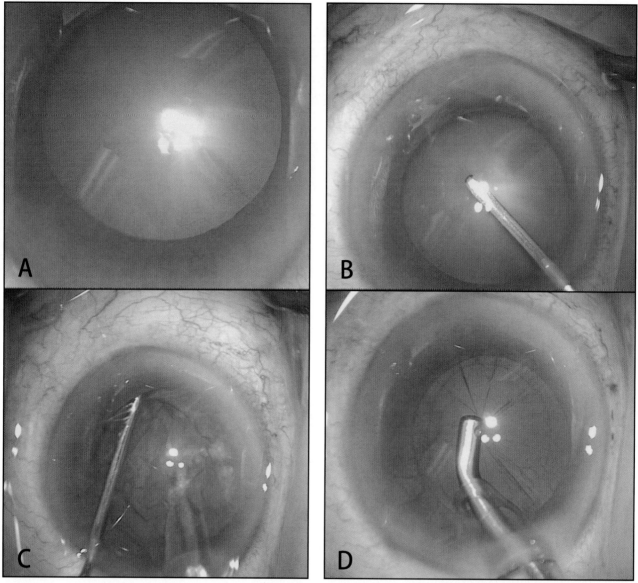

Figure 23-1. Case 1. (A) Eye with pseudoexfoliation. (B) Diffuse zonular weakness creates a lax anterior capsule that dimples rather than being incised by the cystotome. (C) Horizontal chop minimizes lateral and vertical displacement of the nucleus. (D) A lax posterior capsule is much more easily snagged by irrigation/aspiration (I/A) instrumentation.

CAPSULORRHEXIS

The capsulorrhexis step provides the first opportunity to directly assess zonular integrity. The peripheral anterior capsule is normally immobile but will demonstrate "pseudoelasticity" by seemingly stretching as the capsular flap is pulled[12] (see Figure 17-16). This is not true capsular elasticity, but is rather due to the failure of the zonules to immobilize the peripheral lens capsule. Another sign of severe or diffuse zonular weakness is difficulty incising the anterior capsule, as though the cystotome were dull (see Figures 17-17 and 23-1B). If the cystotome tip depresses rather than incises the central anterior capsule,

a halo-shaped light reflex may be noted. These signs represent a lack of zonular circumferential traction that should normally create a taut anterior capsule. Finally, there may be significant movement of the entire lens as the cystotome first perforates and tears the anterior capsule.

As mentioned in Chapter 17, weak zonules significantly increase the risk of a radial anterior capsular tear because of this pseudoelasticity. Because the zonules do not adequately immobilize the anterior capsule, the peripheral capsule moves along with the flap as it is being torn. While a large diameter capsulorrhexis would be helpful for phaco, making a smaller opening reduces the risk of a peripheral extension if one is struggling to control the tear.

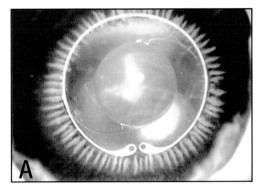 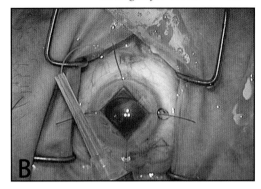

Figure 23-2. (A) Miyake-Apple view of capsular tension ring. (Reprinted with permission of Ophtec, Boca Raton, FL). (B) Morcher preloaded capsular tension ring with disposable plastic injector.

Because use of capsular retractors or a capsular tension ring (CTR) requires a continuous curvilinear capsulotomy, the overriding importance of achieving an intact capsulorrhexis dictates that one should err on the side of a smaller diameter that can be secondarily enlarged after the IOL has been implanted. If pseudoelasticity is noted, one may intentionally make the capsulotomy diameter slightly smaller to improve the odds of successfully achieving a continuous curvilinear capsulotomy (see Figure 16-6). The Brian Little Tear Out Rescue Maneuver is particularly helpful for controlling a tear that wants to move radially because of weak zonules and pseudoelasticity[13] (see Figure 17-18).

HYDRODISSECTION

Upon successful completion of the capsulorrhexis, loose zonules still pose multiple problems for the phacoemulsification and cortical aspiration steps. Because of deficient capsular rotational stability and counter fixation, the nucleus is more difficult to rotate. One should always suspect significant circumferential zonular weakness if, despite proper hydrodissection technique, the nucleus does not rotate easily. Finally, the epinucleus and cortex do not separate as easily from a capsular bag that is loosely anchored.

Normally, we are able to rotate a hydrodissected nucleus with a single instrument because of the counter fixation provided by the capsular bag. However, the rotating instrument (eg, hydrodissection cannula or chopper) must partially push the nucleus against the capsular bag to impart the necessary rotational force. In fact, of all of our surgical maneuvers, the author believes that rotation of either the nucleus or a 3-piece IOL imparts the most force against the capsular bag. This explains why these 2 steps are the most likely to extend a radial anterior capsular tear into the posterior capsule. With pseudoexfoliation, overly forceful efforts to rotate the nucleus may shear already weakened zonules. This may potentially create a large zonular dialysis or dislocate the crystalline lens even prior to insertion of the phaco tip.

One alternative is to use 2 instruments to bimanually rotate the nucleus. In this situation, the second instrument tip, rather than the capsular bag, becomes the counter fixating fulcrum around which to rotate the nucleus. However, when severe zonular laxity is diagnosed during the capsulotomy step and the nucleus cannot be easily rotated following hydrodissection, the safest strategy is to insert capsule retractors as described in the following section. By fixating the capsular bag to the eye wall, capsule retractors will facilitate nuclear rotation and prevent creation of a zonular dialysis in the process.

CAPSULAR TENSION RINGS

Polymethylmethacrylate (PMMA) capsular tension rings (Morcher, FCI Ophthalmics, Marshfield Hills, MA; Ophtec) partially compensate for a weakened zonular apparatus in several ways.[14-27] Using forceps or an injector (Geuder, Ophtec, Boca Raton, FL), the ring can be inserted at any stage following completion of the capsulorrhexis.[28,29] If there is a focal zonular dehiscence or weakness, the ring redistributes mechanical forces, such as that of nuclear sculpting or IOL insertion, to areas of stronger zonular support (see Figure 24-4). However, if the entire circumference of zonules is uniformly weak, this benefit is lost.

A second advantage is that centrifugal pressure applied by the ring makes the flaccid capsular bag tauter (Figure 23-2). This reduces redundant capsule folds, forward trampolining of the posterior capsule, and inward collapsing of the capsular fornices toward the aspirating instrument tip. In the absence of a CTR, the stiff PMMA haptics of a 3-piece foldable IOL can provide some of the same benefits during cortical aspiration. In addition, the IOL optic can block a floppy posterior capsule from vaulting toward the I/A tip in the subincisional area.

The final benefit of a CTR is to counter progressive contractile capsular forces. Postoperatively, centrifugal zonular tension normally resists capsulorrhexis shrinkage as the capsular bag contracts. Therefore, severe capsulophimosis is always a result of deficient zonular counter traction. Excessive or asymmetric capsular contracture can decenter the IOL and further weaken the remaining zonules. This is a likely factor in spontaneous late dislocation of the entire capsular bag in pseudoexfoliation cases.[10,30]

CTRs have 2 important disadvantages. Significant compression is required to implant the ring into the capsular bag because of its larger size. This may stretch the capsulorrhexis and potentially shear zonules by distorting or decentering the bag. Because of this compressive force, CTRs should never be inserted in the presence of an anterior or posterior capsule tear. In addition, insertion with an injector is preferable in order to reduce the forces exerted on the zonules during insertion[28] (see Figure 24-6C-F). A second drawback to CTRs is that they may impede cortical aspiration by pinning and trapping cortex in the capsular fornix. For this reason, surgeons should consider using capsule retractors instead of a CTR to stabilize the bag during phaco. Ideally, CTR insertion can then be delayed until after the cortex has been removed.[28] The Henderson modified CTR (FCI Ophthalmics) has a scalloped contour that facilitates cortical removal following placement[31] (Figure 23-3). If one area of cortex is difficult to remove because the Henderson CTR impinges on it, the ring can be rotated slightly until one of the gaps overlies the cortex. As an alternative to the expensive metal injectors, Morcher makes a preloaded disposable CTR injector (FCI Ophthalmics; see Figure 23-2).

Capsule Retractors

In addition to enlarging a small pupil, flexible iris retractors can be used to support the capsular bag in the presence of extremely loose zonules[32-35] (see Figure 21-8). Merriam first described using self-retaining iris retractors through paracentesis openings to hook and fixate the capsulorrhexis[32] (see Figures 21-8 and 23-4). However, because the hooked ends are very short and flexible, iris retractors may tend to slip off the anterior capsular edge during phaco and will not support the equator of the capsular bag.

Richard J. Mackool, MD designed the Cataract Support System (Impex, FCI Ophthalmics, Marshfield Hills, MA) with capsular hooks that are elongated enough to support the peripheral capsular fornix and not just the capsulorrhexis edge.[36] In this way, the retractors function as artificial zonules to stabilize the entire bag during phaco and cortical clean-up. Unlike CTRs, capsule retractors provide much better support in the anterior-posterior direction and do not trap the cortex. This is because each retractor applies only point pressure to the capsular fornix without ensnaring the cortex. The disposable nylon capsular retractors (MicroSurgical Technology [MST], Redmond, WA) are a newer alternative to the Mackool Cataract Support System (Figures 23-5, 23-6, and 23-7). Instead of a set of 5 retractors

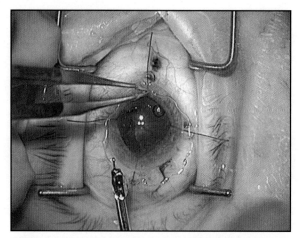

Figure 23-3. Henderson CTR has scalloped contours that make it less likely to pin cortex to the capsular fornix.

with the Mackool system, MST's capsular hooks are packaged 3 to a container (see Figure 23-5A). They feature a double-stranded design that creates a loop at the tip, which is less likely to puncture the equatorial capsule (see Figure 23-5B).

Capsule retractors can be inserted through limbal stab incisions at any stage including midway through the capsulorrhexis step (see Figure 23-7C). By anchoring the bag to the eye wall, the additional anteroposterior support and rotational stability facilitate hydrodissection and nuclear rotation. The self-retaining capsule retractors are also strong enough to center and immobilize a capsular bag that is partially subluxated due to a severe zonular dialysis (see Figure 23-6). They also restrain the peripheral anterior and equatorial capsule from being aspirated and dehisced by the phaco or I/A tip.

As a single strategy for severe zonular deficiency, capsule retractors are significantly more effective than CTRs at preventing posterior capsule rupture. Because CTRs can only redistribute instrument and mechanical forces to the remaining intact zonules, the greater the zonular defect or deficiency is, the less effective a CTR is at stabilizing the bag. However, a CTR can be used in conjunction with capsule retractors, particularly if there is a sizable zonular dialysis. If, after first inserting retractors, the unsupported equatorial regions of the capsular bag tend to collapse inward toward the phaco tip, a CTR can be inserted to distend the equator of the bag to its proper anatomic configuration.

Although the tip of the capsule retractor is dull, it is possible for the hooks to tear the capsulorrhexis margin during surgery. A key objective is to support the capsular bag without excessive tension and stretching of the capsulorrhexis. There is a tendency to overtighten the capsular retractors because the tension is initially adjusted with a soft eye. Inserting the phaco tip with irrigation suddenly displaces the nucleus and capsular bag posteriorly, which

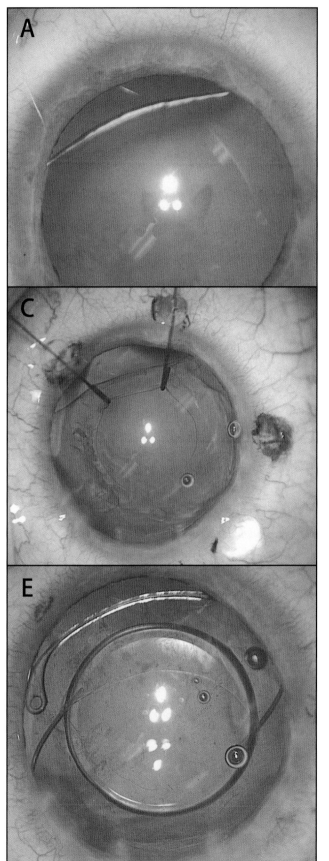

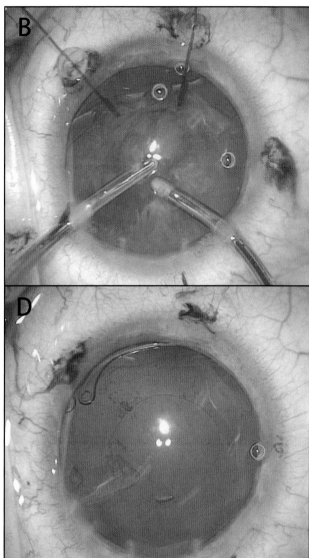

Figure 23-4. Case 2. (A) Eye with traumatic cataract and truncated lens equator due to zonular dialysis. (B, C) Because of focal zonular weakness noted during the capsulotomy, the iris retractors are advanced around the nasal capsulotomy edge to support the capsular bag during aspiration of the soft lens and cortex. (D) After insertion of a CTR, the equator of the bag expands nasally to close the zonular gap. (E) Following insertion of a 3-piece foldable IOL into the ciliary sulcus (with capsulorrhexis-optic capture), there is a new gap peripheral to the CTR nasally.

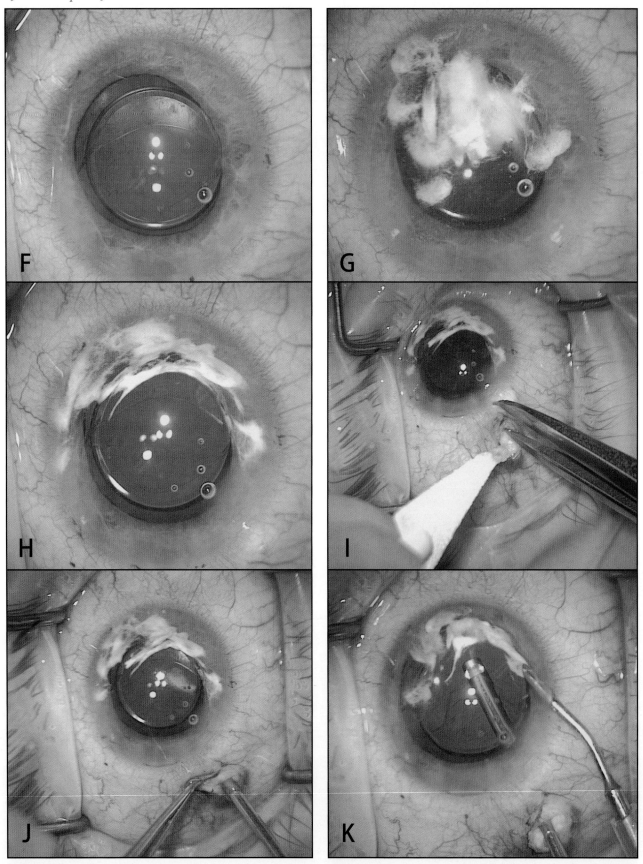

Figure 23-4 (continued). Case 2. (F) After Miochol-E, the pupil fails to constrict nasally (G) and triamcinolone injection reveals a large amount of vitreous that has prolapsed through the zonular dialysis. (H) After pushing the vitreous peripherally with dispersive OVD, (I) a pars plana sclerotomy is made 3.5 mm behind the limbus (J) through which the sleeveless vitrectomy tip is inserted. (K) With a separate self-retaining infusion cannula, the pars plana anterior vitrectomy is performed.

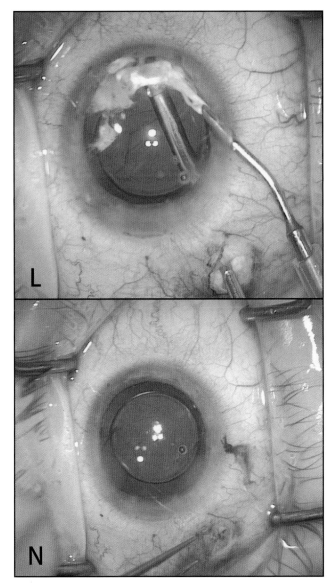

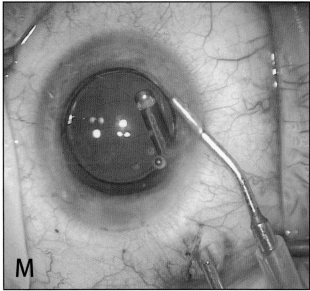

Figure 23-4 (continued). Case 2. (L) Once the vitrector reaches the area of the zonular dialysis, (M) the vitreous is pulled posteriorly behind the IOL and evacuated. (N) After removing the prolapsed vitreous, the peripheral gap beyond the CTR is closed once again.

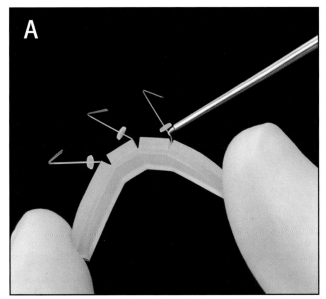

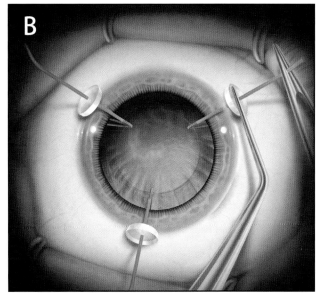

Figure 23-5. (A) MST disposable capsule retractors packaged 3 to a set. (B) The double stranded design creates a smooth loop at the tip which will not puncture the capsular equator. (Reprinted with permission of MST.)

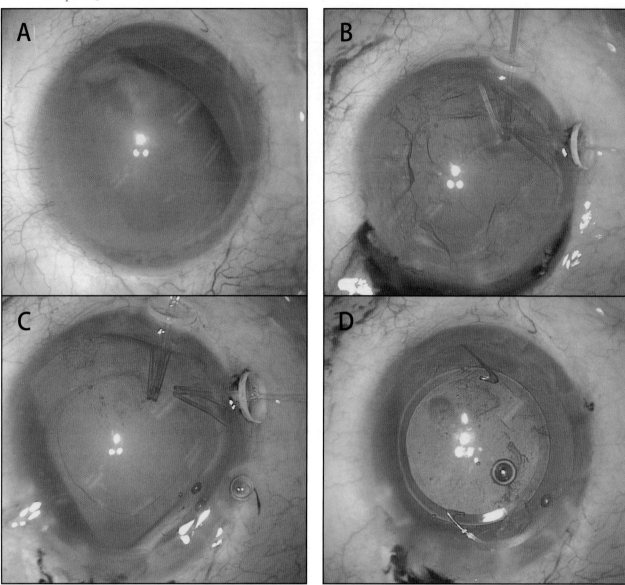

Figure 23-6. Case 3. (A) Different traumatic cataract, but similar to Case 2. (B) Instead of iris retractors, 2 capsule retractors inserted to support the area of the zonular dialysis. (C) The looped tips do not perforate the truncated equator of the bag and, unlike a CTR, do not impede cortical clean-up. (D) A longer 13.5-mm STAAR AQ-2010 V foldable 3-piece silicone IOL is placed in the sulcus with the haptics oriented 90 degrees away from the zonular dialysis. Optic capture prevents capsulorrhexis contraction, assures centration, and prevents the haptics from later rotating into and potentially through the zonular dialysis.

effectively tightens the retractors further (see Figure 23-7E). After inserting the phaco tip, it is therefore important to momentarily assess whether the capsule retractors have become so taut that they tent the capsulorrhexis edge. If so, they should be loosened slightly so that the capsular rim does not tear during phacoemulsification. This is particularly important if the capsulorrhexis diameter is on the small side.

Nuclear Emulsification

Fragile zonules are very prone to further damage during nuclear emulsification and poor capsular bag stability heightens the risk of capsular rupture. Forceful sculpting or rotation of the nucleus may shear zonules in the oppositely located quadrants. Care should be taken to avoid causing excessive nuclear movement with sculpting, chopping, or rotation. Phaco chop significantly reduces the stress placed

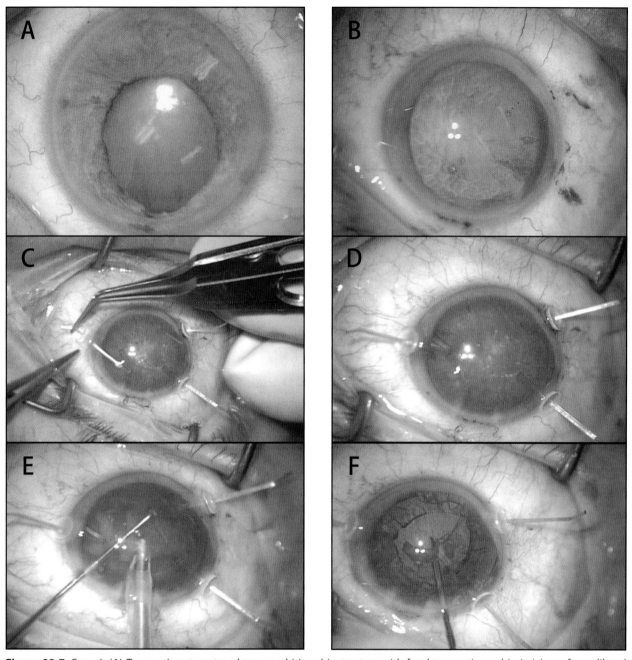

Figure 23-7. Case 4. (A) Traumatic cataract and temporal iris sphincter tear with focal traumatic mydriasis (view of nondilated pupil from temporal side). (B) After topical mydriasis, the microscope is repositioned superiorly to avoid the large zonular dialysis temporally. (C, D) Three MST capsule retractors are placed around the capsulotomy edge to support the capsular bag. (E) With irrigation the capsular bag moves slightly posterior, which increases the tension of the capsule retractors during horizontal phaco chop. (F) Prior to removing the last small fragment, dispersive OVD such as sodium chondroitin sulfate (Viscoat) is used to displace the lax capsule further posteriorly to make it taut and to create a barrier to its being aspirated by the phaco tip.

on the zonules and capsule by replacing sculpting and cracking motions with the manual forces of one instrument pushing inward against another. Because of the centrally directed instrument forces, horizontal chopping is particularly effective at avoiding nuclear tilt or displacement and is this author's preference for weak zonule cases (see Figure 23-1C and Figure 23-7E).

The supracapsular flip technique, as popularized by David C. Brown, MD, FACS, prolapses and flips the endonucleus out of the capsular bag prior to emulsification. If accomplished, this prevents the capsular bag from bearing any of the phaco instrumentation forces. The ease with which this flipping maneuver can be accomplished varies depending on the size of the endonucleus relative to

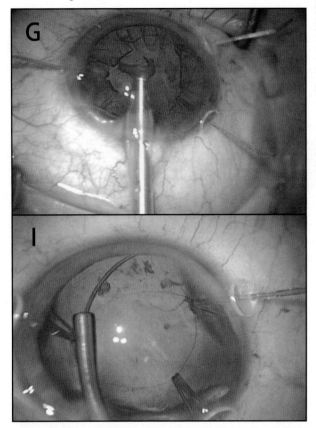

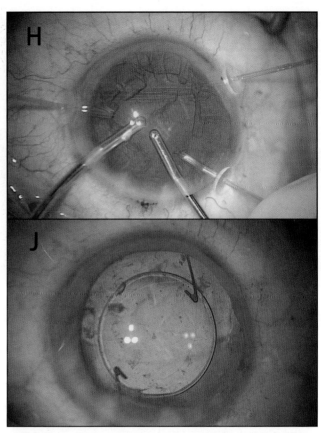

Figure 23-7 (continued). Case 4. (G) A smaller 20-gauge phaco tip is safer in this setting of weak zonules and a lax posterior capsule. (H) Bimanual I/A instrumentation provides excellent maneuverability and access to subincisional cortex, which is not trapped by the iris retractors. This also allows the irrigation and aspiration currents to be dissociated, so that the irrigation (left hand instrument) is kept flowing anterior to the iris and not toward the area of the zonular dialysis. (I) After inflating the capsular bag with OVD, the capsule retractors remain in place until after the CTR is implanted with an injector. The CTR injector tip is kept as far to one side of the capsular bag as possible to minimize lateral displacement of the bag as the ring expands. (J) A 13.5-mm STAAR AQ-2010 V foldable 3-piece silicone IOL is placed in the sulcus with the haptics oriented 90 degrees away from the zonular dialysis. Optic capture prevents capsulorrhexis contraction, assures centration, and prevents the haptics from later rotating into and potentially through the zonular dialysis.

the capsulorrhexis diameter. Using this technique with a nucleus that is too large or a capsulorrhexis that is too small risks further zonular dehiscence. Care must also be taken to avoid endothelial trauma during the nuclear flipping maneuver. With chopping, one should consider bringing larger sections of nucleus out of the capsular bag where they can be subchopped within the supracapsular space. For example, it may be possible to lift each heminucleus out of the capsular bag following the initial bisecting horizontal or vertical chop.

Throughout phaco and cortical clean-up, one should anticipate that deficient centrifugal zonular tension will result in greater posterior capsule laxity. The flaccid posterior capsule will tend to trampoline toward any aspirating tip as the last nuclear fragments, epinucleus, and cortex are removed. Because the nuclear bulk will initially mask this situation, one must be vigilant as more nucleus is

removed. Compared to a standard 19-gauge phaco tip, a smaller-diameter, 20-gauge tip greatly reduces the risk of inadvertently aspirating the peripheral or posterior capsule (see Figure 23-7G). If one suspects or encounters zonular laxity, the aspiration settings can be lowered as progressively more of the nucleus is removed. To slow the pace down, a lower than usual aspiration flow rate is advisable. A preprogrammed vacuum setting that usually avoids postocclusion surge with routine cases may not be safe with a lax posterior capsule that is lacking normal centrifugal zonular tension. Therefore, one should consider decreasing the vacuum to lower than normal levels to prevent trampolining of the capsule. Finally, repeatedly inflating the capsular bag with a dispersive OVD can further restrain a flaccid posterior capsule from vaulting toward the aspirating instrument as the final fragments and epinucleus are aspirated (see Figure 23-7F). Guarding the phaco tip by placing the horizontal chopper tip beneath it is another strategy. These safety measures are especially important if there is no epinuclear shell remaining as the last nuclear fragment is emulsified.

CORTICAL CLEAN-UP

As adherent cortex is aspirated, the usual centrifugal capsular counter fixation afforded by stronger zonules is deficient. Lacing circumferential zonular tension, a lax posterior capsule tends to cling to epinucleus and cortex that is being aspirated, and redundant capsular folds can be easily ensnared by the aspirating instrument or snagged by a capsule polisher (see Figure 23-1D). While removing cortex, inadvertently aspirating the more pliant anterior capsule may cause a zonular dialysis. Effective hydrodissection is crucial because the more easily lens material separates from a floppy capsule, the less likely it is for the capsular folds to be aspirated.

As mentioned previously, continually reinflating the capsular bag with a dispersive OVD is an excellent strategy for removing cortex from a floppy bag. Placing both the anterior and posterior capsule on stretch prevents a pliant posterior capsule from trampolining toward the aspiration port. In this situation, cortical aspiration can be performed either with or without irrigation, also known as dry aspiration. Dispersive agents are preferable to cohesive viscoelastics because they better resist aspiration. Finally, stripping the cortex tangentially rather than radially helps to distribute the tractional force across as large an area of zonules as possible.

Bimanual I/A instrumentation provides several advantages in the presence of weak zonules. The ability to alternate between 2 aspirating ports improves access to the subincisional cortex, which can be particularly challenging to remove if the capsulorrhexis diameter is small and the posterior capsule is lax (see Figure 23-4F). A dual incision system also means that the aspirating port never needs to turn toward the capsular fornix. It can be kept facing the cornea and away from the posterior capsule virtually at all times. Without a constraining infusion sleeve, the surgeon is better able to reach across to the opposite equatorial quadrants where the aspirating port can be safely buried within fluffs of cortex before vacuum builds. This further lessens the risk of aspirating the pliant peripheral or posterior capsule. Finally, in the presence of a zonular dialysis, the ability to dissociate the irrigating and aspirating tips can help to prevent misdirection of irrigating fluid through the zonular defect (see Figure 23-7H).

If capsule retractors are used, placing a CTR can usually be delayed until the cortex has been removed (see

Figure 23-7I). One must be careful not to snag or tear posterior capsular folds with the leading tip of a CTR during its insertion. Fully expanding the capsular bag with OVD prior to injecting the ring is critical for this reason. Brian Little has described the fish tail method of reducing zonular stress when inserting a ring without an injector.[29] As mentioned previously, using an injector has the advantage of introducing the CTR into the capsular bag without excessively stretching the capsulorrhexis.[28] One can either load the ring manually with a reusable metal injector or use a preloaded, disposable plastic injector from Morcher (FCI Ophthalmics). The injector tip should be positioned as far peripherally within the bag as possible in order to minimize lateral displacement of the capsular bag as the ring emerges (see Figure 23-7I). If used, capsular retractors should be left in place to counter the lateral decentering forces of the CTR as it is injected. In fact, an additional advantage of capsular retractors is to reduce the potential for zonular damage caused during insertion of a CTR (see Figure 23-7I). The retractors can then be removed prior to IOL implantation.

REPAIR OF TRAUMATIC IRIS DEFECTS

Traumatic cataracts are frequently associated with traumatic mydriasis, iridodialysis, or even iris tissue defects due to prolapse or excision during primary surgical repair. Because of the associated glare, photophobia, and abnormal contrast sensitivity, cataract surgery affords the opportunity for simultaneous repair of the iris abnormality. There is no artificial iris implant that is FDA approved for use in the United States. However, there is usually sufficient iris tissue present to permit a pupil cerclage procedure in cases of traumatic mydriasis (Figure 23-8 and Figure 23-9).

In lieu of vermiform suture imbrication of the entire pupillary margin, this author has achieved excellent cosmetic and functional results by placing 2 interrupted 10–0 Prolene sutures in the pupillary margin directly opposite each other (see Figure 23-9). These are placed with a McCannel suture technique so that the 2 ends of the suture are externalized through paracentesis incisions. For this technique, MST microforceps are introduced via a paracentesis site to grasp 2 consecutive and generous bites of iris tissue that are approximately 2 to 3 clock hours apart from each other (see Figures 23-8A, 23-8B, 23-9A and 23-9B). A Siepser sliding slip knot is tied so that the newly knotted pupillary margin is not displaced or tented (see Figure 23-8C, 23-8D, and 23-9C). This step is important because of the propensity of the taut iris to tear when it stretched too much. Positioning 2 interrupted 10–0 Prolene sutures in this way usually results in a rounded pupil (see Figure 23-9F).

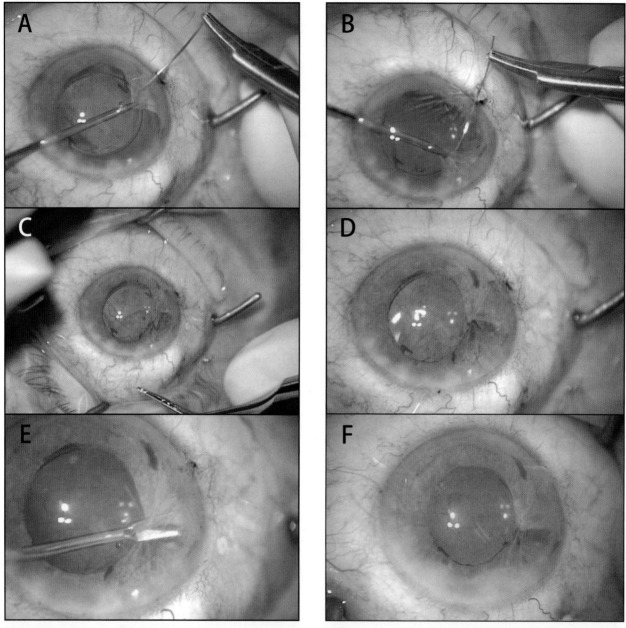

Figure 23-8. Case 4 (continued). (A) Single interrupted suture (10-0 Prolene) repair of traumatic mydriasis. MST microforceps are introduced through a paracentesis site to grasp the pupil edge at the first point to be sutured. (B) A second bite of iris is taken 3 clock hours away. (C, D) The edges are drawn together by a Siepser sliding slip knot. (E) The knot is cut with MST intraocular microscissors. (F) Repair of the focal sphincter rupture restores a rounded pupil shape and a smaller diameter.

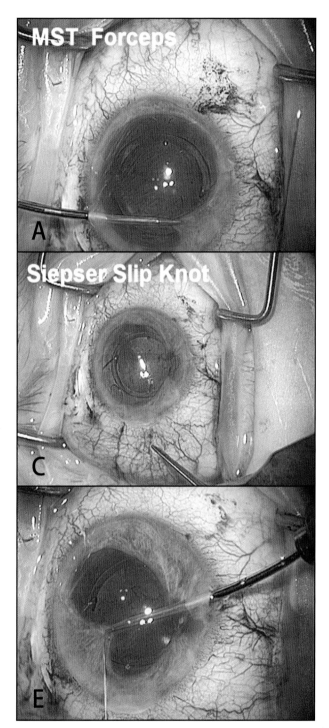
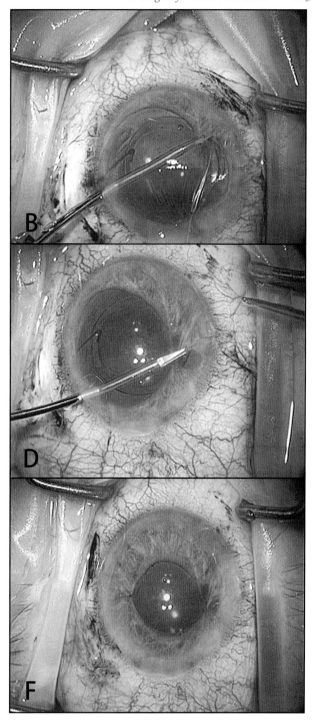

Figure 23-9. Case 5. Interrupted suture (10-0 Prolene) repair of traumatic mydriasis (insertion of a capsule tension segment and implantation of an IOL in the sulcus in this case are shown in Figure 24-8 in the next chapter). (A) MST microforceps are introduced through a paracentesis site to grasp the pupil edge at the first point to be sutured. (B) A second bite of iris is taken 3 clock hours away. (C) The edges are drawn together by a Siepser sliding slip knot. (D) The knot is cut with MST intraocular microscissors. (E) A second 10-0 Prolene interrupted suture is placed opposite to the first in an identical fashion, (F) creating a smaller, rounded pupil.

REFERENCES

1. Osher RH, Cionni RJ, Gimbel HV, Crandall AS. Cataract surgery in patients with pseudoexfoliation syndrome. *Eur J Implant Ref Surg.* 1993;5:46-50.

2. Fine IH, Hoffman RS. Phacoemulsification in the presence of pseudoexfoliation: challenges and options. *J Cataract Refract Surg.* 1997; 23:160-165.

3. Avramides S, Traianidis P, Sakkias G. Cataract surgery and lens implantation in eyes with exfoliation syndrome. *J Cataract Refract Surg.* 1997;23:583-587.

4. Kuchle M, Viestenz A, Martus P, et al. Anterior chamber depth and complications during cataract surgery in eyes with pseudoexfoliation syndrome. *Am J Ophthalmol.* 2000;129:281-185.

5. Shingleton BJ, Heltzer J, O'Donoghue MW. Outcomes of phacoemulsification in patients with and without psuedoexfoliation syndrome. *J Cataract Refract Surg.* 2003;29:1080-1086.

6. Blecher MH, Kirk MR. Surgical strategies for the management of zonular compromise. *Curr Opin Ophthalmol.* 2008;19:31-35. Review.

7. Shingleton BJ, Crandall AS, Ahmed K. Pseudoexfoliation and the cataract surgeon: preoperative, intraoperative, and postoperative issues related to intraocular pressure, cataract, and intraocular lenses. *J Cataract Refract Surg.* 2009;35:1101–1120.

8. Belovay GW, Varma DK, Ahmed II. Cataract surgery in pseudoexfoliation syndrome. *Curr Opin Ophthalmol.* 2010;21(1):25-34. Review.

9. Shingleton BJ, Marvin AC, Heier JS, O'Donoghue MW, Laul A, Wolff B, Rowland A. Pseudoexfoliation: high risk factors for zonule weakness and concurrent vitrectomy during phacoemulsification. *J Cataract Refract Surg.* 2010;36(8):1261-1269.

10. Jahan FS, Mamalis N, Crandall AS. Spontaneous late dislocation of intraocular lens within the capsular bag in psuedoexfoliation patients. *Ophthalmology.* 2001;108:1727-1731.

11. Marques DMV, Marquess FF, Osher RH. Subtle signs of zonular damage. *J Cataract Refract Surg.* 2004;30:1295-1299.

12. Chang DF. Phacoemulsification in high-risk cases. In: Wallace RB, ed. *Multifocal IOLs and Refractive Cataract Surgery.* Chapter 11. Thorofare, NJ: Slack; 2001.

13. Little BC, Smith JH, Packer M. Little capsulorhexis tear-out rescue. *J Cataract Refract Surg.* 2006;32:1420-1422.

14. Nagamato T, Bissen-Miyajima H. A ring to support the capsular bag after continuous curvilinear capsulorhexis. *J Cataract Refract Surg.* 1994;20:417-420.

15. Legler UFC, Witschel BM. The capsular ring: a new device for complicated cataract surgery. *Ger J Ophthalmol.* 1994;3:265.

16. Cionni RJ, Osher RH. Endocapsular ring approach to the subluxed cataractous lens. *J Cataract Refract Surg.* 1995;21:245-249.

17. Gimbel HV, Sun R, Heston JP. Management of zonular dialysis in phacoemulsification and IOL implantation using the capsular tension ring. *Ophthalmic Surg Lasers.* 1997;28:273-281.

18. Menapace R, Findl O, Georgopoulos M, et al. The capsular tension ring: designs, applications, and techniques. *J Cataract Refract Surg.* 2000;26:898-912.

19. Bayraktar S, Altan T, Küçüksümer Y, Yılmaz ÖF. Capsular tension ring implantation after capsulorhexis in phacoemulsification of cataracts associated with pseudoexfoliation syndrome; intraoperative complications and early postoperative findings. *J Cataract Refract Surg.* 2001;27:1620–1628.

20. Gimbel HV, Sun R. Clinical applications of capsular tension rings in cataract surgery. *Ophthalmic Surg Lasers.* 2002;33:44-53.

21. Lee DH, Shin SC, Joo CK. Effect of a capsular tension ring on intraocular lens decentration and tilting after cataract surgery. *J Cataract Refract Surg.* 2002;28:843–846.

22. Jacob S, Agarwal A, Agarwal A, et al. Efficacy of a capsular tension ring for phacoemulsification in eyes with zonular dialysis. *J Cataract Refract Surg.* 2003;29:315–321.

23. Price FW Jr, Mackool RJ, Miller KM, Koch P, Oetting TA, Johnson AT. Interim results of the United States investigational device study of the Ophtec capsular tension ring. *Ophthalmology.* 2005;112:460-465.

24. Hasanee K, Butler M, Ahmed II. Capsular tension rings and related devices: current concepts. *Curr Opin Ophthalmol.* 2006;17:31-41. Review.

25. Hasanee K, Ahmed II. Capsular tension rings: update on endocapsular support devices. *Ophthalmol Clin North Am.* 2006;19:507-519. Review.

26. Boomer JA, Jackson DW. Anatomic evaluation of the Morcher capsular tension ring by ultrasound biomicroscopy. *J Cataract Refract Surg.* 2006;32:846-848.

27. Hasanee K, Butler M, Ahmed II. Capsular tension rings and related devices: current concepts. *Curr Opin Ophthalmol.* 2006;17:31-41. Review.

28. Ahmed IIK, Cionn RJ, Kranemann C, Crandall AS. Optimal timing of capsular tension ring implantation: Miyake-Apple video analysis. *J Cataract Refract Surg.* 2005;31:1809–1813.

29. Angunawela RI, Little B. Fish-tail technique for capsular tension ring insertion. *J Cataract Refract Surg.* 2007;33:767-769.

30. Chang DF. Prevention of bag-fixated IOL dislocation in pseudoexfoliation (letter). *Ophthalmology.* 2002;109:5-6.

31. Henderson BA, Kim JY. Modified capsular tension ring for cortical removal after implantation. *J Cataract Refract Surg.* 2007;33:1688-1690.

32. Merriam JC, Zheng L. Iris hooks for phacoemulsification of the subluxed lens. *J Cataract Refract Surg.* 1997:23:1295-1297.

33. Lee V, Bloom P. Microhook capsule stabilization for phacoemulsification in eyes with pseudoexfoliation-syndrome-induced lens instability. *J Cataract Refract Surg.* 1999; 25:1567-1570.

34. Santoro S, Sannace C, Cascella MC, Lavermicocca N. Subluxated lens: phacoemulsification with iris hooks. *J Cataract Refract Surg.* 2003;29:2269–2273.

35. Sethi HS, Sinha A, Pal N, Saxena R. Modified flexible iris retractor to retract superior iris and support inferior capsule in eyes with iris coloboma and inferior zonular deficiency. *J Cataract Refract Surg.* 2006;32:715-716.

36. Mackool RJ. Capsule stabilization for phacoemulsification (letter). *J Cataract Refract Surg.* 2000;26:629.

Please see companion narrated videos on the accompanying Web site at
www.Healio.com/phacochopvideos

Intraocular Lens Implantation With Abnormal Zonules

David F. Chang, MD

Devices designed to help stabilize the loosened capsular bag during phaco include capsular tension rings (CTR) (Morcher Gmb, Stuttgart, Germany; Ophtec, Netherlands), the Ahmed capsular tension segment (Morcher; FCI Ophthalmics, Marshfield Hills, MA), and capsule retractors.[1-3] Thanks to these devices and techniques such as phaco chop, surgeons are frequently able to preserve the capsular bag despite the challenges posed by weakened zonules (see Figures 23-3 through Figure 23-7). However, this presents the surgeon with a new set of decisions. Is the capsular bag suitable for long-term support of an intraocular lens (IOL)? Which IOL should be used? Is a CTR or other implantable device, such as a Cionni ring or capsular tension segment, necessary? The same questions are particularly important for eyes with pseudoexfoliation because of the increasing incidence of late spontaneous dislocation of the capsular bag due to progressive zonular weakening.[4-14]

In 2001, Jahan, Mamalis, and Crandall reported their initial series of patients with pseudoexfoliation who presented with late spontaneous dislocation of the capsular bag[4] (Figures 24-1 and 24-2). The original case series was composed of 8 PMMA IOLs and 1 plate haptic silicone IOL that dislocated between 5 to 10 years after the original surgery. Soon after, this author published the first report of late spontaneous 3-piece silicone IOL dislocation in pseudoexfoliation syndrome (PXF) patients.[5]

During the initial postoperative period, the capsulorrhexis always constricts until this contracting force is counterbalanced by the centrifugal capsular tension of the zonules. Therefore, excessive capsulorrhexis contraction or capsulophimosis usually indicates diffuse zonular weakness and is typical in these cases of late bag-IOL dislocation[15-17] (see Figures 24-2B and 24-2C). However, it also seems likely that extensive anterior capsule fibrosis and contraction exerts excessive centripetal strain on the already weakened zonules in these eyes.[5] This vicious cycle may progressively worsen zonular integrity beyond that which was observed intraoperatively.

Given that the capsulorrhexis technique was not widely adopted until the early 1990s, and given the 5- to 10-year latency for this complication, it made sense that the increasing frequency of bag-IOL dislocation was not seen until a decade later. Complicating any evaluation of preventive measures is the fact that dislocation may take more than 10 years to occur. However, it is possible to make rational choices based on our knowledge of IOL design and materials, and that is one objective of this chapter. One should conceptualize zonular weakness as representing a continuum of severity rather than being a single uniform condition. This concept is equally important whether one is considering phaco technique or long term IOL fixation. Conceptually, there are 4 clinical scenarios that one can consider as representing the spectrum of mild to weak zonulopathy.

Chang DF.
Phaco Chop and Advanced Phaco Techniques: Strategies for Complicated Cataracts, Second Edition (pp 267-276).
© 2013 SLACK Incorporated.

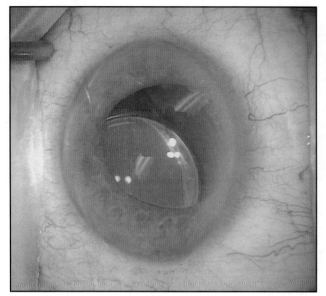

Figure 24-1. Delayed bag-IOL dislocation in an eye with pseudoexfoliation. The peripheral edge of the bag can be seen at the far right end of the pupil.

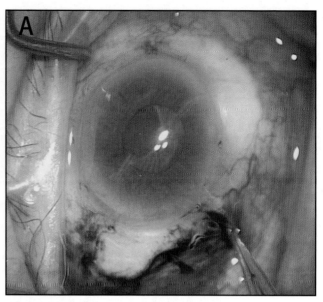

Figure 24-2. (A) Delayed bag-IOL dislocation in an eye with pseudoexfoliation.

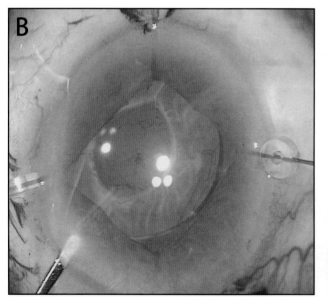

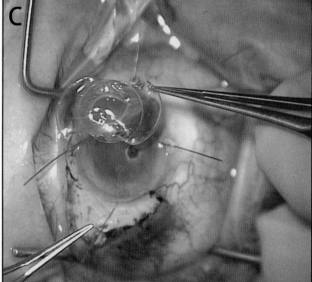

Figure 24-2 (continued). (B, C) Note the capsulorrhexis contraction with this 3-piece silicone IOL.

OPTION 1: PSEUDOEXFOLIATION WITH NO EVIDENCE OF ZONULOPATHY

Should every patient with pseudoexfoliation receive a CTR? Because of the likelihood of progressive loss of zonules over time, the author recommends placing a CTR whenever an eye with pseudoexfoliation exhibits any degree of zonulopathy during surgery. However, many pseudoexfoliation patients exhibit no zonular laxity during surgery and, in these cases, a CTR is unnecessary. When a CTR is not used, there are several surgical and IOL design objectives that make sense with pseudoexfoliation in order to reduce the risk of capsular contraction, progressive zonular traction, and late bag-IOL dislocation.

Thorough cortical clean-up is certainly important in these eyes. While circumferential anterior capsular overlap of the optic edge is desirable, an excessively small diameter capsulorrhexis must be avoided in these patients. Following IOL implantation, a small capsulorrhexis can be secondarily enlarged if necessary. After obliquely cutting one edge with a long intraocular scissors, one retears the opening under viscoelastic. This technique is illustrated in Chapters 16 and 17 (see Figures 16-4, 16-5, 16-6, 17-12, and 17-14). To reduce the likelihood of capsulorrhexis contraction, the rationale for enlarging the diameter out to or beyond the optic edge in eyes with weak zonules or pseudoexfoliation was also discussed in Chapter 16 (Figure 24-3). As an alternative to enlarging a small diameter capsulorrhexis, one could make relaxing incisions in the CCC edge after placing the IOL in the bag.

Since hydrophobic acrylic IOLs are associated with less anterior capsule fibrosis compared to silicone IOLs, it is this author's opinion that the former material is preferable for PXF eyes[16,18] (see Figure 24-3). Three-piece designs with broad, stiff PMMA haptics are able to exert the maximum centrifugal tension against the capsular equator (Figure 24-4). In this author's opinion, they are preferable to the soft, floppy single-piece haptics for this reason. Finally, one should specifically examine the anterior capsule reaction during the early postoperative period in patients with pseudoexfoliation. If one already sees signs of early contracture and fibrosis, prophylactic YAG relaxing cuts in the capsulorrhexis edge should be considered.[19]

Occasionally, the zonules may appear reasonably intact and a 3-piece IOL is inserted. However, if a round capsulorrhexis becomes ovalized following insertion of a 3-piece IOL, this indicates zonular laxity (see Figure 24-4A). The longitudinal expansion of the capsular bag by the stiff 3-piece haptics is usually counterbalanced by zonular traction 90 degrees from this axis. However, if the zonules are diffusely weak, the lack of this counter-traction usually results in an ovalized capsulotomy. At this point, a CTR can still be implanted into the capsular bag to stabilize the capsular bag (see Figure 24-4B-D).

OPTION 2: MILD TO MODERATE ZONULAR WEAKNESS

In any eye where intraoperative signs of zonular laxity are noted, placement of a CTR would be prudent. The goals would be to prevent capsulophimosis, reduce progressive centripetal zonular stress caused by capsulorrhexis contraction, and avoid IOL decentration caused by asymmetric capsular fibrosis.[1-3] Because of expected progressive zonular loss, even mild evidence of zonulopathy should warrant CTR placement in eyes with pseudoexfoliation. Clearly, a CTR alone will not always prevent late bag-IOL dislocation[20-22] (Figure 24-5). However, should this complication occur years later, the presence of a CTR may afford the surgical option of suture fixating the ring to the sclera.[22] Even following insertion of a CTR, a small capsulorrhexis diameter should still be avoided. In eyes with weaker zonules,

the capsulorrhexis will exhibit a sphincter-like effect that is stronger with a smaller diameter opening. For this reason, my personal preference even following CTR insertion is still to secondarily enlarge the capsulorrhexis diameter out to the edge of the optic in eyes with pseudoexfoliation (see Figure 24-3).

If there is a small (< 3 clock hour) zonular dialysis associated with otherwise strong zonular support in the remaining quadrants, a CTR alone should restore excellent IOL support and fixation. The CTR effectively redistributes the capsular forces to the entire circumferential zonular ligament and essentially recruits the remaining stronger zonules to help compensate for a focal area of abnormality. If a 3-piece IOL is used, orienting one haptic toward the quadrant of weakness adds the compressive force of the haptic to that of the CTR in resisting capsule contraction and further zonular dehiscence.

OPTION 3: SEVERE FOCAL OR DIFFUSE ZONULAR INSTABILITY

There are numerous situations where a ring alone may not provide sufficient long-term capsular support. These would include eyes with severe, diffuse circumferential weakness or a larger zonular dialysis. Although associated first and most commonly with pseudoexfoliation, delayed bag-IOL dislocation can occur with virtually any eye manifesting zonular abnormalities, such as trauma,[6-9,12] uveitis,[6,7,9] and retinitis pigmentosa.[8-12] Prior vitrectomy appears to be the next most common risk factor after pseudoexfoliation.[7-9,12] Suture fixating a bag stabilizing device can be considered (see Option 4), but this technique is time consuming and surgically demanding, and requires that the device be available in the operating room.

In this author's opinion, an under-utilized option is to place a 3-piece foldable IOL in the ciliary sulcus (Figure 24-6). With saccadic lateral eye movements, there is a certain amount of IOL inertial displacement force that is transmitted to the zonular complex if the lens is encased by the capsular bag. One would expect that these lateral saccadic forces continually strain the nasal and temporal zonules to some degree. In the setting of diffuse and significant zonular weakness, this cumulative strain may contribute to eventual dislocation of the bag-IOL complex. The rationale of sulcus placement of 3-piece IOLs is that the haptics will lie in contact with and transmit lateral IOL inertial displacement forces directly to the ciliary body, instead of the zonules.

If there is no optic capture, the capsulorrhexis will aggressively constrict in the absence of an intracapsular IOL. This may avulse the remaining weakened zonules and result in a dehisced and crumpled mass of capsule suspended in the visual axis. Therefore, if sulcus placement

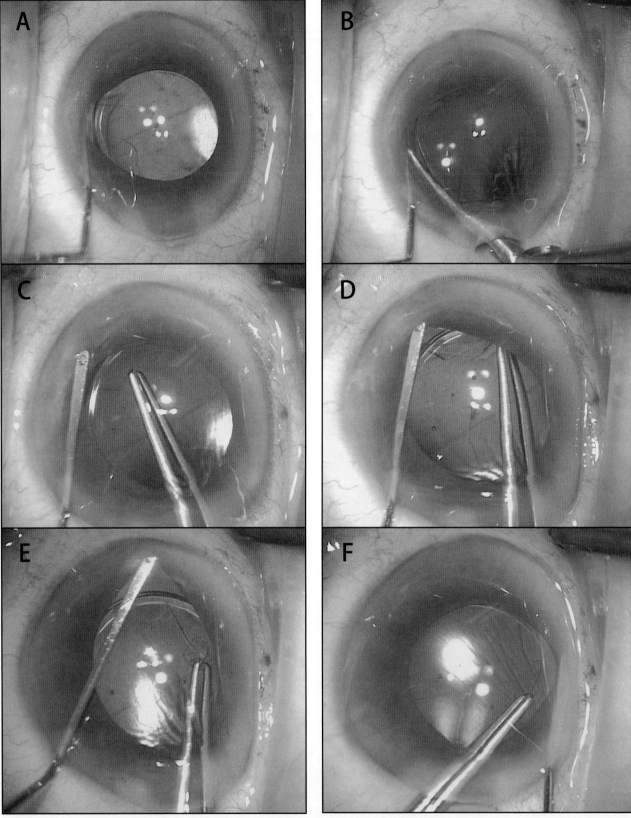

Figure 24-3. Continuation of Case 1 from Chapter 23 (see Figure 23-1). (A) After implantation of a CTR and 3-piece hydrophobic acrylic IOL, the decision is made to enlarge the capsulotomy diameter to the optic edge. (B) An oblique cut in the capsulorrhexis edge is made with curved tip Uthoff-Gills scissors (Katena, Denville, NJ). A Lester hook is used to retract the pupil to expose the peripheral IOL edge. (C-H) Capsule forceps are used to secondarily enlarge the capsulorrhexis diameter out to or beyond the IOL optic edge.

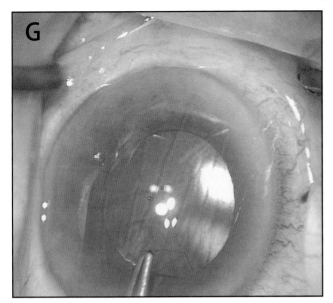

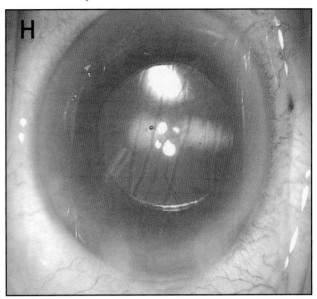

Figure 24-3 (continued). Continuation of Case 1 from Chapter 23 (Figure 23-1). (C-H) Capsule forceps are used to secondarily enlarge the capsulorrhexis diameter out to or beyond the IOL optic edge.

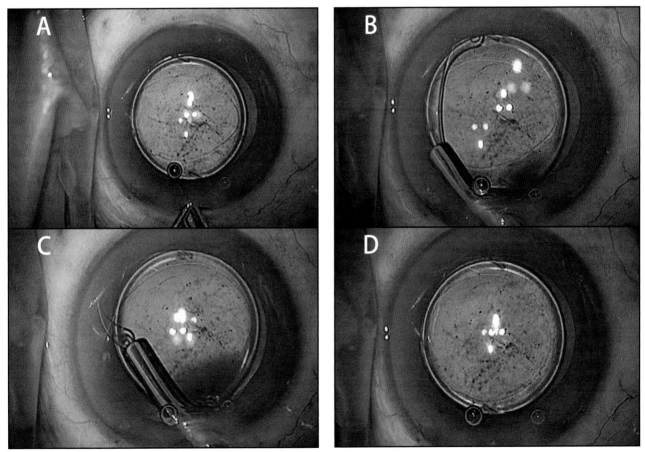

Figure 24-4. Case 2. (A) After implantation of a 3-piece hydrophobic acrylic IOL, the formerly round capsulorrhexis has become oval. (B, C) A CTR is implanted with the injector tip kept as far to one side of the capsulotomy as possible. (D) The capsulorrhexis becomes round, indicating that the CTR has produced evenly distributed centrifugal tension against the capsular equator.

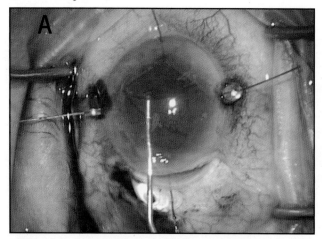

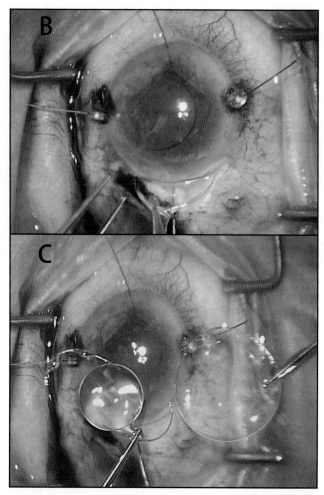

Figure 24-5. Case 3. (A) Late bag-IOL dislocation of a 3-piece foldable IOL with a CTR in the bag. (B) As the subluxated CTR is grabbed and extracted, the IOL separates and is left behind. (C) Part of the capsular bag remains draped around the CTR.

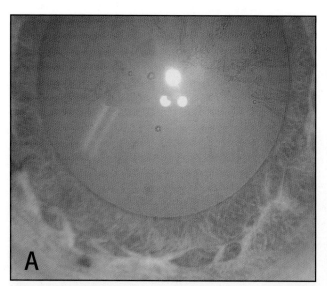

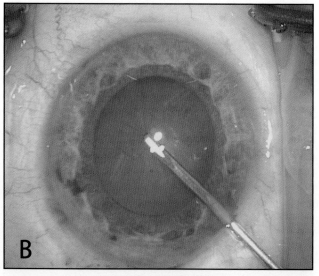

Figure 24-6. Case 4. (A) Pseudoexfoliation material is visible on the peripheral anterior capsule. (B) Dimpling and folds of the anterior capsule with the cystotome tip indicates diffuse zonular weakness contributing to a lax anterior capsule.

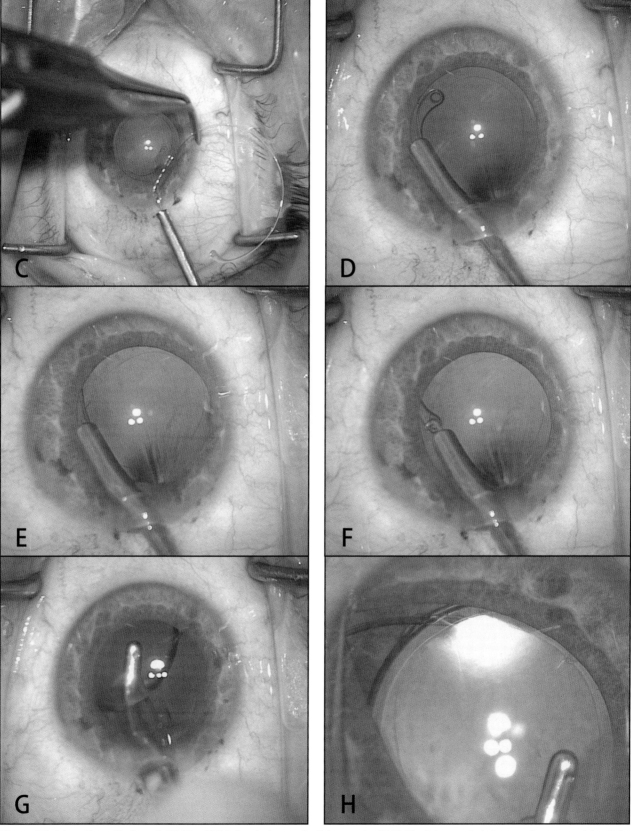

Figure 24-6 (continued). Case 4. (C) The CTR is loaded onto the injector tip. (D-F) The injector tip is kept as far to one side of the capsulotomy as possible to minimize lateral stress on the zonules as the ring expands. (G) Following placement of the haptics and IOL in the ciliary sulcus, and prior to capturing the optic with the capsulorrhexis, the I/A tip is used to remove as much OVD from within the capsular bag as possible. (H) The optic of this 3-piece acrylic IOL in the sulcus is captured by the capsulorrhexis, and this is confirmed by retracting the pupil at the optic-haptic junction.

is elected because of severe zonular weakness, this author still implants a CTR to prevent this from occurring (see Figure 24-6D-F). Capsulorrhexis capture of the IOL optic can also be considered as a measure to prevent capsulophimosis (see Figure 24-6H). With pseudoexfoliation, there is also the risk of an occult zonular dialysis that is hidden from the surgeon's view by the iris. Therefore, an additional benefit of optic capture with sulcus IOL placement is to prevent late rotation of one haptic through a potential zonular dialysis resulting in delayed postoperative IOL subluxation (see Figures 23-4E, 23-6D, 23-7J, 23-9A, and 24-6H).

Surgeons typically gain experience with this method when the posterior capsule has a defect. When the capsular bag is intact and inflated with OVD, however, optic/capsulorrhexis capture will often trap OVD behind the optic. The distended capsular bag may produce a myopic shift due to the more anterior axial optic location. Once the IOL haptics are positioned in the sulcus, it is therefore advisable to carefully evacuate some of this OVD with the I/A instrument prior to capturing the optic with the capsulorrhexis (see Figure 24-6G). If anterior optic displacement because of capsular bag OVD distention is noted postoperatively, it can be easily remedied. One or 2 Nd:YAG laser shots to the posterior capsule will break the capsulorrhexis block, allowing the distended capsular compartment to empty.

The typical 13.0 mm overall length foldable IOL may be too short for eyes with a corneal diameter of 12.0 mm or greater. STAAR Surgical manufactures a 13.5-mm foldable silicone IOL (model AQ-2010 V; Monrovia, CA) which is the author's preference for sulcus placement without optic capsulorrhexis capture (see Figures 23-6D, 23-7J, and 24-8D). The posterior vaulting of the AQ 2010 V elastimide haptics and the rounded anterior edge of its optic lessen the risk of posterior chafing of the iris. This IOL also has very low spherical aberrations, should there be any postoperative decentration. Single-piece acrylic IOLs are not only too short for sulcus placement, but they have thicker, sharp-edged haptics that can cause posterior iris chafing and pigment dispersion (Figure 24-7). If the optic is not captured, the IOL power should be reduced by 0.5 to 1.0 diopters from that calculated for capsular bag placement.[23]

OPTION 4: SEVERE ZONULAR INSTABILITY—TILTED OR DECENTERED CAPSULAR BAG

With up to 3 to 4 clock hours of zonular dialysis, the capsular bag is usually neither tilted nor decentered. However, with a larger dialysis or more extensive zonular loss, there will often be tilting or decentration of the capsular bag. Although it may be possible by using capsule retractors to preserve the bag following phaco, this poses a separate problem of adequate long-term capsular fixation of the IOL.

It is for these cases that the Cionni modified CTR or the Ahmed capsular segment (CTS) (Morcher GmbH; FCI Ophthalmics) were designed.[24-31] Both devices are FDA approved. CTSs merge the concept of a Cionni ring and a capsule retractor (Figure 24-8). The Ahmed CTS is a partial ring with a hole for temporary or permanent fixation.[26,27] By hooking this hole, a single iris retractor can support the segment during surgery. Lacking a pointed tip, these broad segmental retractors will not tear the capsulorrhexis during phaco. Following surgery, the CTS can either be removed or sutured to the sclera to provide permanent capsular bag support. Along the lines of the CTS, Ehud Assia, MD designed the "capsular anchor" for scleral suture fixation of one quadrant of the capsular bag.[32] This is positioned and sutured to the sclera prior to phaco and left permanently in place for long-term bag fixation. At the time of this writing, the capsular anchor is not FDA approved.

There are a variety of techniques used for scleral suture fixation of an intracapsular Cionni ring or Ahmed segment. The same techniques used for scleral suture fixation of IOL haptics, such as the Hoffman pocket, can be used here as well.[33] The author's personal preference is to make a half-thickness scleral groove approximately 1.5 mm posterior to the limbus at the desired site for a scleral suture. One should thread a double-armed 9-0 Prolene suture (FCI Ophthalmics) through the eyelet of the Cionni ring or CTS prior to inserting and maneuvering it into the capsular bag (Figure 24-8A). A 25-gauge disposable guide needle is introduced ab externo through the base of the half-thickness scleral groove (Figure 24-8B). The guide needle is passed through the ciliary sulcus, between the iris and the anterior capsule, and into the pupillary space. The Prolene needle is docked into its lumen so that it can be backed out externally through the scleral groove. The second of the double-armed Prolene needles is similarly guided out through the base of the scleral groove so that it exits approximately 1 mm away from the first needle. Once tied, the trimmed knot lies within the half thickness scleral groove so that it will not erode through the overlying conjunctiva. One must avoid tying the knot so tightly that the ring or segment peaks or distorts the edge of the capsulorrhexis (Figure 24-8C).

If the capsular bag support is deemed sufficient following the sutured support device, the intended IOL may be placed into the capsular bag. As an alternative, sulcus fixation with or without capsulorrhexis capture of the optic can be considered.

PREMIUM REFRACTIVE INTRAOCULAR LENSES

Accommodating, multifocal, and toric IOLs are much less forgiving of tilt and decentration. Furthermore, weak zonules and postoperative capsular contraction with an accommodating IOL, such as the Crystalens

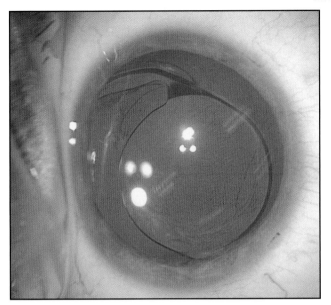

Figure 24-7. Single-piece multifocal acrylic IOL with one haptic in the bag (as seen in top of the figure) and the optic and second haptic in the sulcus.

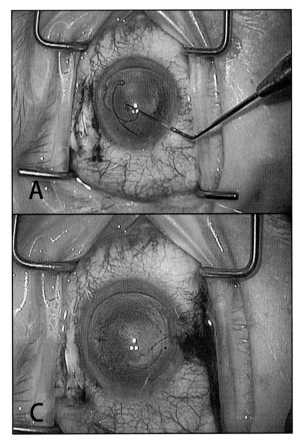
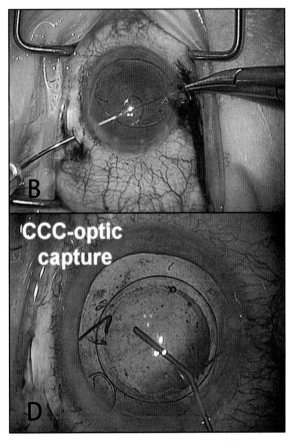

Figure 24-8. Continuation of Case 5 from Chapter 23 (see Figure 23-9). (A) There is a large traumatic zonular dialysis in the superotemporal quadrant in this left eye. An Ahmed CTS is inserted to support the weakened quadrant. After a double-armed 9-0 Prolene suture has been threaded through the eyelet, the CTS is inserted into the anterior chamber. (B) Because the scleral suture site must be located in the superotemporal quadrant, each long transchamber needle is first externalized through a paracentesis site located directly across from the intended scleral fixation site, where a half-thickness scleral groove has been made 1.5 mm behind the limbus. A 25-gauge guide needle is passed ab externo through the base of the scleral groove, behind the iris, and anterior to the anterior capsule. (C) This will guide the ab interno 9-0 Prolene needle out through the base of the scleral groove. After the second of the double-armed Prolene needles is passed in an identical fashion, but 1 mm adjacent to the first pass, the knot is tied so that it drops within the half thickness groove. (D) It must not be over-tightened or there will be excessive tenting of the capsulorrhexis. A STAAR AQ-2010 13.5-mm long 3-piece silicone IOL is placed in the sulcus and the optic is captured by the capsulorrhexis. The CTS is visible in the superotemporal quadrant.

(Bausch + Lomb, Rochester, NY) can cause deformation of the optic and a Z-syndrome with haptic buckling. With significant zonular abnormality, the conservative approach would be to avoid implanting these IOLs for these concerns. With mild zonular abnormality or with pseudoexfoliation without any clinical zonulopathy noted during surgery, the decision is less straightforward.

Because of the high associated risk of progressive zonulopathy, this author chooses not to implant accommodating IOLs, such as the Crystalens, in any eyes with pseudoexfoliation. If there is no evidence of zonulopathy, one might still consider concomitant use of a CTR if one is to implant a multifocal or toric IOL in an eye with pseudoexfoliation.[34] Finally, one must be careful when considering multifocal or toric IOL implantation in any eye displaying mild zonular weakness. Even with a CTR, tilt of a diffractive multifocal IOL can be associated with higher order aberrations that can compromise optical quality despite good Snellen acuity.

REFERENCES

1. Blecher MH, Kirk MR. Surgical strategies for the management of zonular compromise. *Curr Opin Ophthalmol.* 2008;19:31-35.
2. Shingleton BJ, Crandall AS, Ahmed K. Pseudoexfoliation and the cataract surgeon: preoperative, intraoperative, and postoperative issues related to intraocular pressure, cataract, and intraocular lenses. *J Cataract Refract Surg.* 2009;35:1101–1120.
3. Belovay GW, Varma DK, Ahmed II. Cataract surgery in pseudoexfoliation syndrome. *Curr Opin Ophthalmol.* 2010;21(1):25-34.
4. Jahan FS, Mamalis N, Crandall AS. Spontaneous late dislocation of intraocular lens within the capsular bag in psuedoexfoliation patients. *Ophthalmology.* 2001;108:1727-1731.
5. Chang DF. Prevention of bag-fixated IOL dislocation in pseudoexfoliation (letter). *Ophthalmology.* 2002;109:5-6.
6. Gross JG, Kikame GT, Weinberg DV. In-the-bag intraocular lens dislocation: the dislocated in-the-bag lens study group. *Am J Ophthalmol.* 2004;137(4):630–635.
7. Gimbel HV, Condon GP, Kohnen T, et al. Late in-the-bag intraocular lens dislocation: incidence, prevention, and management. *J Cataract Refract Surg.* 2005;31:2193–2204.
8. Hayashi K, Hirata A, Hayashi H. Possible predisposing factors for in-the-bag and out-of-the-bag intraocular lens dislocation and outcomes of intraocular lens exchange surgery. *Ophthalmology.* 2007;114:969–975.
9. Davis D, Brubaker J, Espandar L, et al. Late in-the-bag spontaneous intraocular lens dislocation: evaluation of 86 consecutive cases. *Ophthalmology.* 2009;116:664–670.
10. Shingleton BJ, Crandall AS, Ahmed K. Pseudoexfoliation and the cataract surgeon: preoperative, intraoperative, and postoperative issues related to intraocular pressure, cataract, and intraocular lenses. *J Cataract Refract Surg.* 2009;35:1101–1120.
11. Jakobsson G, Zetterberg M, Lundström M, et al. Late dislocation of in-the-bag and out-of-the-bag intraocular lenses: ocular and surgical characteristics and time to lens repositioning. *J Cataract Refract Surg.* 2010;36:1637–1644.
12. Matsumoto M, Yamada K, Uematsu M, et al. Spontaneous dislocation of in-the-bag intraocular lens primarily in cases with prior vitrectomy. *Eur J Ophthalmol.* 2012;22:363-367.
13. Mönestam EI. Incidence of dislocation of intraocular lenses and pseudophakodonesis 10 years after cataract surgery. *Ophthalmology.* 2009;116:2315-2320.
14. Pueringer SL, Hodge DO, Erie JC. Risk of late intraocular lens dislocation after cataract surgery, 1980-2009: a population-based study. *Am J Ophthalmol.* 2011;152:618-623.
15. Davison JA. Capsule contraction syndrome. *J Cataract Refract Surg.* 1993;19:582-589.
16. Hayashi H, Hayashi K, Nakao F, Hayashi F. Reduction in the area of the anterior capsule opening after polymethylmethacrylate, silicone, and soft acrylic intraocular lens implantation. *Am J Ophthalmol.* 1997;123:441-447.
17. Hayashi H, Hayashi K, Nakao F, Hayashi F. Anterior capsule contraction and intraocular lens dislocation in eyes with pseudoexfoliation syndrome. *Br J Ophthalmol.* 1998;82:1429-1432.
18. Werner L, Pandey SK, Escobar-Gomez M, et al. Anterior capsule opacification; a histopathological study comparing different IOL styles. *Ophthalmology.* 2000;107:463–471.
19. Hayashi K, Yoshida M, Nakao F, Hayashi H. Prevention of anterior capsule contraction by anterior capsule relaxing incisions with neodymium:yttrium-aluminum-garnet laser. *Am J Ophthalmol.* 2008;146:23-30.
20. Lorente R, de Rojas V, Vazquez de Parga P, et al. Management of late spontaneous in-the-bag intraocular lens dislocation: retrospective analysis of 45 cases. *J Cataract Refract Surg.* 2010;36:1270–1282.
21. Werner L, Zaugg B, Neuhann T, Burrow M, Tetz M. In-the-bag capsular tension ring and intraocular lens subluxation or dislocation: a series of 23 cases. *Ophthalmology.* 2012;119:266-271.
22. Ahmed II, Chen SH, Kranemann C, Wong DT. Surgical repositioning of dislocated capsular tension rings. *Ophthalmology.* 2005;112:1725-1733.
23. Suto C, Hori S, Fukuyama E, Akura J. Adjusting intraocular lens power for sulcus fixation. *J Cataract Refract Surg.* 2003;29:1913-1917.
24. Cionni RJ, Osher RH, Marques DMV, et al. Modified capsular tension ring for patients with congenital loss of zonular support. *J Cataract Refract Surg.* 2003;29:1668–1673.
25. Moreno-Montañés J, Sainz C, Maldonado MJ. Introperative and postoperative complications of Cionni endocapsular ring implantation. *J Cataract Refract Surg.* 2003;29:492–497.
26. Hasanee K, Butler M, Ahmed II. Capsular tension rings and related devices: current concepts. *Curr Opin Ophthalmol.* 2006;17:31-41.
27. Hasanee K, Ahmed II. Capsular tension rings: update on endocapsular support devices. *Ophthalmol Clin North Am.* 2006;19:507-519.
28. Blecher MH, Kirk MR. Surgical strategies for the management of zonular compromise. *Curr Opin Ophthalmol.* 2008;19:31-35.
29. Chee SP, Jap A. Management of traumatic severely subluxated cataracts. *Am J Ophthalmol.* 2011;151:866-871.
30. Vasavada AR, Praveen MR, Vasavada VA, Yeh RY, Srivastava S, Koul A, Trivedi RH. Cionni ring and in-the-bag intraocular lens implantation for subluxated lenses: a prospective case series. *Am J Ophthalmol.* 2012;153:1144-1153.
31. Buttanri IB, Sevim MS, Esen D, Acar BT, Serin D, Acar S. Modified capsular tension ring implantation in eyes with traumatic cataract and loss of zonular support. *J Cataract Refract Surg.* 2012;38:431-436.
32. Assia EI, Ton Y, Michaeli A. Capsule anchor to manage subluxated lenses: Initial clinical experience. *J Cataract Refract Surg.* 2009;35(8):1372–1379.
33. Hoffman RS, Fine IH, Packer M. Scleral fixation without conjunctival dissection. *J Cataract Refract Surg.* 2006;32:1907-1912.
34. Lee DH, Shin SC, Joo CK. Effect of a capsular tension ring on intraocular lens decentration and tilting after cataract surgery. *J Cataract Refract Surg.* 2002;28:843–846.

Please see companion narrated videos on the accompanying Web site at
www.Healio.com/phacochopvideos

25

Phaco in Highly Myopic Eyes

David F. Chang, MD

Whether performed for cataracts or refractive lens exchange, phacoemulsification in highly myopic eyes presents several challenges. Because these eyes are already at increased risk of pseudophakic retinal detachment, avoiding posterior capsular rupture is critical.[1] It is therefore important to understand the operative difficulties unique to these eyes and how to overcome them. Along with vitreous syneresis, myopic eyes tend to develop nuclear and oil drop cataracts at a younger age than the general population.[2-6] Some have hypothesized that vitreous syneresis allows more oxygen from the choroid to reach the hypoxic lens, and that this may be the primary cause of the myopic nuclear cataract.[7]

INTRAOCULAR LENS SELECTION

The first challenge in myopic eyes is proper IOL power selection.[8] Although the advantages of noncontact biometry are widely acknowledged, myopic eyes (> 26 mm long) pose the unique problem of how to measure the appropriate axial length in eyes with a staphyloma.[9] Immersion ultrasound typically locates the posterior-most point of the globe, but will not measure the distance to the fovea if it is located on the slope of the staphyloma. Partial coherence interferometry, such as with the IOL Master (Carl Zeiss Meditec, Dublin, CA) or Lenstar (Haag Streit USA, Mason, OH), are noncontact biometric technologies that specifically measure the distance from the cornea to the fovea and are the preferred biometric methodology for highly myopic eyes.

The IOL formulae are generally less accurate for eyes with extremely long or short axial lengths. Assuming that the axial length measurement is accurate, many lens formulae assume certain linear relationships between axial length and effective lens position (ELP). Holladay has shown that this assumption of a deeper ELP in increasingly longer eyes is not always correct; his proprietary Holladay 2 formula uses other parameters besides axial length to predict ELP.[10] Hoffer has shown that, of the modern regression formulae, the SRK/T formula is more accurate in long eyes compared to the Hoffer Q or Holladay 1 formulae.[11]

Extremely myopic eyes may require very low or even negative power IOLs. Fortunately, several manufacturers now provide lens powers in the minus to low plus range. Even if the calculated power is very low or zero, it is still advisable to implant a posterior chamber IOL. Once it becomes shrinkwrapped by the capsular bag, the IOL will reduce the chance of capsular fibrosis and opacification

Chang DF.
Phaco Chop and Advanced Phaco Techniques: Strategies for Complicated Cataracts, Second Edition (pp 277-282).
© 2013 SLACK Incorporated.

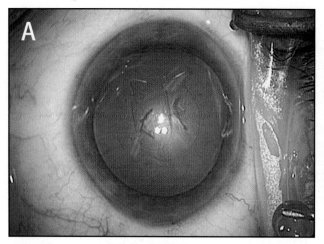 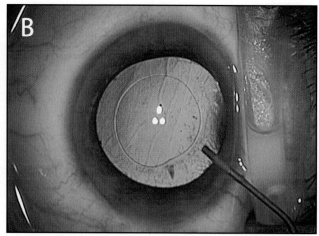

Figure 25-1. In a highly myopic eye with a large diameter cornea, a conscious effort is made to make a capsulorrhexis that appears to be smaller than usual. (A) View prior to hydrodissection. (B) View after cortical clean-up.

and will serve as a barrier to vitreous prolapse should a YAG capsulotomy ever be necessary.[12] The SRK/T formula tends to lead to a hyperopic overcorrection when negative-powered IOLs are implanted, and one should generally aim for a slightly more myopic target refraction.[13]

ANESTHESIA AND INCISIONS

Because of the elongated globe and decreased scleral thickness, the increased risk of scleral perforation is an important concern with any regional injection anesthetic in high myopes.[14] Using a peribulbar technique alone does not negate this risk. Topical anesthesia, with or without intracameral lidocaine supplementation, has the obvious benefit of avoiding a blind needle injection in these eyes. Topical anesthesia, however, will not block the pain induced by lens iris diaphragm retrodisplacement syndrome (LIDRS), which causes significant stretching of uveal tissues.[15] Avoiding and reversing LIDRS, as described in the following paragraphs, is important if one is to employ topical anesthesia.

Proper incision architecture can be more difficult to attain in myopic eyes because of the thinner peripheral cornea and reduced scleral rigidity. A clear corneal tunnel must be appropriately long in order to be self-sealing. The surgeon must therefore avoid the tendency to penetrate Descemet's membrane too soon when the peripheral cornea is thinner than usual. Use of an interrupted suture should always be considered if the integrity of a clear corneal incision is in doubt at the conclusion of surgery.

CAPSULORRHEXIS

The difficulty of controlling the anterior capsule flap if the anterior chamber becomes shallow during the capsulorrhexis step is well recognized. The same is true, however, if the anterior chamber becomes excessively deep, such as in a highly myopic or vitrectomized eye. The amount of ophthalmic viscosurgical device (OVD) needed to adequately pressurize the globe prior to creating the incision will often displace the lens much farther posteriorly than normal. In this situation, the capsular flap often tends to veer peripherally as the capsulorrhexis is performed, presumably due to excessive zonular traction. These traction vectors are directed both anteriorly and peripherally when the lens is posteriorly displaced by OVD or irrigation infusion.

Aside from avoiding complications such as capsular rupture, an intact capsulorrhexis that circumferentially overlaps the IOL optic edge for all 360 degrees is the most important anatomic consideration for minimizing the risk of retinal detachment. Along with thorough cortical clean-up and a truncated IOL optic edge, an overlapping capsulorrhexis significantly reduces the probability of capsular opacification requiring a YAG capsulotomy.[12,16] The latter, in turn, elevates the risk of retinal detachment, particularly in young myopic men.[1]

Proper capsulorrhexis sizing is difficult, however, because surgeons usually rely solely on visual clues to gauge the appropriate diameter. Because of the larger corneal diameter and anterior segment of a myopic eye, surgeons unintentionally tend to make a larger diameter capsulorrhexis in these patients. If the capsulorrhexis extends beyond the optic edge, the lens epithelial cell blocking capsular bend described by Nishi will not occur.[16] Parallax also makes it difficult to perfectly center the capsulorrhexis.

Recognizing this, one obvious advantage of a femtosecond laser capsulotomy is the ability to program and automate a specific size and diameter. For a manual technique, one solution is to err on making the primary capsulorrhexis on the small side (Figure 25-1). Following IOL implantation, the diameter can always be enlarged but not reduced.

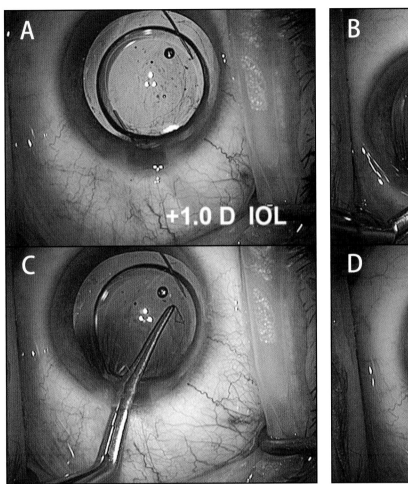

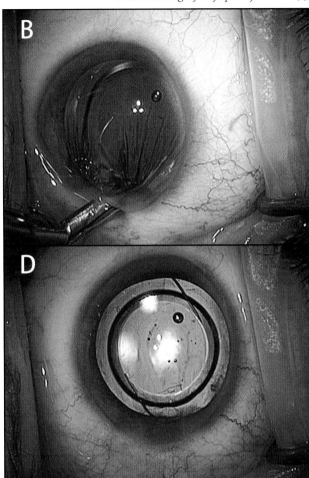

Figure 25-2. Same eye as in Figure 25-1. (A-D) Small diameter capsulorrhexis is enlarged with forceps after creating a new flap with an oblique microscissors cut.

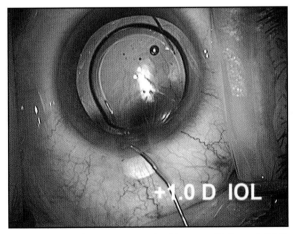

Figure 25-3. Same eye as in Figures 25-1 and 25-2. Because of the excessive anterior chamber depth in this highly myopic eye, some OVD is burped out of the anterior chamber prior to initiating a secondary capsulorrhexis enlargement.

A short oblique cut with capsule scissors creates a new flap that can be grasped with forceps (Figure 25-2). The cut should be oblique, rather than radial, to better incline the resulting flap to tear in a circumferential direction. Curved Uthoff-Gills capsulotomy scissors with blunt tips (Katena K4-5126; Katena Eye Instruments, Denville, NJ) have the perfect shape for creating an initial curved cut to either side of the phaco incision. If the anterior chamber is extremely deep, it helps to burp out some OVD so that the capsulorrhexis becomes more level with, and not posterior to, the iris plane (Figure 25-3).

LENS IRIS DIAPHRAGM RETRODISPLACEMENT SYNDROME

Initially described in 1994 by Wilbrandt, the LIDRS is commonly encountered as soon as the irrigation fluid infuses the anterior chamber during phacoemulsification in high myopes and in vitrectomized eyes.[17] Robert J. Cionni, MD used intraoperative endoscopy to elegantly show that LIDRS is caused by reverse pupillary block as the iris becomes circumferentially pinned against the lens by

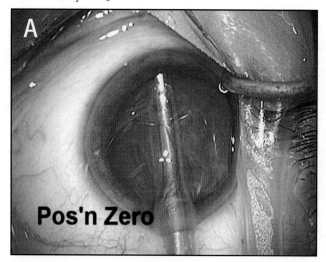 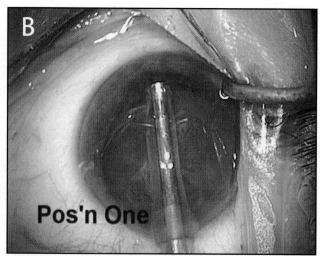

Figure 25-4. (A) In order to prevent LIDRS, the phaco tip lifts the contraincisional iris edge while in FP0. (B) This allows irrigation to immediately flow into the posterior chamber when FP1 is activated.

the hydrostatic infusion pressure.[15] Lifting the iris pupillary margin off of the lens with an instrument tip breaks the pupillary block and allows equilibration of the hydrostatic forces anterior and posterior to the iris.

Although the pupil initially widens due to hydrostatic mydriasis, the excessive anterior chamber deepening from LIDRS causes sudden discomfort for patients under topical anesthesia and exerts significant traction on the zonules. Nuclear emulsification is more difficult with an excessively deepened anterior chamber because the instruments and phaco tip must approach the lens from a much steeper angle. If the reverse pupillary block abruptly breaks during phacoemulsification, the pupil will suddenly constrict, creating a pupil diameter that is often much smaller than it was preoperatively. Cionni hypothesized that this might be due to prostaglandin release caused by the excessive ciliary body stretching.

To prevent LIDRS, one can insert the phaco tip into the OVD-filled anterior chamber while in foot pedal position 0 (FP0). Next, the surgeon lifts the iris in the contraincisional nasal quadrant using the phaco tip before initiating inflow with FP1 (Figure 25-4). Alternatively, one can simply lift the pupil edge with a second instrument before initiating irrigation inflow. Either maneuver can also be utilized following the onset of LIDRS to gradually break the reverse pupillary block. These steps allow irrigation fluid to circulate into the posterior chamber, thereby equilibrating the hydrostatic forces both in front of and behind the iris. The hydrostatically widened pupil will then gradually constrict as the pupillary block is broken.

PHACO AND INTRAOCULAR LENS INSERTION TECHNIQUE

It is difficult to sculpt a nuclear trough with an excessively deep anterior chamber. Recognizing and managing LIDRS is therefore particularly important for the divide-and-conquer or stop and chop phaco techniques. The smaller nuclear and oil droplet cataracts typical of younger, high myopes are well suited for both chopping and supracapsular flipping techniques.

To minimize the clear corneal incision size while injecting the IOL, it is important to have a relatively firm globe. Because of the increased volume of the anterior segment, there is frequently insufficient OVD remaining by this stage to tense the globe (Figure 25-5A). An alternative to opening a new vial of OVD is to inject saline into the back of the capsular bag in the presence of a dispersive or retentive OVD (Figure 25-5B). Because the latter will not burp out of the eye, the globe will become firmer which should facilitate insertion of the injector tip.

STEROID RESPONSE RISK

In 2011, the author published a retrospective study analyzing risk factors for a steroid response following uncomplicated cataract surgery.[18] A chart review was performed for all 1642 patients who had undergone cataract surgery during a 2-year period in a single-surgeon practice. In addition to a topical fluoroquinolone and NSAID, all patients

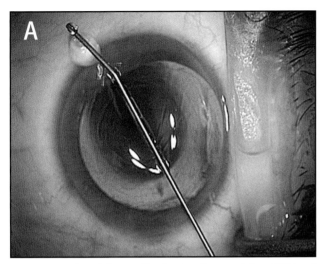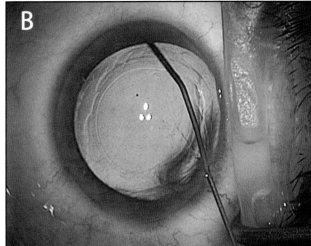

Figure 25-5. (A) Globe is still soft after the remaining OVD has been injected. (B) Globe becomes tense after balanced salt solution injected into the back of the capsular bag is trapped by the retentive OVD.

Table 25-1.
CUMULATIVE STEROID RESPONDERS BY AGE AND AXIAL LENGTH GROUP

AGE	< 25.0 MM	≥ 25.0 MM	≥ 27.0 MM	≥ 29.0 MM	ALL EVENTS < .0001
40 to 54 years	(2/53) **3.8%**	(9/63) **14.3%**	(6/35) **17.1%**	(5/14) **35.7%**	(11/116) **9.5%**
55 to 64 years	(3/150) **2.0%**	(10/128) **7.8%**	(3/49) **6.1%**	(1/11) **9.1%**	(13/278) **4.7%**
≥65 years	(7/955) **0.7%**	(8/264) **3.0%**	(4/39) **10.3%**	(1/7) **14.3%**	(15/1219) **1.2%**
All events < .0001	(12/1158) **1.0%**	(27/455) **5.9%**	(13/123) **10.6%**	(7/32) **21.9%**	(39/1613) **2.4%**

Table 25-2.
STEROID RESPONDER RISK: ODDS RATIOS

AGE	< 25.0 MM	25.0 TO 27.0 MM	27.0 TO 29.0 MM	≥ 29.0 MM
40 to 54 years	3.8%, **4.1x**	10.0%, **7.9x**	5.3%, **15.8x**	35.7%, **46.1x**
55 to 64 years	2.0%, **2.5x**	8.9%, **5.2x**	5.3%, **9.7x**	9.1%, **31.8x**
≥65 years	0.7%, **1**	1.8%, **2.4x**	9.4%, **5.4x**	14.3%, **14.4x**

were routinely treated with topical 1% prednisolone acetate. A steroid response was defined as an IOP of at least 28 mm Hg that had risen by at least 25% from the preoperative baseline, and then fell by at least 25% after cessation of topical steroid. Any IOP elevation during the first 72 hours postoperatively was excluded, as well as any rise associated with an intraoperative complication.

Overall, 2.4% of patients were steroid responders and 85% of these had no prior history of glaucoma or ocular hypertension (Table 25-1). However, there was a statistically significant increase in steroid response risk with both increasing axial length and decreasing age. Combining both risk factors generated the highest risk—patients younger than 55 years with an axial length of at least 29 mm had a 46-fold increased risk of a steroid response (Table 25-2). A number of patients from this latter group had dangerously high IOP elevations within the first week of treatment.

As a result of this study, one might consider using a "weaker" steroid such as loteprednol etabonate 0.5% and, at the very least, avoiding difluprednate 0.05% in higher myopes. Particularly with patients younger than 65 years with an axial length of at least 25 mm, closer IOP monitoring might be advisable if topical steroids are used postoperatively.

REFERENCES

1. Lois N, Wong D. Pseudophakic retinal detachment. *Surv Ophthalmol.* 2003;48:467-487.
2. Kaufman BJ, Sugar J. Discrete nuclear sclerosis in young patients with myopia. *Arch Ophthalmol.* 1996;114:1178-1180.
3. Chen SN, Lin KK, Chao AN, et al. Nuclear sclerotic cataract in young patients in Taiwan. *J Cataract Refract Surg.* 2003;29:983-988.
4. Tuft SJ, Bunce C. Axial length and age at cataract surgery. *J Cataract Refract Surg.* 2004;30:1045-1048.
5. Lin HY, Chang CW, Wang HZ, Tsai RK. Relation between the axial length and lenticular progressive myopia. *Eye.* 2005;19:899-905.
6. Kubo E, Kumamoto Y, Tsuzuki S, Akagi Y. Axial length, myopia, and the severity of lens opacity at the time of cataract surgery. *Arch Ophthalmol.* 2006;124:1586-1590.
7. Harocopos GJ, Shui YB, McKinnon M, et al. Importance of vitreous liquefaction in age-related cataract. *Invest Ophthalmol Vis Sci.* 2004;45:77-85.
8. Pierro L, Modorati G, Brancato R. Clinical variability in keratometry, ultrasound biometry measurements, and emmetropic intraocular lens power calculation. *J Cataract Refract Surg.* 1991;17:91-94.
9. Bose LT, Moshegov CN. Comparison of the Zeiss IOL Master and applanation A-scan ultrasound biometry for intraocular lens calculations. *Clin Experiment Ophthalmol.* 2003;31:121-124.
10. Hoffer KJ. The Hoffer Q formula: a comparison of theoretic and regression formulas. *J Cataract Refract Surg.* 1993;19:700-712. ERRATA 1994;20:677 and2007;33:2-3.
11. Hoffer KJ. Clinical results using the Holladay 2 intraocular lens power formula. *J Cataract Refract Surg.* 2000;26:1233-1237.
12. Ram J, Pandey SK, Apple DJ, et al. Effect of in-the-bag intraocular lens fixation on the prevention of posterior capsule opacification. *J Cataract Refract Surg.* 2001;27:367-370.
13. MacLaren RE, Sagoo MS, Restori M, Allan BD. Biometry accuracy using zero- and negative-powered intraocular lenses. *J Cataract Refract Surg.* 2005;31:280-290.
14. Gadkari SS. Evaluation of 19 cases of inadvertent globe perforation due to periocular injections. *Indian J Ophthalmol.* 2007;55:103-107.
15. Cionni RJ, Barros MG, Osher RH. Management of lens-iris diaphragm retropulsion syndrome during phacoemulsification. *J Cataract Refract Surg.* 2004;30:953-956.
16. Nishi O, Nishi K, Wickstrom K. Preventing lens epithelial cell migration using intraocular lenses with sharp rectangular edges. *J Cataract Refract Surg.* 2000;26:1543-1549.
17. Wilbrandt HR, Wilbrandt TH. Pathogenesis and management of the lens-iris diaphragm retropulsion syndrome during phacoemulsification. *J Cataract Refract Surg.* 1994;20:48-53.
18. Chang DF, Tan JJ, Tripodis Y. Risk Factors for steroid response among cataract patients. *J Cataract Refract Surg.* 2011;37:675-681.

26

Phaco Within the Crowded Anterior Segment

David F. Chang, MD

The crowded anterior segment presents one of the most challenging situations for the phaco surgeon. Whether because of a short axial length, a larger lens, or a combination of both factors, these hyperopic eyes present with narrow angles and shallow anterior chambers that complicate multiple surgical steps. A properly constructed clear corneal incision may be more difficult to achieve due to peripheral iridocorneal apposition or proximity. These eyes often have posterior synechiae and a miotic pupil, and yet reduced corneal clearance for performing a pupilloplasty or inserting pupil expansion devices. Because of the anterior iris location, there is an increased chance of iris prolapse and of instrument trauma to the iris, both of which cause intraoperative pupillary constriction. The capsulorrhexis is more difficult to control because the increased convexity of the anterior capsule tends to steer the tear peripherally. Finally, because of the decreased working space, nuclear emulsification is carried out in much closer proximity to the cornea. This markedly increases the risk of endothelial cell loss, particularly if the nucleus is brunescent.[1]

Hyperopic eyes with short axial lengths may be more predisposed to suprachoroidal hemorrhage. Sudden shallowing of the chamber during phaco, accompanied by a tense globe, may also indicate fluid misdirection or a suprachoroidal effusion. If a suprachoroidal hemorrhage is suspected, surgery should be halted and the incision should be secured. Intraoperative indirect ophthalmoscopy may confirm the suspected diagnosis. In the case of fluid misdirection or a suprachoroidal effusion, surgery can eventually be resumed or completed once the eye is no longer firm.

GENERAL STRATEGIES

Sufficient chamber depth can usually be achieved by using appropriate ophthalmic viscoelastic devices (OVDs). Digital massage or intravenous (IV) mannitol can be combined if necessary. A high molecular weight cohesive agent is able to maximally flatten the central anterior lens surface. Dispersive OVDs exhibit superior retention in the face of wound manipulation. The "soft shell" technique, as originally described by Steve A. Arshinoff, MD, FRCSC, combines a cohesive agent to maximally expand space and a dispersive agent to coat the cornea and block any egress via the incision[2] (see Figure 17-7). Sodium hyaluronate 2.3% (Healon 5) is maximally cohesive and retentive, and is also well suited for this purpose.[3,4] However, because Healon 5 will not ooze out of the paracentesis sites to decompress the

Chang DF.
Phaco Chop and Advanced Phaco Techniques: Strategies for Complicated Cataracts, Second Edition (pp 283-286).
© 2013 SLACK Incorporated.

globe, it is possible to disrupt the zonules by over-inflating the anterior segment with this OVD.

One must also be careful not to overinflate the anterior segment to the point of causing iris prolapse. Typically, surgeons deepen the anterior chamber by injecting OVD first distally and then progressively more proximally as the cannula is withdrawn from the eye. This can cause OVD to get behind the subincisional iris, causing the iris stroma to prolapse through the incision. Attempts to mechanically reposit the iris via the clear corneal incision will usually not succeed because of the persistent pressure gradient caused by OVD trapped behind the iris stroma. Instead, the anterior chamber must be decompressed by burping a large amount of OVD out through a separately located paracentesis incision. Only then can a cyclodialysis spatula be used through an adjacent paracentesis site to sweep the prolapsed iris back into the eye. To avoid iris prolapse, the best measure is to first inject OVD proximally over the subincisional iris. By first depressing this section of the iris and pupil and being careful not to overinflate the globe, iris prolapse through the incision should not occur.

Pars Plana Vitreous Tap

Occasionally, eyes at the far extreme of the shallow chamber spectrum are encountered. In these cases, viscoelastic injection may be unable to adequately deepen the chamber without first causing iris prolapse or a dangerously firm globe. In these situations, performing a vitreous tap prior to OVD injection can expand the chamber to a safer depth (Figure 26-1). This author was the first to report using a vitrectomy cutter for this technique in a series of eyes with unusually crowded chambers.[5]

Anticipating this possibility preoperatively, a peribulbar or retrobulbar block should be considered. Some OVD is first injected into the anterior chamber until the globe starts to become slightly firm. Typically the anterior chamber will remain shallow. Following a conjunctival cut-down incision and adequate hemostasis, a disposable 19-gauge microvitreoretinal (MVR) blade (Alcon Laboratories, Fort Worth, TX) is used to make a pars plana sclerotomy located 3.0 mm behind the limbus (see Figures 26-1B and 26-1C). The MVR blade must be aimed posteriorly toward the optic nerve to avoid hitting the crystalline lens. An automated vitrectomy cutter without infusion is inserted and

advanced several millimeters into the vitreous cavity until the tip is visible through the pupil. If the nucleus precludes visualization, making a measured mark on the side of the vitrectomy shaft can prevent the tip from being advanced too far[6] (see Figure 26-1D). Using a vitrectomy cutter for the tap is preferable to a needle and syringe; this helps the surgeon avoid vitreous traction or blindly searching for a fluid pocket. Care must be taken not to force the vitrector through too small a sclerotomy and to aim it posteriorly enough to avoid hitting the lens.

Removing only a few tenths of a milliliter of vitreous will soften the eye. An OVD is immediately injected through a limbal paracentesis to deepen the anterior chamber. This injection should be initiated quickly enough to lessen the potential for a suprachoroidal hemorrhage. Care must be taken to avoid over-softening the globe by extracting too much vitreous. While operating the vitrectomy handpiece, the surgeon should intermittently palpate the globe to see if it is softening (see Figure 26-1D). It is best to err on the side of removing insufficient vitreous volume. If the anterior chamber still does not deepen, the vitreous tap can be repeated. The sclerotomy is left open until the conclusion of the case, when it is then closed with a single, interrupted 8-0 Vicryl suture (see Figure 26-1H).

If available, small gauge vitrectomy instruments can be introduced directly through a pars plana sclerotomy without the need for a separate peritomy.[7] Some of these systems employ a 25-gauge vitrector, which is inserted via a pars plana trochar placed directly through the conjunctiva and sclera. Because of uncertain and abnormal anatomic landmarks, this vitreous tap technique should not be used with nanophthalmic eyes with an axial length shorter than 21 mm.

Although a standard manual extracapsular extraction (ECCE) approach is an option in these eyes, a small incision may be preferable for 2 reasons. First of all, these eyes often have coexisting glaucoma and may have had or may require a trabeculectomy. Second, a small incision provides greater safety in hyperopic eyes at increased risk of a suprachoroidal hemorrhage or effusion. Thus, in the rare situation where the anterior chamber cannot be sufficiently deepened with a cohesive viscoelastic alone, an automated, pars plana vitreous tap can provide enough working space for the pupilloplasty, capsulorrhexis, phaco, and foldable IOL steps to be performed through the safety of a small incision.

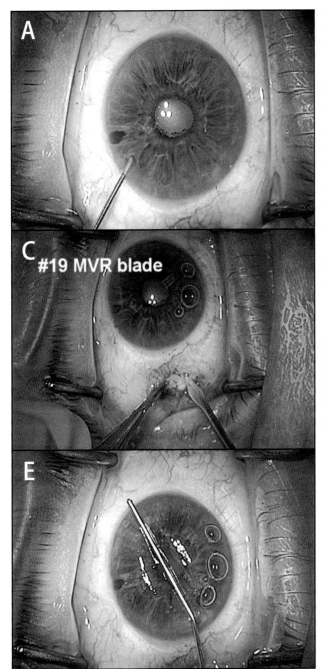

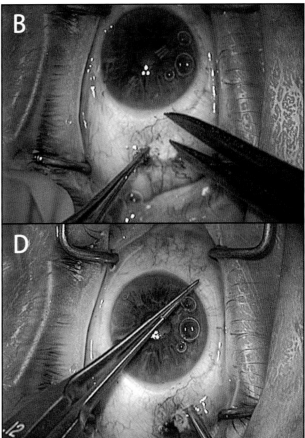

Figure 26-1. Crowded anterior chamber with nearly flat anterior chamber and a brunescent cataract. The pupil is fixed with posterior synechiae and a prior laser iridotomy is visible. (A) After injecting only a small amount of OVD, the eye is already rock hard. (B) Calipers are used to mark the location of a pars plana sclerotomy 3.5 mm posterior to the limbus in an oblique quadrant. (C) A disposable 19-gauge MVR blade is used to make the sclerotomy, while being sure to aim posteriorly enough to avoid the hitting the lens. (D) An automated vitrectomy probe without infusion is used to remove a small amount of vitreous while periodically palpating the ocular pressure to avoid over-softening. (E) Following the automated vitreous tap, the eye is soft enough to allow normal chamber deepening with OVD.

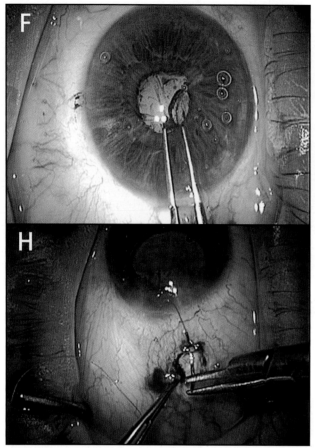
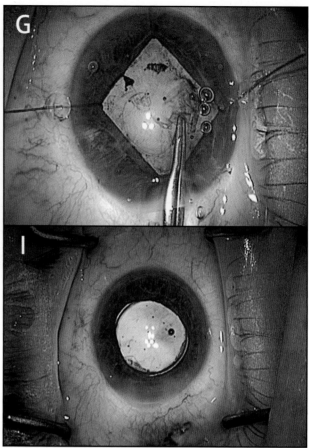

Figure 26-1 (continued). Crowded anterior chamber with nearly flat anterior chamber and a brunescent cataract. The pupil is fixed with posterior synechiae and a prior laser iridotomy is visible. (F) With adequate anterior chamber depth, the peripupillary membrane can be peeled away with capsule forceps. (G) Placement of iris retractors and the capsulotomy can be performed without the constraints or impediments of an overly shallow anterior chamber. (H) An interrupted 8-0 Vicryl suture is used to close the pars plana sclerotomy. (I) Appearance at the conclusion of surgery.

REFERENCES

1. Walkow T, Anders N, Klebe S. Endothelial cell loss after phacoemulsification: relation to preoperative and intraoperative parameters. *J Cataract Refract Surg.* 2000;26:727-732.
2. Arhsinoff SA. Dispersive-cohesive viscoelastic soft shell technique. *J Cataract Refract Surg.* 1999;25:167-173.
3. Arhsinoff SA. Using BSS with viscoadaptives in the ultimate softshell technique. *J Cataract Refract Surg.* 2002;28:1509-1514.
4. Dick HB, Krummenauer F, Augustin AJ, Pakula T, Pfeiffer N. Healon 5 viscoadaptive formulation: comparison to Healon and Healon GV. *J Cataract Refract Surg.* 2001;27:320-326.
5. Chang DF. Pars Plana Vitreous Tap for Phaco in the Crowded Eye. *J Cataract Refract Surg.* 2001;27:1911-1914.
6. Mackool RJ. Pars plana vitreous tap for phacoemulsification in the crowded eye. *J Cataract Refract Surg.* 2002;28:572-573.
7. Hilton GF, Josephberg RG, Halperin LS, et al. Office-based sutureless transconjunctival pars plana vitrectomy. *Retina.* 2002;22:725-732.

Please see companion narrated videos on the accompanying Web site at
www.Healio.com/phacochopvideos

27

Strategies for Managing Posterior Capsule Rupture

David F. Chang, MD

During phacoemulsification, avoiding posterior capsule rupture is continually on the ophthalmologist's mind. However, once this unexpected and infrequent complication occurs, the surgeon must immediately recognize it and make a series of critical decisions under stressful circumstances. Proper advance preparation requires each cataract surgeon to anticipate and think through how he or she would handle a number of different hypothetical clinical situations. Specifically, every cataract surgeon should have a game plan for when and how to perform an anterior vitrectomy following posterior capsule rupture. Such advance planning helps one to respond with greater confidence and less trepidation.

This chapter will review the goals, the indications, and the techniques. Understanding and mentally rehearsing these strategies will better prepare cataract surgeons to remain calm under pressure and to make correct decisions amidst the stress of an unexpected complication.

INCIDENCE OF POSTERIOR CAPSULE RUPTURE AND VITREOUS LOSS

Thirteen studies of vitreous loss rates in nonresident series published during the decade between 1999 and 2009 are listed in Table 27-1.[1-13] Excluding the exceptionally low rate of 0.2% by Howard V. Gimbel, MD, MPH, FRCSC, FACS,[5] the vitreous loss rates consistently range from 1 to 4%. Table 27-2 lists 8 studies of vitreous loss rates among residency programs that were published from 2002 to 2010.[14-21] With the exception of one study, these rates consistently range from 3% to 6%. The best current published data on vitreous loss rates come from 3 recent studies of large patient populations. Narendran and coauthors' 2009 report on the Cataract National Dataset audit of 55,567 operations from the United Kingdom reported a 1.9% rate of vitreous loss.[22] Greenberg and coauthors' 2010 study of cataract surgery performed in 45,082 patients at the United States Veterans Administration Hospital had a vitreous loss rate of 3.5%.[23] Finally, in 2011, Lundstrom and coauthors reported on all cataract surgeries performed at the 52 centers that compose the Swedish National Register during the period from 2002 to 2009.[24] From a total of 602,533 cataract procedures, the incidence of capsule complications was 2.1%. Assuming that the Greenberg data would have included many resident surgeries, it appears that 2% is a representative estimate of the capsule complication rate for large populations of nonresident surgeons.

Chang DF.
Phaco Chop and Advanced Phaco Techniques: Strategies for Complicated Cataracts, Second Edition (pp 287-307).

Table 27-1.

Vitreous Loss Rates in Nonresident Series Published During the Decade Between 1999 and 2009

AUTHOR	PUBLISHED	% VITREOUS LOSS	STUDY SIZE
Desai[1]	1999	4.4%	18,454
Martin[2]	2000	1.3%	3000
Lundström[3]	2001	2.2%	2731
Ionides[4]	2001	2.9%	1420
Gimbel[5]	2001	0.2%	18,470
Tan[6]	2002	3.6%	2538
Chan[7]	2003	1.1%	8230
Androudi[8]	2004	4.0%	543
Hyams[9]	2005	2.0%	1364
Ang[10]	2006	1.1%	2727
Zaidi[11]	2007	1.1%	1000
Mearza[12]	2009	2.7%	1614
Agrawal[13]	2009	1.6%	6564

Table 27-2.

Vitreous Loss Rates in Resident Series Published During the Decade Between 2002 and 2010

AUTHOR	PUBLISHED	% VITREOUS LOSS	STUDY SIZE
Blomquist[14]	2002	4.5%	1400
Dooley[15]	2006	4%	100
Bhagat[16]	2007	5.4%	755
Pot[17]	2008	1.3%	982
Rutar[18]	2009	3.1%	320
Lee[19]	2009	4.9%	226
Carricondo[20]	2010	6.1%	261
Blomquist[21]	2010	3.2%	1833

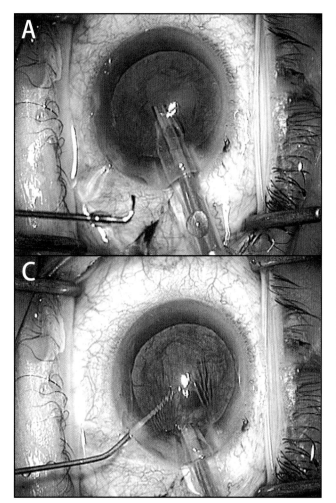
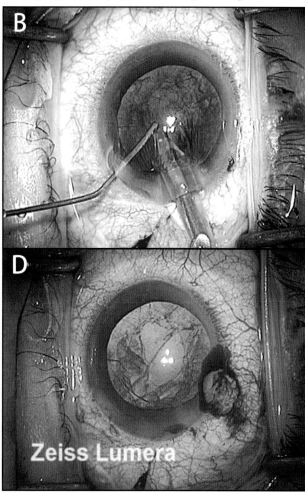

Figure 27-1. Case 1. Polar cataract with posterior capsular rupture. (A) Once a posterior capsular tear is suspected or recognized, the phaco tip is kept in place with irrigation flow (FP1) while the second instrument is withdrawn. Note the irrigation flow through the sideport incision. (B) As OVD sodium chondroitin sulfate (Viscoat) is injected through the sideport incision, the phaco tip remains in place while moving to FP0 to allow the OVD to accumulate. (C) Once the anterior chamber is filled with OVD, the phaco tip is withdrawn. (D) Because the anterior chamber remains inflated, there is no vitreous prolapse through the posterior capsular rent, which is now visible using the enhanced red reflex setting of the microscope.

AVOIDING VITREOUS LOSS FOLLOWING POSTERIOR CAPSULE RUPTURE

In many instances when the posterior capsule tears, it is possible to avoid rupturing the hyaloid face. Caught unexpectedly by surprise, the surgeon must avoid the natural reflex to immediately withdraw the phaco tip upon recognizing a posterior capsular defect. Like pulling one's hand away from a hot stove, there is a natural reflex to suddenly withdraw the phaco or irrigation/aspiration (I/A) tip out of the eye. However, this abruptly unplugs the incision and allows the anterior chamber to collapse. The sudden posterior pressure gradient will rupture an intact anterior hyaloid face and vitreous will prolapse along with the rest of the exiting fluid toward the incision, expanding the capsular rent in the process.

This undesirable cascade of events can be averted by filling the anterior chamber with ophthalmic viscosurgical device (OVD) prior to removing the phaco tip (Figure 27-1). As OVD is injected through the sideport opening, the surgeon moves from foot pedal position 1 (FP1) to 0 (FP0) (see Figure 27-1B). Once the chamber is filled with OVD, the posterior capsule cannot bulge forward once the incision is unplugged (see Figures 27-1C and 27-1D). If one resumes phacoemulsification or cortical clean-up, the same maneuver must be repeated whenever any irrigating instrument is removed (see Figure 27-1G).

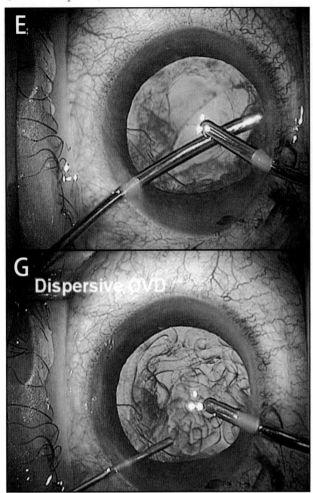

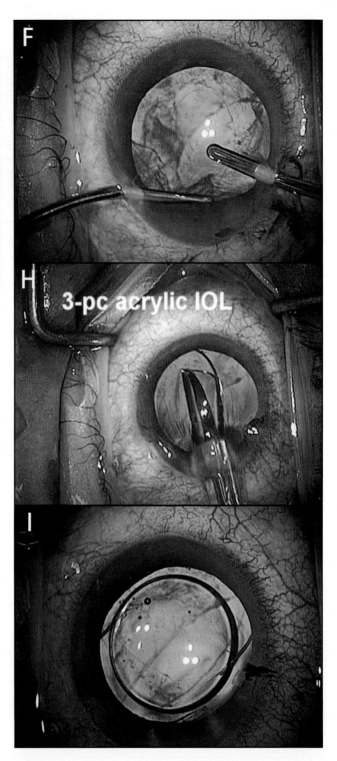

Figure 27-1 (continued). Case 1. Polar cataract with posterior capsular rupture. (E) Bimanual I/A instrumentation is used to remove the cortex and allows dissociation of the irrigation and aspiration fluid counter-currents. The irrigation handpiece (right hand) is kept in the anterior chamber so that the inflow is aimed away from the posterior capsular opening. (F) Bimanual I/A also facilitates access to the subincisional cortex. (G) OVD is injected through the sideport incision prior to removing the irrigating handpiece. (H) A 3-piece acrylic IOL is placed in the ciliary sulcus. (I) The optic is captured by the capsulorrhexis. Vitreous has not prolapsed through the posterior capsular defect which is visible behind, and blocked by the IOL optic.

EARLY RECOGNITION OF POSTERIOR CAPSULE OR ZONULAR RUPTURE

It is much easier to remove the nucleus while it remains anterior to any posterior capsule defect. Therefore, early recognition of posterior capsule rupture is the key to avoiding a dropped nucleus. One must often rely on indirect clues to recognize a posterior capsular defect because the iris and the nucleus obscure the zonular and posterior capsular anatomy. Sudden deepening of the chamber with momentary expansion of the pupil (Figure 27-2), the transitory appearance of a clear red reflex in the periphery, and the inability to rotate a previously mobile nucleus can all indicate capsular or zonular rupture. More obvious and ominous signs would be excessive tipping or lateral mobility of the nucleus or partial posterior descent of the nucleus.

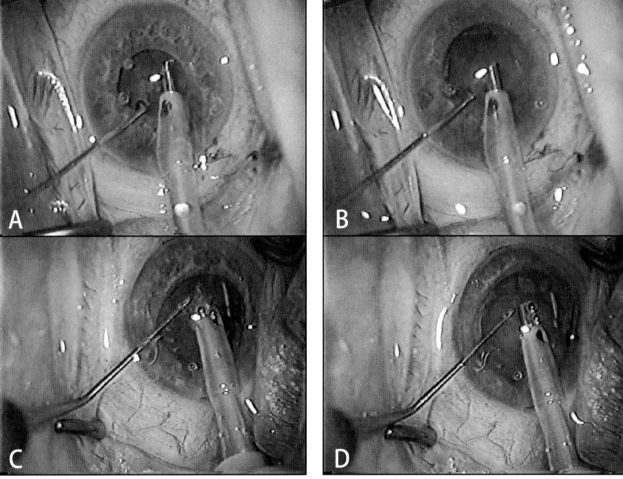

Figure 27-2. (A, B) Momentary anterior chamber and pupil expansion due to zonular dialysis caused by surge. (C, D) Second case showing the same sign.

Although resuming phaco is tempting, doing so in the presence of an occult posterior capsular defect will invariably expand the defect and increase the risk of descending retained lens material. Phaco relies on high irrigation inflow to inflate the anterior chamber. This inflow, the phaco tip, and the second instrument all approach the nucleus from above. It is because of the underlying support of the posterior capsule that this surgical system is both safe and effective. However, routine maneuvers that are safely performed above an intact capsule become potentially treacherous once the posterior capsule has ruptured.

Fluctuations in chamber depth and surgical maneuvers such as nuclear rotation, sculpting, and cracking will tend to expand any posterior capsular defect. The vitreous face may be ruptured by the infusion stream or by slight postocclusion surge that an intact capsule would have normally shielded. The downwardly directed infusion and instrumentation forces will tend to propel the nucleus posteriorly against or through the rent. The large phaco tip diameter makes it hard to selectively aspirate nucleus but not prolapsing vitreous. Therefore, the likelihood of a dropped nucleus increases the longer the capsular breach goes undetected.

At whatever point a posterior capsular defect is suspected or diagnosed, the surgeon must consider any coincident risk factors before deciding on a strategy. If only small, soft nuclear fragments remain and there is no vitreous prolapse, continuing phaco over a temporary scaffold (see the following section) may be considered. However, with a larger mass of remaining nucleus—particularly if brunescent or with concomitant pseudoexfoliation, weak zonules, a small pupil, or poor visibility—it may be prudent to convert to a large incision manual extracapsular cataract extraction (ECCE) (Figure 27-3). Because the zonular or capsular defect often remains concealed beneath the residual nucleus, the temptation to resume phaco is frequently strong. However, the best opportunity to remove the entire nucleus is before it descends through or below the posterior capsular plane.

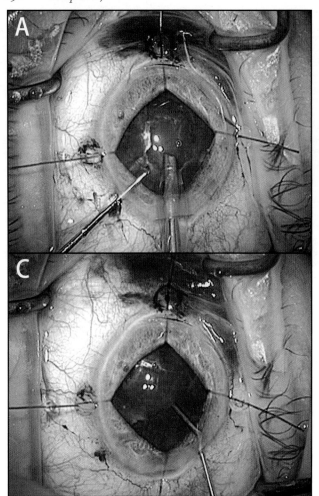
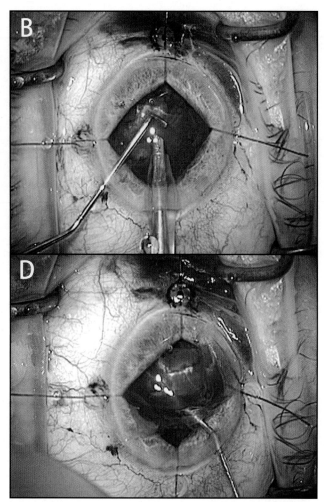

Figure 27-3. Case 2. Pseudoexfoliation with posterior capsular rupture; converted to ECCE. (A) Phacodonesis is noted during sculpting of a brunescent cataract in this eye with pseudoexfoliation. (B) Excessive lateral displacement and posterior tilting of the nucleus raises suspicion of posterior capsule rupture and zonular dialysis. (C) OVD is injected behind the nucleus for support. (D) The OVD cannula is used via the paracentesis incision to levitate the remaining nucleus into the anterior chamber.

CONVERTING TO A LARGE INCISION MANUAL EXTRACAPSULAR CATARACT EXTRACTION

When converting to a manual ECCE, it is preferable to make a new incision superiorly (see Figure 27-3E). This provides better protection for the larger incision, improves comfort because of less lid margin movement across the sutures, and avoids the irregular wound architecture associated with extending the shelved temporal clear corneal incision. The latter can be abandoned and left unsutured because it is inherently self-sealing. Creation of the new incision can usually be done under topical anesthesia supplemented with a local subconjunctival injection of lidocaine. Alternatively, a posterior sub-Tenon's injection of 2% lidocaine can be made with a curved 23-gauge blunt-tipped Simcoe cannula. Through a tiny, inferior fornix conjunctival buttonhole, the cannula is advanced alongside the globe into the posterior sub-Tenon's space (Figure 27-4). Anesthetic is slowly injected until retrograde flow causes ballooning of the inferior conjunctiva.

If the capsulorrhexis diameter is smaller than the remaining nucleus, it should be cut with one or more radial relaxing cuts along the superior margin. The large ECCE incision is made with corneal scissors following a diamond blade limbal groove (Figure 27-3E). The incision size should be generous enough to permit use of an irrigating lens loop. Because of the risk of forcibly expelling vitreous, bimanual expression should be avoided if a posterior capsular rent is present or suspected. A generous amount of dispersive OVD should be placed both behind and in front of the nucleus, and tipping up the superior pole of the nucleus with OVD facilitates sliding the lens loop beneath (Figure 27-3F and 27-3G). The irrigating lens loop is attached to a 3-mL syringe with balanced salt solution, and after it cradles the nucleus, it is withdrawn slowly like

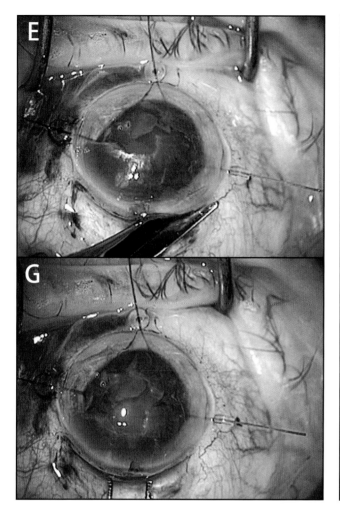

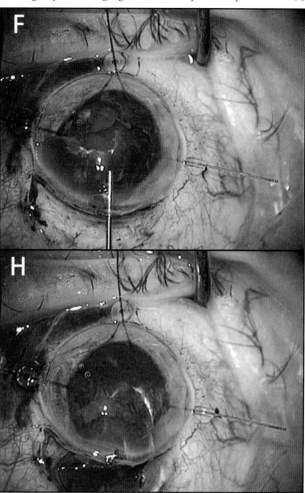

Figure 27-3 (continued). Case 2. Pseudoexfoliation with posterior capsular rupture; converted to ECCE. (E) The temporal clear corneal incision is abandoned and the microscope repositioned. A superior limbal incision is created for a manual ECCE extraction of the remaining nucleus. (F) OVD is placed above the nucleus to protect the endothelium. (G) A serrated irrigating lens loop is advanced beneath the superior pole of the nucleus. (H) The nucleus is extracted by placing pressure against the posterior lip of the incision to avoid compressing the nucleus against the corneal endothelium.

a kitchen spatula. The resistance of the incision will usually cause the nucleus to slide off. One must avoid the instinct to lift and drag the nucleus against the cornea, resulting in excessive endothelial cell loss. Instead, the backside of the lens loop should press against the posterior scleral lip of the incision (see Figure 27-3H). This counterintuitive action will generate slight posterior pressure and create a large enough gap in the incision to deliver the nucleus as the lens loop is withdrawn.

ESTABLISHING PRIORITIES

How far the nucleus initially descends through a capsular defect will depend on the vitreous anatomy. If the vitreous is too liquefied or the eye has undergone a prior vitrectomy, the nucleus will sink back to the retina too

rapidly to allow any response by the surgeon. Alternatively, the nucleus may partially descend onto an intact hyaloid face. Such slight posterior displacement can be very subtle. Finally, if the hyaloid face is ruptured, the nucleus may tip or partially descend until it is suspended and supported by formed vitreous. In these latter 2 situations, a rescue technique may be possible.

Surgeons should mentally rehearse how to manage a partially descending nucleus. In formulating a game plan one should consider the clinical consequences of several different scenarios. Understandably, the surgeon dreads having to refer a disappointed patient for additional surgery following a complication. However, assuming that a vitreoretinal colleague is not simultaneously available in the same operating suite, leaving a dropped nucleus behind is not a disastrous complication if managed properly. This does require the inconvenience of a subsequent posterior vitrectomy to remove the retained nucleus, but the outcome

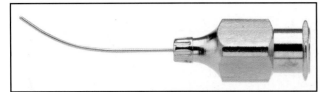

Figure 27 4. Sub Tenon's cannula for injecting anesthetic via inferior fornix conjunctival cut down. (Reprinted with permission of Katena Products.)

is generally favorable following timely referral to the vitreo-retinal surgeon.[25]

Although tempting, the worst tactic for recovering a partially descended nucleus is to try to chase and spear it with the phaco tip.[26] Lacking the normal capsular barrier, the posteriorly directed irrigation flow will flush more vitreous forward, expanding the rent and propelling the nucleus away. Attempting to emulsify or aspirate the nucleus may ensnare vitreous into the large diameter phaco tip. Applying suction and ultrasound following vitreous incarceration can produce a giant retinal tear. Regardless of the vitreoretinal surgeon's expertise, repair of a retinal detachment associated with a giant retinal tear is complicated and carries a very high risk of proliferative vitreoretinopathy.

The subsequent strategies in this chapter are considered advanced techniques and may not be appropriate for the skill set or comfort zone of many good cataract surgeons. Therefore, each individual surgeon must weigh his or her comfort and confidence in performing these maneuvers against the very acceptable option of allowing the nucleus to drop. In this case, no one would criticize a surgeon for simply closing the eye following an anterior vitrectomy and implantation of an IOL, prior to referral to a vitreoretinal colleague.

WHICH OPHTHALMIC VISCOSURGICAL DEVICE?

The varied properties and types of OVDs beg the question: which agent is best for managing use following posterior capsular rupture? Dispersive agents, such as Viscoat or sodium hyaluronate 3% (Healon EndoCoat), are very retentive. They better resist aspiration and are less apt to be burped out of the eye with slight pressure at the incision site. These properties make dispersive OVDs ideal following posterior capsule rupture, where the objective may be to block a zonular defect, partition space, or to support lens material on the verge of descending. Of course, when one needs to quickly inflate the anterior chamber prior to removing the phaco tip, whatever OVD is on the instrument tray should be used.

At the conclusion of surgery, one should not aggressively aspirate the OVD in the posterior chamber if the capsule

is ruptured, particularly if the vitreous face is intact. Fortunately, the smaller size and molecular weight of dispersive agents makes a prolonged and protracted pressure spike less likely when small quantities are retained.[27-29] The inability to aggressively and thoroughly aspirate OVD in the posterior chamber is a significant drawback to choosing maximally cohesive agents, such as sodium hyaluronate 2.3% (Healon 5) or sodium hyaluronate 1.4% (Healon GV) in the setting of posterior capsular rupture. Because of their larger molecular weight, residual amounts of these agents will produce the most severe and most prolonged pressure spikes.[27-30] In the presence of any posterior capsular or zonular defect, it is generally safer to first constrict the pupil with acetylcholine chloride (Miochol-E) prior to aspirating OVD in the anterior chamber.

RESCUING A PARTIALLY DESCENDED NUCLEUS—THE VISCOAT POSTERIOR-ASSISTED LEVITATION TECHNIQUE

If one elects to retrieve a partially descended nucleus, a safer alternative to aspirating it with the phaco tip is to elevate the nucleus into the pupillary plane or anterior chamber from below. It may be possible to inject OVD beneath the nucleus via a limbal incision (see Figures 27-3C and 27-3D). There may be several obstacles to accomplishing this, however. First, the pupil or capsulorrhexis diameter may be quite small (and which may have predisposed the eye to capsular rupture in the first place). A small pupil or capsulorrhexis can impede elevation of a large nucleus and make it particularly difficult for an OVD cannula to maneuver behind it. Prolapsed vitreous will further hinder such attempts to inject OVD beneath the nucleus. The nucleus may suddenly sink if these maneuvers induce further vitreous loss and prolapse.

Charles Kelman, MD popularized the posterior-assisted levitation, or "PAL" technique, in which a metal spatula, inserted through a pars plana sclerotomy, is used to levitate the nucleus into the anterior chamber from below.[31-37] Compared to the phaco incision, a pars plana sclerotomy provides a much better instrument angle for getting behind the lens. Richard B. Packard, MD, FRCS and this author subsequently published the results of using Viscoat and the Viscoat cannula to support and levitate the nucleus—the so-called Viscoat PAL technique[32] (Figures 27-5 to 27-9). The authors specifically recommended Viscoat because it is a dispersive agent and it is packaged with the narrowest gauge cannula.

After opening the conjunctiva and applying light cautery, a disposable microvitreoretinal (MVR) blade (Alcon Laboratories, Fort Worth, TX; Katena Eye Instruments, Denville, NJ) is used to make a pars plana sclerotomy located 3.5 mm behind the limbus (see Figures 27-5A,

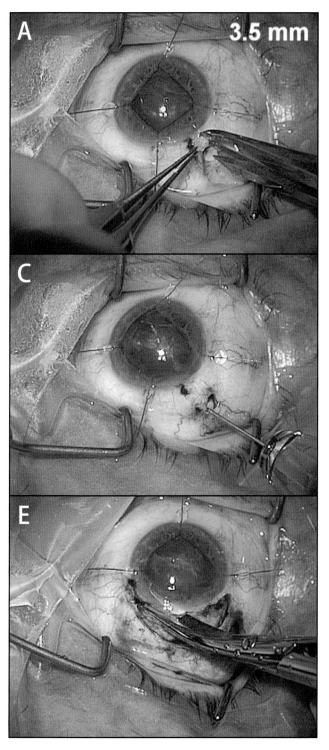

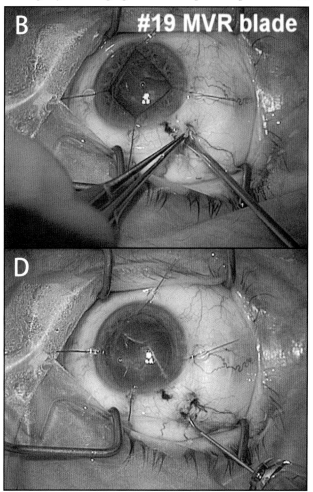

Figure 27-5. Case 3. Viscoat PAL with anterior chamber IOL. Because of excessive nuclear movement, the microscope has been repositioned in order to convert to a manual ECCE. (A) Calipers are used to locate the site for a pars plana sclerotomy 3.5 mm posterior to the limbus in an oblique quadrant. (B) A pars plana sclerotomy is made with a #19 disposable MVR blade. (C, D) With the Viscoat PAL technique, the OVD cannula is used to elevate the nucleus into the anterior chamber. (E) After removing the superior iris retractor, a generous superior limbal incision is made with corneal scissors.

27-5B, and 27-6A). An oblique quadrant should be selected, and these steps can be performed under topical anesthesia. The Viscoat cannula is then advanced and aimed behind the nucleus under direct visualization. The first step is to inject a bolus of dispersive OVD behind the nucleus to provide immediate supplemental support (see Figure 27-8). Periodic palpation of the globe confirms that over inflation has not occurred.

If the nucleus is subluxated laterally, directing OVD toward the region beneath it will often buoy the nucleus toward a more central position. This is preferable to blindly probing with a metal spatula. One should not attempt to float the nucleus into the anterior chamber using a massive infusion of OVD alone. Unlike using liquid perfluorocarbon in a vitrectomized cavity, an excessive injection of OVD may over-inflate the globe and cause vitreous expulsion through the sclerotomy.

Instead, the cannula tip itself should be used to mechanically prop and levitate the nucleus into the anterior chamber (see Figures 27-5C-D, 27-6B-C, and 27-9). Small aliquots of additional OVD can be injected to help in the

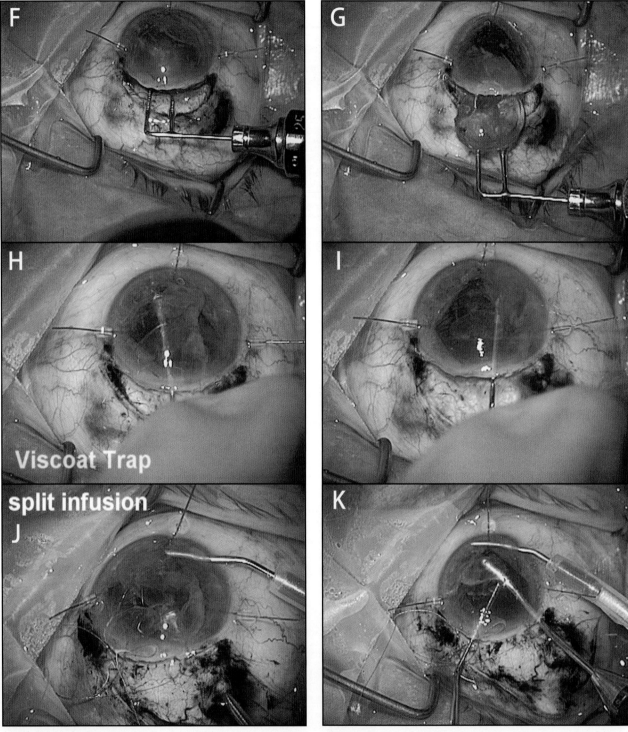

Figure 27-5 (continued). Case 3. Viscoat PAL with anterior chamber IOL. Because of excessive nuclear movement, the microscope has been repositioned in order to convert to a manual ECCE. (F, G) Serrated irrigating lens loop is used to extract the nucleus manually. (H, I) Residual epinucleus is elevated toward the cornea and suspended with Viscoat, which is used to fill the anterior chamber. (J) Pars plana anterior vitrectomy is performed with separate split infusion via a limbal self-retaining cannula inferiorly. Residual epinucleus is removed with bimanual I/A instrumentation. (K) A Lester hook is poised to stuff the epinucleus into the 0.3-mm aspirating port.

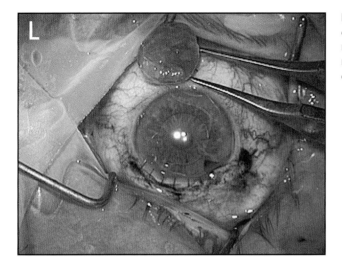

Figure 27-5 (continued). Case 3. Viscoat PAL with anterior chamber IOL. Because of excessive nuclear movement, the microscope has been repositioned in order to convert to a manual ECCE. (L) Anterior chamber IOL is placed following pupil constriction with Miochol-E and a peripheral iridectomy.

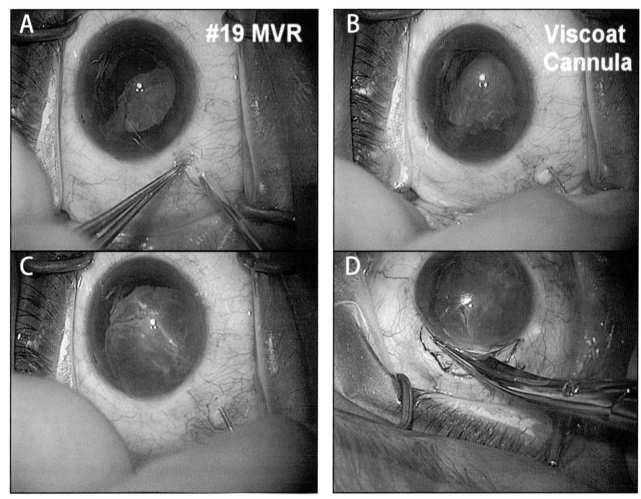

Figure 27-6. Case 4. Viscoat PAL with posterior chamber IOL. (A) Following posterior capsule rupture with a large heminucleus present, a pars plana sclerotomy is made with a #19 disposable MVR blade 3.5 mm behind the limbus under topical anesthesia. (B) Viscoat is injected behind the nucleus to support it and the tip is used to manipulate the lens fragment. (C) The Viscoat cannula tip is used to elevate the nucleus into the anterior chamber. (D) The microscope is repositioned and a superior limbal incision is made for manual extraction.

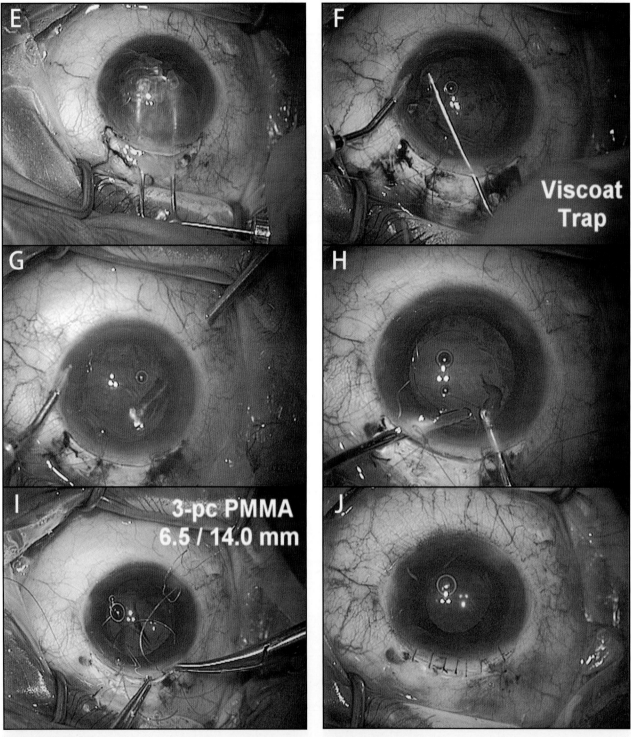

Figure 27-6 (continued). Case 4. Viscoat PAL with posterior chamber IOL. (E) Serrated irrigating lens loop is used to extract the nucleus manually. (F) Viscoat Trap is used to suspend lens fragment against the cornea. (G) Bimanual anterior vitrectomy is performed through the pars plana sclerotomy, along with split infusion via a limbal self-retaining cannula. The incision has been partially closed with 2 interrupted 8-0 Vicryl sutures. (H) Bimanual I/A instrumentation is used to remove the cortex. Capsulorrhexis remains intact. (I) Three-piece PMMA IOL (6.5 mm; 14.0 mm overall length) is inserted into the ciliary sulcus. (J) Incision is closed with interrupted 10-0 nylon sutures.

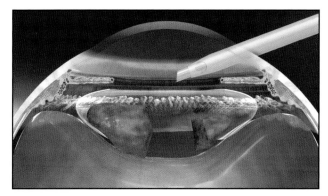

Figure 27-7. Chopped nuclear fragments partially descend onto the vitreous face following posterior capsular rupture.

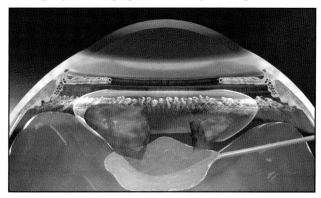

Figure 27-8. Viscoat is injected via a pars plana sclerotomy behind the descending nuclear fragments to provide immediate supplemental support.

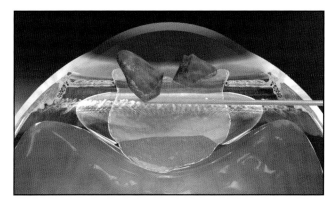

Figure 27-9. The Viscoat cannula is used to carefully lift the fragments into the anterior chamber.

elevation and maneuvering of the nucleus. A small capsulorrhexis or pupil will stretch to accommodate the levitation of a greater diameter nucleus. Using dispersive OVD to first support and reposition the nucleus prior to definitive manual levitation is the major advantage of the Viscoat PAL variation. Because there is no aspiration involved, these PAL maneuvers should minimize iatrogenic vitreous traction and reduce the chance of touching the retina with a metal spatula tip.

Once a fragment descends into the mid- or posterior vitreous cavity, it is dangerous to blindly fish for it with any instrument. One should abandon the dropped nucleus and concentrate on removing the residual epinucleus and cortex while preserving as much capsular support as possible. A thorough anterior vitrectomy must be performed prior to inserting the IOL. Since the vitreoretinal surgeon will later use a 3-port fragmatome and vitrectomy technique to remove any retained nucleus, it is preferable to insert an IOL through the cataract incision during the initial surgery, if possible.

Managing Posterior Capsule Rupture and Residual Lens Material—Nuclear Scaffold

Any residual nucleus retrieved with the Viscoat PAL technique can be removed using 1 of 2 techniques: resuming phaco over a temporary scaffold (eg, Sheet's glide or the Agarwal 3-piece IOL technique), or converting to a large incision manual ECCE. If the remaining nucleus or fragments can be elevated into the anterior chamber with a dispersive OVD, one can consider inserting a scaffold to serve as an artificial posterior capsule. Marc A. Michelson, MD first described using a trimmed Sheet's glide through the phaco incision to serve as a temporary scaffold to prevent lens material from dropping posteriorly.[38] Use of a scaffold will also shield the phaco tip from aspirating vitreous from below. The incision should be widened slightly to accommodate the phaco tip above and alongside the glide. Maneuvers made with the phaco tip should be minimized to avoid simultaneously moving the glide.

More recently, Kumar and Agarwal described using a 3-piece foldable IOL as a temporary scaffold, particularly if the capsulorrhexis is intact.[39] After the nuclear material is first elevated into the anterior chamber, the foldable IOL is injected and the optic is allowed to open beneath the residual nucleus. The lead haptic can be positioned over the nasal iris or an intact capsulorrhexis and the trailing haptic is kept protruding through the clear corneal incision. Phaco can now be resumed above the IOL optic, which provides the desired barrier between the vitreous cavity and the residual lens material. Because nuclear scaffold techniques require the surgeon to perform anterior chamber phaco, the size and density of the nucleus must be considered prior to

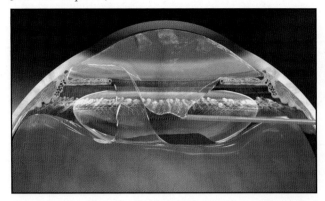

Figure 27-10. Following anterior vitreous prolapse, the residual lens fragments are elevated toward the cornea where they are trapped by filling the anterior chamber with Viscoat.

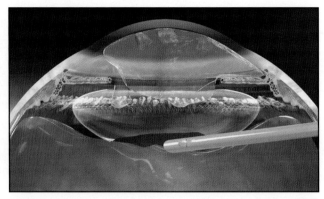

Figure 27-11. The sleeveless vitrectomy cutter is introduced via a pars plana sclerotomy and is kept behind the plane of the capsulorrhexis and pupil. This severs the transpupillary bands but keeps the vitrectomy separated from the partitioned anterior chamber. The self-retaining infusion cannula (not shown) is placed through a limbal stab incision.

using these strategies. One should also readjust the phaco machine parameters. Lowering the irrigating bottle height slightly and reducing the aspiration flow rate (eg, to 20 to 22 cc/min) will slow the pace down. The vacuum should be decreased (eg, 100 to 125 mm Hg) in order to eliminate the degree of postocclusion surge.

MANAGING VITREOUS LOSS AND RESIDUAL LENS MATERIAL—THE "VISCOAT TRAP"

At some point during this sequence, the phaco or irrigation/aspiration (I/A) tip may ensnare prolapsing vitreous. To avoid vitreous traction, the surgeon must stop to perform an anterior vitrectomy before extraction of the remaining lens material can be resumed. The most common practice is to place a separate self-retaining irrigating cannula though a limbal paracentesis and to insert the vitrectomy probe through the phaco incision. However, there are multiple drawbacks to this approach. First, the phaco incision is too large for the sleeveless vitrectomy instrument. This leaking incision affords poor chamber stability and allows both irrigation fluid and vitreous to prolapse externally alongside the vitrector shaft. Second, performing the vitrectomy in the anterior chamber will tend to draw more posteriorly located vitreous forward. Finally, as more and more vitreous exits the eye through either the cutting instrument or the incision, the residual lens material that it was supporting will sink down toward the retina. It bears repeating that once the posterior capsule is open, it is the vitreous that is preventing the remaining nucleus and epinucleus from descending.

This author has proposed a strategy called the *Viscoat Trap* which, when combined with a pars plana anterior vitrectomy, can prevent this undesirable chain of events.[33] The first step is to use a dispersive OVD (such as Viscoat

or Healon EndoCoat) to levitate any mobile lens fragments up toward the cornea (Figure 27-5H-I and Figure 27-6F). Next, one completely fills the anterior chamber with OVD (Figure 27-10). Even though vitreous has already prolapsed forward, injecting OVD should not exert traction on the retina. The dispersive OVD can now support and trap the residual lens material in the anterior chamber as the vitreous is excised from below.

The Viscoat Trap is so named because of the need to employ a dispersive OVD. To effectively "trap" lens material, the OVD should be maximally retentive so that it is less easily burped out of the eye through incisional manipulation. In addition, dispersive OVDs better resist aspiration by a nearby I/A or vitrectomy port. Finally, the smaller size and molecular weight of dispersive agents makes a prolonged and protracted pressure spike less likely when small amounts are retained.[27-30]

BIMANUAL PARS PLANA ANTERIOR VITRECTOMY

Vitreoretinal specialists typically enter the pars plana 3.0 mm behind the limbus with the MVR blade oriented perpendicularly to the scleral surface (Figure 27-11). However, because the anterior segment surgeon orients the MVR blade tangentially and aims toward the posterior chamber, an entry site 3.5 mm posterior to the limbus is appropriate (Figure 27-12C). A disposable #19 MVR blade will create an adequately sized opening for most anterior vitrectomy cutters and should be advanced until it is visualized through the pupil (Figure 27-12D). This maneuver can be performed under topical anesthesia. As described by Scott E. Burk, MD, PhD, staining prolapsed vitreous with a triamcinolone suspension to improve visibility is an option.

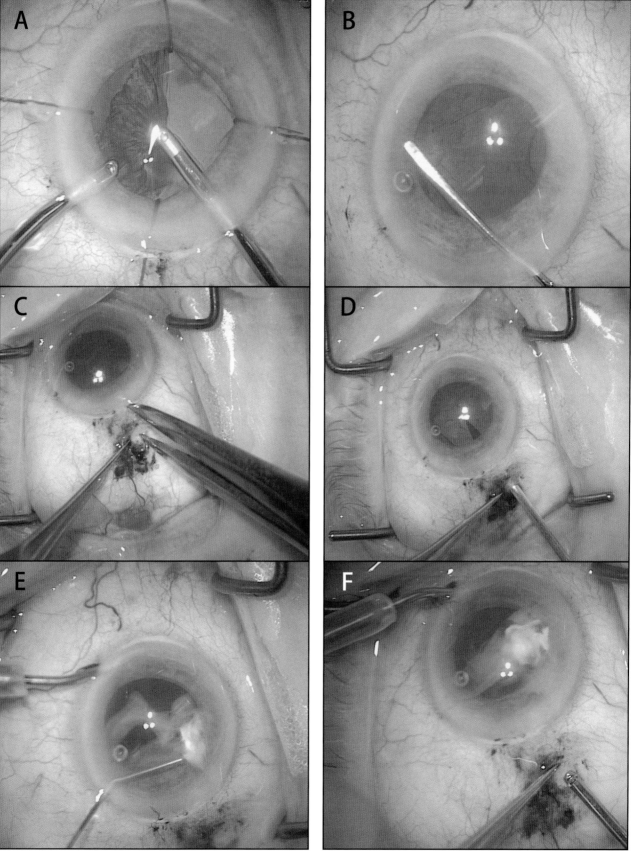

Figure 27-12. Case 5. (A) There are virtually no intact zonules in this eye with pseudoexfoliation. (B) Vitreous prolapse through a large zonular dialysis is noted. (C) A pars plana sclerotomy is made 3.5 mm behind the limbus (D) with a #19 disposable MVR blade angled toward the center of the pupil. (E) Triamcinolone is used to stain the prolapsing vitreous. (F) With a split, self-retaining limbal infusion cannula, the sleeveless vitrectomy tip is introduced through the sclerotomy.

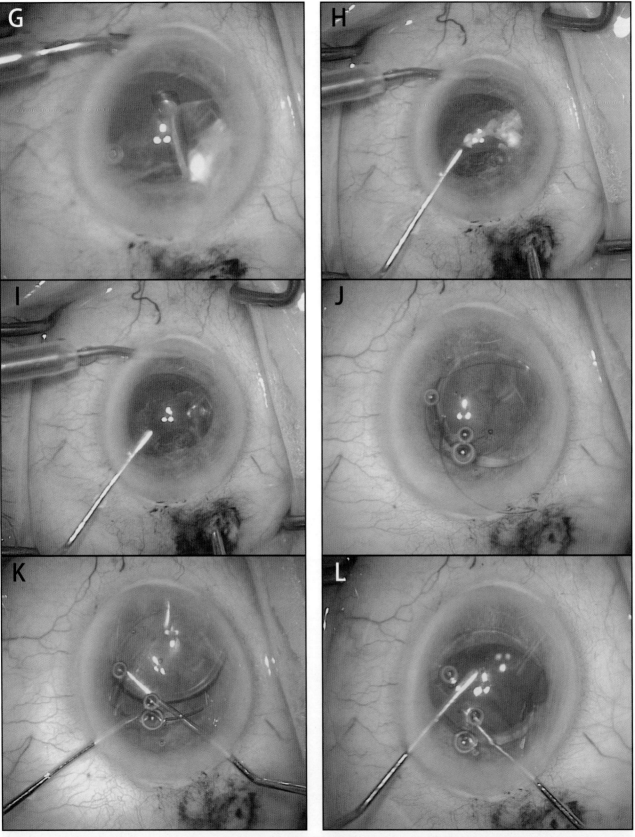

Figure 27-12 (continued). Case 5. (G) Using a high cutting rate, the tip is kept anterior enough to be visualized through the microscope. (H, I) The prolapsed vitreous is pulled back into the vitreous cavity, rather than forward and toward a corneal incision. (J) After removing the entire capsular bag, the IOL optic is unfolded in the anterior chamber with one haptic in the posterior chamber. (K) The second haptic is placed behind the iris (L) while keeping one hook behind the optic to prevent it from falling back.

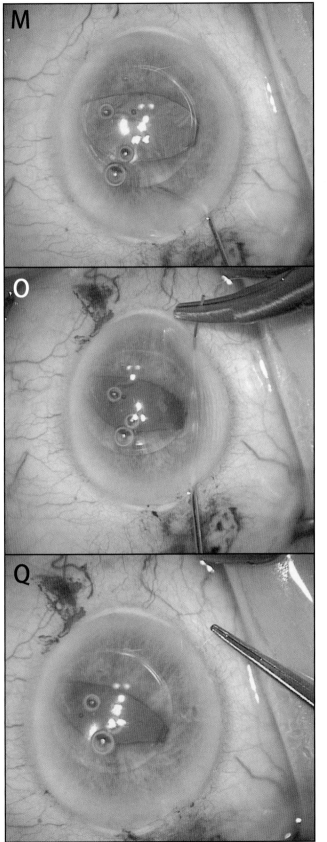

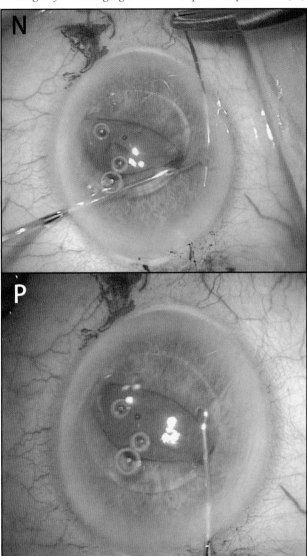

Figure 27-12 (continued). Case 5. (M) Miochol-E constricts the pupil to maintain optic capture. (N) A 10-0 Prolene suture on a curved CIF needle is used to snare one haptic for a McCannel suture. Lifting the optic-haptic junction with a hook elevates the haptic into the iris stroma. (O) The OVD cannula is used to guide the CIF needle out through a paracentesis site. (P) A Jaffe-Knolle hook (Katena Eye Instruments, Denville, NJ) pulls the distal suture through the same paracentesis site. (Q) A Siepser sliding slip knot is placed by pulling the opposite ends of the suture.

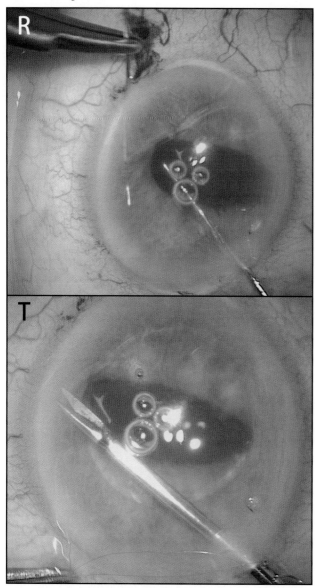

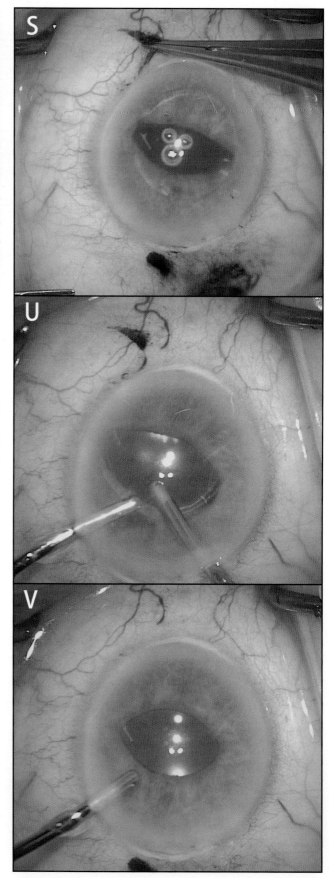

Figure 27-12 (continued). Case 5. (R, S) The steps are repeated for the second haptic. (T) The knot is trimmed intracamerally with intraocular microscissors. (U) During bimanual I/A removal of the OVD, the optic is reposited behind the iris (V) leaving a pupil that is slightly peaked by the 2 knots.

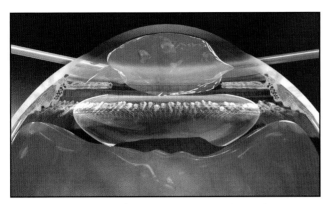

Figure 27-13. Bimanual I/A instrumentation is used to remove residual cortex following the anterior vitrectomy.

However, the author finds that it is usually unnecessary in the presence of retained lens material unless there is vitreous prolapsing through a zonular dialysis (Figure 27-12E).[39] A self-retaining irrigating cannula is placed through an angled limbal paracentesis and directed away from the pupil (Figure 27-12F). The sleeveless vitrectomy shaft is inserted through the pars plana sclerotomy until the tip can be visualized in the retropupillary space (see Figure 27-5J, 27-6G, and 27-12F-I). If it does not pass through the incision easily, it is important to slightly enlarge the opening rather than to force entry.

Utilizing low flow and vacuum settings (and as high a cutting rate as possible to minimize vitreous traction), a thorough anterior vitrectomy is performed. One should focus posteriorly enough with the microscope to keep the tip under direct visualization at all times. One should attempt to keep the vitrectomy tip behind the plane of the pupil if possible. While any transpupillary bands of vitreous will still be severed, this will avoid removing the dispersive OVD that fills the anterior chamber (see Figure 27-11). When properly performed, one will see that the anteriorly trapped lens fragments remain immobilized as the vitrectomy is being carried out from below (see Figure 27-5J). This is because 2 separate chambers have been formed by the OVD partition, such that the anterior chamber is isolated from the vitrectomized posterior chamber.

Using a pars plana sclerotomy is an under-utilized option when performing an anterior vitrectomy. The principles of anterior vitrectomy technique are the same—one must not aspirate vitreous without cutting it, one should keep the vitrectomy tip under direct microscopic visualization, and one should not attempt to retrieve lens material that is in the posterior vitreous cavity. The main advantage is that using a properly sized sclerotomy will decrease incisional leak and vitreous prolapse and should provide a better fluidic seal. Unlike with a limbal incision, the vitrector need not traverse the anterior chamber and disrupt the Viscoat partition; it will not draw more vitreous forward into the anterior chamber (see Figures 27-12H and 27-12I). Performing the vitrectomy posterior to the plane of the pupil and capsulorrhexis also decreases the chance of inadvertently cutting either structure. If the capsulorrhexis is preserved, a foldable posterior chamber IOL may still be implanted in the ciliary sulcus. The sclerotomy can be closed with a single interrupted 8-0 Vicryl suture.

Following the retropupillary anterior vitrectomy, one can resume aspiration of the remaining cortex or epinucleus trapped in the Viscoat-filled anterior chamber (Figure 27-13). Once the capsule or zonules have ruptured, bimanual I/A instrumentation is ideal for epinuclear and cortical extraction for several reasons (see Figure 27-5K and Figure 27-6H). The absence of an infusion sleeve permits placement of the aspirating tip as far peripherally as is necessary to preferentially block the 0.3 mm opening with cortex. Access to subincisional cortex is improved. The tighter paracentesis incisions better restrain vitreous from prolapsing compared to using the phaco incision. Finally, this is a lower flow fluidic system compared to coaxial I/A. This permits the surgeon to work in "slow motion" by lowering the irrigation bottle and decreasing the aspiration flow and vacuum settings. If the aspirating ports again become entangled with vitreous, one can repeat the Viscoat Trap maneuver followed by additional pars plana anterior vitrectomy. Bimanual cortical I/A can then be resumed.

EMERGENCY PREPAREDNESS

Posterior capsule rupture and vitreous loss necessitates a stressful departure from the surgical routine for both surgeons and their staff in the operating room. Anticipating these difficulties, one can prepare for this contingency in several ways. First, one can assign a machine memory setting to preprogram parameters for an "emergency." These might include a decreased bottle height, aspiration flow rate (20 to 22 cc/min), and vacuum limit (100 to 125 mm Hg). This can avoid the need for nursing personnel to urgently and manually adjust the settings in the face of posterior capsule rupture.

Second, as advocated by Louis D. "Skip" Nichamin, MD and this author, the OR can prepackage special instruments in a "contingency" kit that is kept sterile in a separate, autoclavable container. This avoids the need to urgently search for a seldom-used instrument amidst the stress of an unexpectedly complicated procedure. Based on the scenarios discussed in this chapter for converting to an ECCE or performing a vitrectomy, one might choose to collect a sub-Tenon's cannula, corneal scissors, an irrigating lens loop, a self-retaining limbal infusion cannula, and a bimanual I/A handpiece set. This author has arranged for such a "contingency" set to be commercially available (Chang Contingency Kit, Katena Products) (Figure 27-14). Vitrectomy instrumentation, disposable MVR blades,

Sheet's glides, triamcinolone, and larger syringes of dispersive OVDs—such as Viscoat or Healon EndoCoat—should also be available in the room.

CONCLUSION

Posterior capsule rupture with nucleus present is a precipitous and intimidating complication that tests a surgeon's ability to operate under pressure. Cautious adherence to these principles will reduce the chance of dropping the nucleus following posterior capsular rupture. However, there is a potentially fine line dividing maneuvers that are reasonable and safe from those that are overly aggressive or dangerous. Cataract surgeons must be honest in assessing their own level of comfort and expertise. Timely surgical management of a dropped nucleus by a vitreoretinal surgeon at a later date is always preferable to overstepping this fine line.[37] Many surgeons will not be comfortable using the PAL technique or a pars plana sclerotomy for the anterior vitrectomy. Other surgeons may not be comfortable or experienced enough to convert to a manual ECCE. It is perfectly acceptable to insert an IOL following an anterior vitrectomy and to leave all residual lens material behind to be removed later by a vitreoretinal specialist.

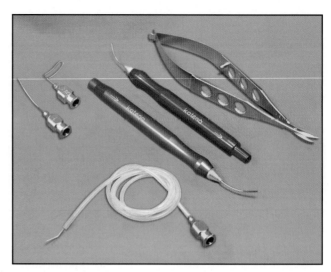

Figure 27-14. Chang Contingency Kit. (Reprinted with permission of Katena Products.)

REFERENCES

1. Desai P, Minassian DC, Reidy A. National cataract surgery survey 1997-1998: a report of the results of the clinical outcomes. *Br J Ophthalmol.* 1999;83:1336–1340.
2. Martin KR, Burton RL. The phacoemulsification learning curve: per-operative complications in the first 3000 cases of an experienced surgeon. *Eye.* 2000;;14(Pt 2):190-195.
3. Lundström M, Barry P, Leite E, Seward H, Stenevi U. 1998 European Cataract Outcome Study: report from the European Cataract Outcome Study Group. *J Cataract Refract Surg.* 2001;27:1176–1184.
4. Ionides A, Minassian D, Tuft S. Visual outcome following posterior capsule rupture during cataract surgery. *Br J Ophthalmol.* 2001;85:222-224.
5. Gimbel HV, Sun R, Ferensowicz M, Anderson Penno E, Kamal A. Intraoperative management of posterior capsule tears in phacoemulsification and intraocular lens implantation. *Ophthalmology.* 2001;108:2186–2189; discussion, 2190–2192.
6. Tan JHY, Karwatowski WSS. Phacoemulsification cataract surgery and unplanned anterior vitrectomy: is it bad news? *Eye.* 2002;16:117–120.
7. Chan FM, Mathur R, Ku JJ, et al. Short-term outcomes in eyes with posterior capsule rupture during cataract surgery. *J Cataract Refract Surg.* 2003;29:537-541.
8. Androudi S, Brazitikos PD, Papadopoulos NT, Dereklis D, Symeon L, Stangos N. Posterior capsule rupture and vitreous loss during phacoemulsification with or without the use of an anterior chamber maintainer. *J Cataract Refract Surg.* 2004;30:449-452.
9. Hyams M, Mathalone N, Herskovitz M, Hod Y, Israeli D, Geyer O. Intraoperative complications of phacoemulsification in eyes with and without pseudoexfoliation. *J Cataract Refract Surg.* 2005;31:1002-1005.
10. Ang GS, Whyte IF. Effect and outcomes of posterior capsule rupture in a district general hospital setting. *J Cataract Refract Surg.* 2006;32:623-627.
11. Zaidi FH, Corbett MC, Burton BJ, Bloom PA. Raising the benchmark for the 21st century--the 1000 cataract operations audit and survey: outcomes, consultant-supervised training and sourcing NHS choice. *Br J Ophthalmol.* 2007;91:731-736.
12. Mearza AA, Ramanathan S, Bidgood P, Horgan S. Visual outcome in cataract surgery complicated by vitreous loss in a district general hospital. *Int Ophthalmol.* 2009;29:157-160.
13. Agrawal V, Upadhyay J. Indian Cataract Risk Stratification Study group. Validation of scoring system for preoperative stratification of intra-operative risks of complications during cataract surgery: Indian multi-centric study. *Indian J Ophthalmol.* 2009;57:213-215.
14. Blomquist PH, Rugwani RM. Visual outcomes after vitreous loss during cataract surgery performed by residents. *J Cataract Refract Surg.* 2002;28:847-852.
15. Dooley IJ, O'Brien PD. Subjective difficulty of each stage of phacoemulsification cataract surgery performed by basic surgical trainees. *J Cataract Refract Surg.* 2006;32(4):604-608.
16. Bhagat N, Nissirios N, Potdevin L, et al. Complications in resident performed phacoemulsification cataract surgery at New Jersey Medical School. *Br J Ophthalmol.* 2007;91:1315–1317.
17. Pot MC, Stilma JS. Low complication rate with cataract operations carried out by registrars in ophthalmology. *Ned Tijdschr Geneeskd.* 2008;8;152(10):563-568.
18. Rutar T, Porco TC, Naseri A. Risk factors for intraoperative complications in resident-performed phacoemulsification surgery. *Ophthalmology.* 2009;116:431-436.
19. Lee JS, Hou CH, Yang ML, Kuo JZ, Lin KK. A different approach to assess resident phacoemulsification learning curve: analysis of both completion and complication rates. *Eye.* 2009;23:683-687.
20. Carricondo PC, Fortes AC, Mourao Pde C, Hajnal M, Jose NK. Senior resident phacoemulsification learning curve (corrected from cure). *Arq Bras Oftalmol.* 2010;73:66-69.
21. Blomquist PH, Sargent JW, Winslow HH. Validation of Najjar-Awwad cataract surgery risk score for resident phacoemulsification surgery. *J Cataract Refract Surg.* 2010;36:1753-1757.
22. Narendran N, Jaycock P, Johnston RL, et al. The Cataract National Dataset electronic multicentre audit of 55,567 operations: risk stratification for posterior capsule rupture and vitreous loss. *Eye* (Lond). 2009;23(1):31-37.

23. Greenberg PB, Tseng VL, Wu WC, et al. Prevalence and predictors of ocular complications associated with cataract surgery in United States Veterans. *Ophthalmology.* 2011;118(3):507-514.

24. Lundstrom M, Behndig A, Kugelberg M, et al. Decreasing rate of capsule complications in cataract surgery. *J Cataract Refract Surg.* 2011;37:1762-1767.

25. Scott IU, Flynn HW Jr, Smiddy WE, et al. Clinical features and outcomes of pars plana vitrectomy in patients with retained lens fragments. *Ophthalmology.* 2003;110:1567-1572.

26. Lu H, Jiang YR, Grabow HB. Managing a dropped nucleus during the phacoemulsification learning curve. *J Cataract Refract Surg.* 1999;25:1311-1312.

27. Burke S, Sugar J, Farber MD. Comparison of the effects of two viscoelastic agents, Healon and Viscoat, on postoperative intraocular pressure after penetrating keratoplasty. *Ophthalmic Surg.* 1990;21:821-826.

28. Probst LE, Hakim OJ, Nichols BD. Phacoemulsification with aspirated or retained Viscoat. *J Cataract Refract Surg.* 1994;20:145-149.

29. Torngren L, Lundgren B, Madsen K. Intraocular pressure development in the rabbit eye after aqueous exchange with ophthalmic viscosurgical devices. *J Cataract Refract Surg.* 2000;26:1247-1252.

30. Sihota R, Saxena R, Agarwal HC. Intravitreal sodium hyaluronate and secondary glaurcoma after complicated phacoemulsification. *J Cataract Refract Surg.* 2003;29:1226-1227.

31. Kelman C. New PAL method may save difficult cataract cases. *Ophthalmology Times.* 1994;19:51.

32. Chang DF, Packard RB. Posterior assisted levitation for nucleus retrieval using Viscoat after posterior capsule rupture. *J Cataract Refract Surg.* 2003;29:1860-1865.

33. Chang DF. Managing residual lens material after posterior capsule rupture. *Techniques in Ophthalmology.* 2003;1(4):201-206.

34. Lifshitz T, Levy J. Posterior assisted levitation: long-term follow-up data. *J Cataract Refract Surg.* 2005;31:499-502.

35. Por YM, Chee SP. Posterior-assisted levitation: outcomes in the retrieval of nuclear fragments and subluxated intraocular lenses. *J Cataract Refract Surg.* 2006;32:2060-2063.

36. Schutz JS, Mavrakanas NA. Posterior-assisted levitation in cataract surgery. *Curr Opin Ophthalmol.* 2010;21:50-54.

37. Arbisser LB, Charles S, Howcroft M, Werner L. Management of vitreous loss and dropped nucleus during cataract surgery. *Ophthalmol Clin North Am.* 2006;19(4):495-506. Review.

38. Michelson MA. Use of a Sheets' glide as a pseudoposterior capsule in phacoemulsification complicated by posterior capsule rupture. *Eur J Implant Surg.* 1993;570-572.

39. Kumar DA, Agarwal A, Prakash G, Jacob S, Agarwal A, Sivagnanam S. IOL Scaffold technique for posterior capsular rupture. *J Refract Surg.* 2012;28(5):314-315.

40. Burk SE, Da Mata AP, Snyder ME, et al. Visualizing vitreous using Kenalog suspension. *J Cataract Refract Surg.* 2003;29:645-651.

**Please see companion narrated videos on the accompanying Web site at
www.Healio.com/phacochopvideos**

28

Intraocular Lens Implantation Following Posterior Capsule Rupture

David F. Chang, MD

The management of posterior capsular rupture and vitreous loss was discussed in the preceding chapter. Following posterior capsular rupture, there may be a number of potential options for intraocular lens (IOL) fixation. These will depend on the size and location of the capsular or zonular defect and the type of IOL contemplated. Even if the patient will require a subsequent vitreoretinal procedure for a dropped nucleus, it is generally permissible to implant an IOL following a thorough anterior vitrectomy. This chapter will discuss a variety of scenarios and options.

SMALL POSTERIOR CAPSULAR DEFECT

It still may be feasible to place a single-piece hydrophobic acrylic IOL in the capsular bag if there is a small posterior capsular rent which does not extend to the periphery. It may be possible to avoid extending the capsular rent during IOL implantation because the single-piece haptics open so gradually, which permits some IOL rotation prior to their full extension. The same is generally not true for 3-piece foldable IOLs, whose stiff haptics will rapidly extend any noncircular rent as the IOL is rotated into position.

As conceived by Howard V. Gimbel, MD, MPH, FRCSC, FACS, a posterior capsulorrhexis can be considered if the capsular rent is localized without peripheral extension[1] (Figures 28-1 and 28-2). A dispersive ophthalmic viscosurgical device (OVD) should be placed anterior and posterior to the rent to help immobilize it and to displace the hyaloid face posteriorly. Because the retrocapsular OVD will not be aspirated out, a dispersive agent is less likely to cause a protracted intraocular pressure (IOP) elevation. Locating a free capsule flap is not always possible, but the capsule forceps can grasp one edge of the defect in an attempt to round it off. Because the posterior capsule is so thin, it behaves with the characteristic elasticity of a pediatric anterior capsule. This makes it difficult to control the progression of the advancing tear unless the Brian Little Tear Out Rescue Maneuver is employed.[2] The advantage of a posterior capsulorrhexis is the ability to securely fixate a single or 3-piece IOL within the capsular bag (see Figures 28-1G and 28-2G).

POSTERIOR CAPSULE DEFECT WITH INTACT CAPSULORRHEXIS

If the capsulorrhexis is intact and of an appropriate diameter, a 3-piece foldable or nonfoldable posterior

Chang DF.
*Phaco Chop and Advanced Phaco Techniques: Strategies for
Complicated Cataracts, Second Edition* (pp 309-329).
© 2013 SLACK Incorporated.

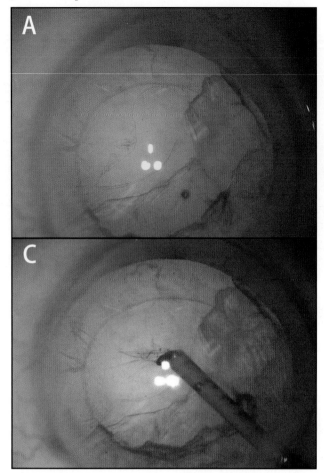

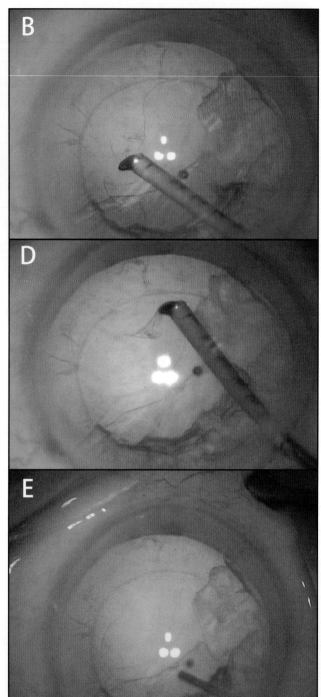

Figure 28-1. Case 1. (A) This posterior capsular tear without vitreous prolapse became visible during the cortical clean-up. (B) Seibel capsulorrhexis forceps (MicroSurgical Technology [MST], Redmond, WA) have the advantage of fitting through a paracentesis incision. (C-E) By grasping one edge of the torn posterior capsule, the tear is rounded off.

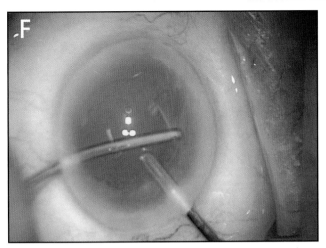
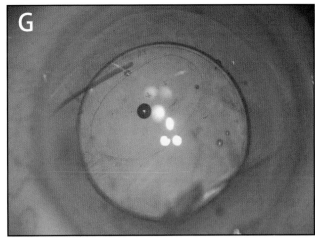

Figure 28-1 (continued). Case 1. (F) The posterior continuous curvilinear capsulotomy prevents extension of the posterior capsule defect during cortical I/A. (G) A 3-piece foldable IOL has been placed within the capsular bag and the optic blocks the posterior capsulorrhexis opening.

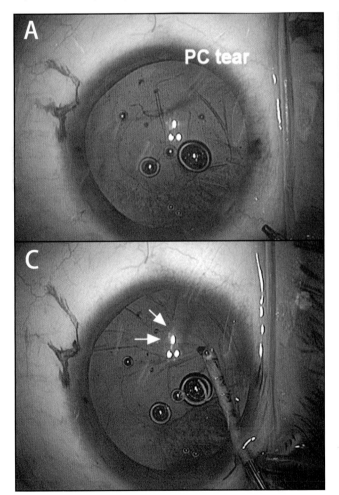
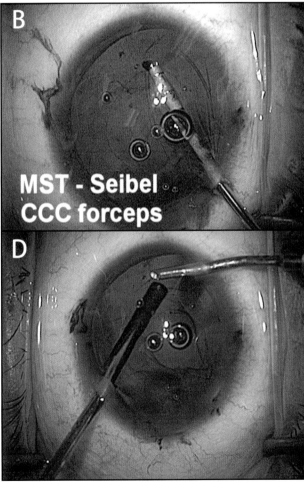

Figure 28-2. Case 2. (A) This posterior capsular tear without vitreous prolapse became visible during the cortical clean-up. (B, C) By grasping one edge of the torn posterior capsule with MST Seibel capsule forceps, the tear is rounded off (arrows show the curvilinear edge of the tear). (D) A biaxial anterior vitrectomy is performed through a limbal incision with a separate self-retaining infusion cannula. Because of the posterior capsulorrhexis, the rent does not expand.

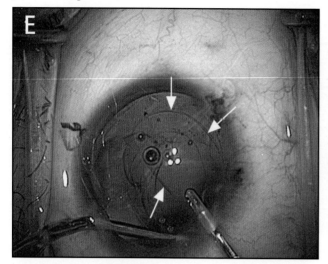

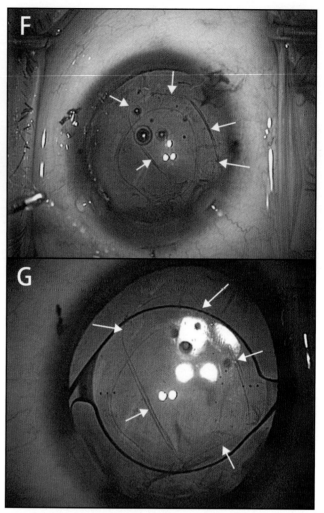

Figure 28-2 (continued). Case 2. (E) Following the anterior vitrectomy, the residual cortex is removed with bimanual I/A instrumentation. (F) The posterior continuous curvilinear capsulotomy is outlined with arrows and can be seen distinctly separate from the anterior capsulorrhexis. (G) The posterior capsulorrhexis facilitates placement of the intended toric IOL into the capsular bag.

chamber IOL should generally be placed in the ciliary sulcus (Figure 28-3). After the haptics are first positioned in the sulcus, the optic should be captured behind the capsulorrhexis, if possible.[1,3] Particularly with a larger diameter ciliary sulcus, relying on optic capture instead of the overall haptic length will assure better centration (Figure 28-4). First one side of the optic is tilted back and beneath the capsular rim before repeating the same maneuver for the other side (Figure 28-3E-G). This maneuver can be more challenging following a vitrectomy, however, and may not be possible if the capsulorrhexis diameter is too large, too small, or decentered. With optic capture, the optic still rests behind the anterior capsule and there is generally no need to adjust the power of the IOL (Figure 28-3G).

In another situation, it may be possible that the posterior capsule tears as a single-piece acrylic IOL is injected into the bag. Particularly if there is no vitreous prolapse, the surgeon may be reluctant to rotate or exchange the IOL at this point. If so, one option is to perform reverse optic capture, where the haptics are left in the capsular equator, but the optic is prolapsed forward through the capsulorrhexis (Figure 28-5). Because the thicker single-piece haptics remain behind the anterior capsule, the risk of iris chafing is low in this situation. It may be possible to achieve reverse optic capture with a 3-piece posterior chamber IOL as well, but the posterior angulation of the haptics makes it difficult.

POSTERIOR CAPSULE DEFECT WITH TORN CAPSULORRHEXIS

If the capsulorrhexis is also torn, there may still be enough remaining peripheral capsular support to safely position the posterior chamber IOL in the ciliary sulcus (Figure 28-6). Amidst the stress of managing an unexpected complication, it may be tempting to use the same foldable posterior chamber IOL that was planned for the capsular bag. This is not recommended for several reasons. First, single-piece acrylic IOLs should never be placed in the sulcus, as discussed later in this chapter.

Second, moving the axial IOL position slightly forward changes the effective power of the lens. Therefore, the IOL power should be decreased by approximately 0.5 to 1.0 diopter (D) to compensate for this change in position.[4-6] The higher the IOL dioptric power, the greater the compensatory reduction in sulcus placement power should be. Therefore, for IOL powers in the low to high 20s, 1.0 D should be subtracted.

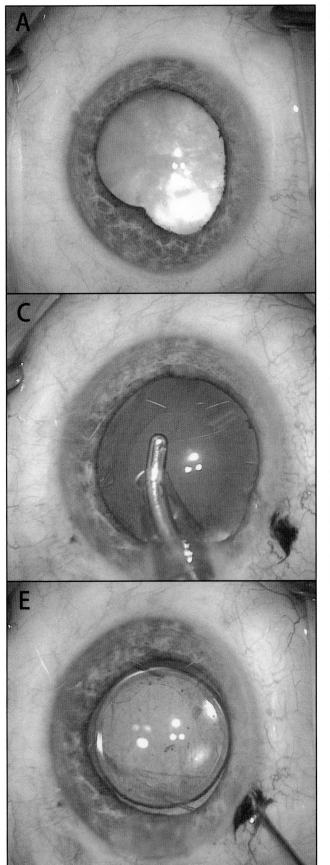

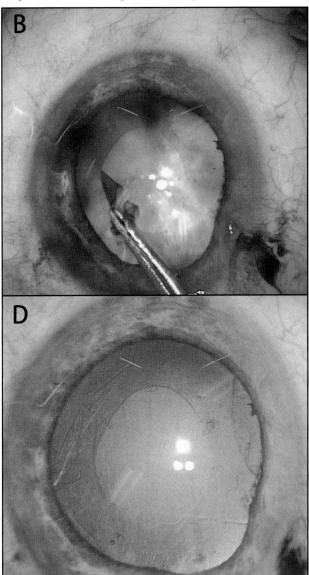

Figure 28-3. Case 3 (this is the same eye as Case 2 from Chapter 17; see Figure 17-9). (A) This patient developed a rapid onset white lens within several weeks of a vitrectomy to remove an epiretinal membrane. (B) Because a posterior capsular tear caused by the vitrectomy instrumentation is suspected, care is taken to make the capsulotomy diameter 5.0 mm or less. (C) As the white lens material is aspirated, the torn posterior capsule becomes visible. (D) Although some of the lens material has descended posteriorly, and IOL can be inserted into the ciliary sulcus because of sufficient peripheral capsular support. (E) A 3-piece acrylic IOL has been placed into the sulcus.

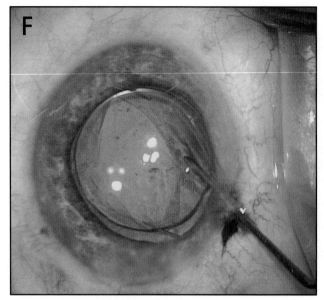
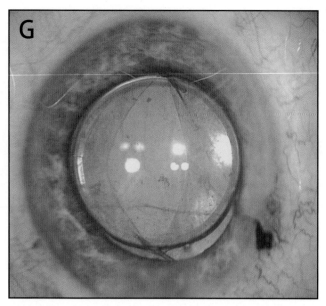

Figure 28-3 (continued). Case 3 (this is the same eye as Case 2 from Chapter 17; see Figure 17-9). (F) Optic capture is achieved by first displacing the left side of the optic behind the capsulotomy edge (G) followed by the right-hand side of the optic.

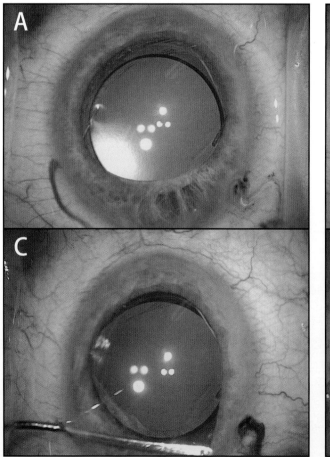
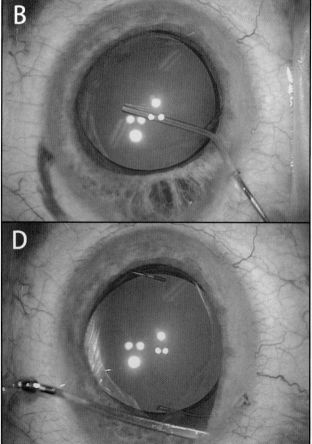

Figure 28-4. Case 4. This patient was referred because of a symptomatic "sunset syndrome." The IOL that had been placed in the ciliary sulcus was initially centered, but subluxated presumably through a zonular dialysis. (A) The IOL is manually repositioned and although the posterior capsule is open, there appears to be circumferential peripheral capsular support. (B) One edge of the IOL is displaced posteriorly with a cannula. (C) After capturing the other side of the optic, a Lester hook is used to confirm that the optic is behind the peripheral capsular rim. (D) Because the capsular opening is not symmetrically round, the IOL is rotated to maximize the capsular overlap of the IOL optic edge.

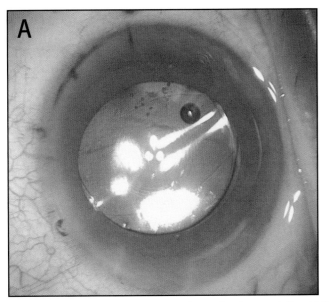
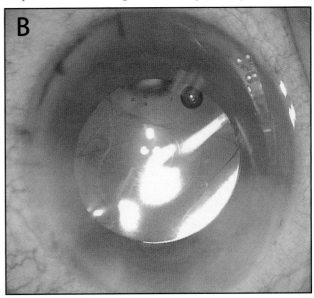

Figure 28-5. Reverse optic capture of a single-piece multifocal IOL. (A) Following insertion of a multifocal IOL, the posterior capsule tore. The optic was prolapsed forward through the capsulorrhexis, while leaving both haptics behind the anterior capsule. This creates an oval shaped anterior capsular opening behind the IOL optic with truncated edges where the single-piece haptics tuck beneath the capsulotomy edge. (B) Focusing slightly posteriorly, the tear in the posterior capsule becomes visible.

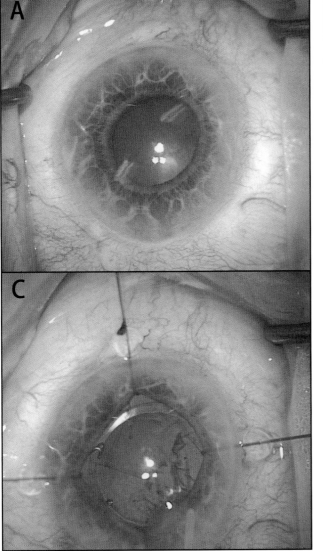
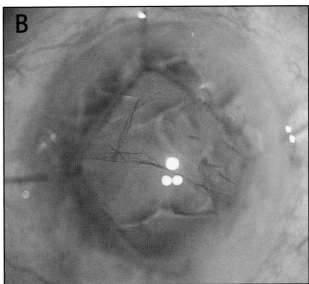

Figure 28-6. Case 5. (A) This eye with pseudoexfoliation has a brunescent lens and dilates poorly. (B) During cortical clean-up, a posterior capsular rent is noticed and as much cortex as possible was removed. There is a wraparound tear of the sub-incisional anterior capsule that extends into the posterior capsule, precluding any possibility of capsulorrhexis optic capture. (C) The longer AQ-2010 IOL (STAAR Surgical) has been implanted into the ciliary sulcus, and the haptics are oriented away from the sizable subincisional anterior and posterior capsular defect.

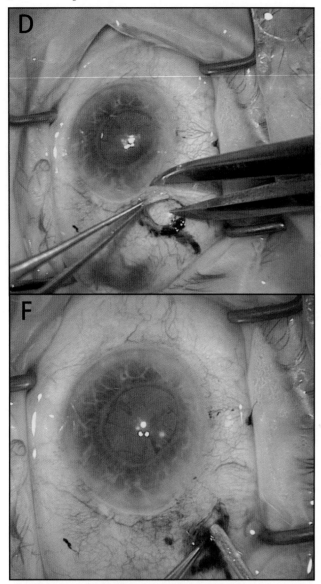

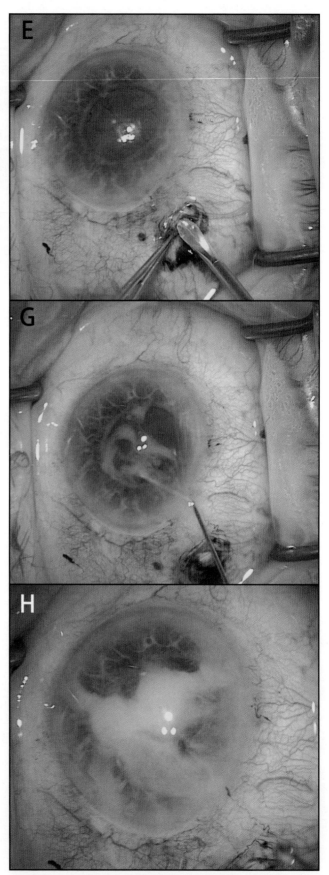

Figure 28-6 (continued). Case 5. (D-F) Because of vitreous presenting at the incision, a pars plana sclerotomy is performed with a 19-gauge microvitreoretinal (MVR) blade (Alcon Laboratories, Fort Worth, TX) 3.5 mm behind the limbus in an oblique quadrant. The tip of the blade is visualized through the pupil. (G, H) Triamcinolone is injected into the anterior chamber to stain the prolapsing vitreous strands. A pars plana anterior vitrectomy is performed with a limbal split self-retaining infusion cannula.

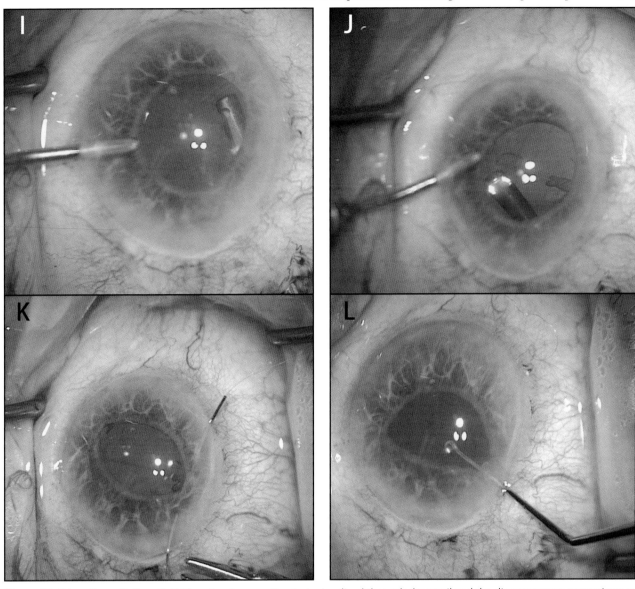

Figure 28-6 (continued). Case 5. (I) The vitrectomy cutter tip is visualized through the pupil and the disappearance or persistence of the triamcinolone is monitored. (J) Performing the anterior vitrectomy through the pars plana incision prevents more vitreous from being drawn into the anterior chamber where strands can get ensnared alongside the IOL. The triamcinolone has disappeared, confirming that no vitreous prolapse remains. Because of the large subincisional capsular defect, it is decided to fixate one haptic to the iris with a 10-0 polypropylene McCannel suture. (K) The optic has been prolapsed through the Miochol-E-constricted pupil and a curved CIF needle has captured the haptic with a bite of peripheral iris stroma. (L) After tying the knot with a Siepser sliding slip knot, the optic is reposited back into the posterior chamber.

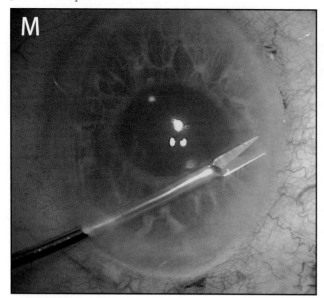
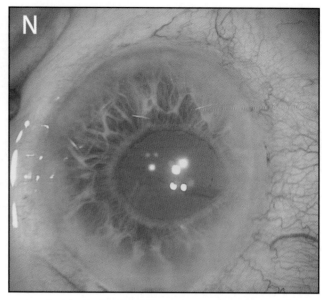

Figure 28-6 (continued). Case 5. (M) MST intraocular microscissors are used to cut the knot. (N) The suture causes a slight distortion of the pupil, but will prevent the IOL from rotating enough for the haptic to subluxate through the subincisional zonular defect.

Finally, nearly all foldable lenses are <13.0 mm long, which is too short for the ciliary sulcus in some eyes. Although the lens may center well in the operating room, if it is too short it can eventually rotate and subluxate peripherally over time. Studies by Liliana Werner, MD, PhD elucidate one mechanism whereby an IOL that initially centers well within the sulcus could later become decentered. Using ultrasound biomicroscopy to measure the sulcus in autopsy eyes, she found that the diameter of the sulcus can vary from 1 meridian to another.[7] In other words, the sulcus plane may be more oval rather than circular. With eye rubbing, one might imagine an IOL eventually rotating into the longest diameter meridian, causing it to become decentered.

Studies by Werner and others have also shown that there is no reliable way to gauge the sulcus diameter according to external landmarks.[7-10] Nevertheless, it is helpful to measure the white-to-white corneal diameter intraoperatively with calipers. If it measures 11.5 mm or less, a standard 13.0 mm long foldable IOL will probably center well within the ciliary sulcus. At 12.0 mm or larger, the author would select the 13.5 mm AQ-2010 foldable IOL (STAAR Surgical, Monrovia, CA) if capsulorrhexis optic capture were not an option, for the reasons discussed in the following paragraphs.

INTRAOCULAR LENS SELECTION FOR CILIARY SULCUS PLACEMENT WITHOUT OPTIC CAPTURE

There are situations in which both the anterior and posterior capsules are torn, but sufficient capsular support remains to support a posterior chamber IOL in the ciliary sulcus. A wraparound anterior capsular tear that extends into the posterior capsule is an example (Figure 28-6B). Single-piece acrylic IOLs should never be placed into the ciliary sulcus.[11] The overall length of this IOL is too short for sulcus placement, and the thicker, sharp-edged haptics can cause posterior iris chafing, pigment dispersion, and iris transillumination defects. Chronic uveitis, pigmentary glaucoma, microhyphema (UGH) syndrome and cystoid macular edema may result until the offending IOL is removed.[11-15] In the largest published retrospective study of complications of single-piece acrylic IOLs in the ciliary sulcus, the most common complication was lens decentration, which frequently resulted in symptomatic edge glare.[11]

In contrast, 3-piece posterior chamber IOLs have the advantage of thin, posteriorly angulated C-shaped haptics. Ideally, the anterior optic surface should be smooth and have rounded edges to prevent iris chafing, should any posterior iris contact occur. In the absence of suturing or capsulorrhexis capture, proper IOL centration requires adequate capsular support and lateral stability within the ciliary sulcus; IOLs shorter than 13.0 mm should not be used. Polymethylmethacrylate (PMMA) posterior chamber

IOLs with 6.5 mm optics and a 14 mm overall length fulfill these criteria but require a much larger incision.

Among foldable IOLs currently available in the United States, only the STAAR Surgical silicone AQ-2010 V has a 13.5 mm-long haptic-to-haptic length in the 5- to 30-D power range (Figure 28-6K). Its rounded anterior edge, 10-degree haptic angulation, and slightly larger 6.3-mm optic diameter are additional advantages of this platform. This lens also has a very low amount of spherical aberration (SA), which is also desirable for a sulcus IOL. Surgical facilities can purchase a backup consignment of these IOLs from the manufacturer for a reasonable cost. One potential disadvantage of silicone IOLs, however, is the compromise in surgical visibility should silicone oil or expansile gas ever be required for vitreoretinal surgery.[16,17]

Among foldable, 3-piece hydrophobic acrylic IOLs, the MA 50 model (Alcon Laboratories, Fort Worth, TX) has a 6.5-mm diameter optic but has a square anterior optic edge and an overall haptic length of only 13.0 mm. This IOL has been associated with pigment dispersion following piggy-back implantation in the sulcus and the sharp anterior edge of this optic is therefore undesirable in this location.[18-22] The Sensar (Abbott Medical Optics [AMO], Santa Ana, CA) has a rounded anterior optic edge and would be a preferable 3-piece hydrophobic acrylic IOL for sulcus placement.

Negatively aspheric IOLs have become popular as a means of reducing overall ocular SA and improving contrast sensitivity. However, because these IOLs have higher amounts of negative SA (to offset the positive SA from the cornea), they will actually induce more unwanted higher order aberrations (HOA) if they become tilted or decentered by more than 0.5 mm.[23-25] For this reason, based on the potential induction of spherical and other HOA, it is inadvisable to implant a negatively aspheric IOL in the sulcus if centration within +0.5 to 0.8 mm cannot be achieved.

A torn posterior capsule should preclude implantation of an accommodating IOL and may not permit proper alignment of a toric IOL. However, placement of a 3-piece multifocal IOL in the sulcus may be an option, particularly if proper centration can be achieved with capsulorrhexis capture of the optic. However, multifocal IOLs are much less forgiving of any tilt and decentration, and sulcus placement therefore carries a greater risk of refractive power surprise, unwanted images, and HOA.

PREVENTING AND MANAGING SUBLUXATION OF A POSTERIOR CHAMBER INTRAOCULAR LENS IN THE SULCUS

Despite adequate residual capsular support, a posterior chamber IOL placed in the sulcus may subsequently become subluxated either because of insufficient overall length or the presence of a zonular dialysis. Lacking the option of capsulorrhexis capture of the optic, this complication can be prevented or later surgically managed by suture fixation of one or both haptics to the iris.

With sufficient peripheral capsular support, a single 10-0 polypropylene McCannel iris suture capturing one of the haptics will often suffice to prevent the lens from rotating or decentering[26] (Figure 28-6K-N). This technique is described in the following paragraphs and can be employed at the time of initial surgery or to later refixate a subluxated sulcus IOL as a secondary procedure.

INTRAOCULAR LENS FIXATION IN THE ABSENCE OF ADEQUATE CAPSULAR SUPPORT—ANTERIOR VERSUS POSTERIOR CHAMBER INTRAOCULAR LENSES

If capsular support is insufficient, the surgeon must decide between suture fixation of a posterior chamber IOL or implantation of an anterior chamber IOL. Scleral suture fixation can be performed with a variety of different techniques and sutures.[27-30] To reduce the long-term risk of suture breakage, 9-0 is preferable to 10-0 polypropylene.[31] Gore-tex sutures (W. L. Gore & Associates, Flagstaff, AZ) have also been used. All of these techniques must address the potential problems of external exposure of the polypropylene knot and of IOL tilt and decentration.[32] The glued scleral flap-haptic tunnel technique popularized by Amar Agarwal, MS, FRCS, FRCOphth employs intrascleral tunnels to fixate each IOL haptic rather than sutures.[33]

McCannel iris suture fixation of the haptics requires only paracentesis incisions and avoids the need to dissect scleral tunnels, grooves, or flaps.[26,34-37] (see Figures 27-12, 28-7, and 28-8). In addition, recent UBM studies show excellent centration and alignment when this method of fixation is used.[37] If a 3-piece foldable IOL is used, the original phaco incision may not need to be enlarged. Following sulcus implantation, the IOL optic is prolapsed anteriorly and captured by the pupil (Figure 28-7B). The latter is then further constricted with acetylcholine (Miochol-E) (see Figure 27-12M). One or both haptics are sutured to the peripheral iris stroma using a modified McCannel technique with a sliding internal Siepser slip knot as initially described by this author[26,36,38] (see Figures 27-12, 28-7, 28-8). A 10-0 polypropylene suture with a long curved needle such as the CTC-6 (#9090G-SD; Ethicon, Somerville, NJ) is used to secure each haptic to the iris (see Figures 27-12N, 27-12R and Figure 28-7C-F). Slightly lifting the optic with a second instrument imprints the haptic

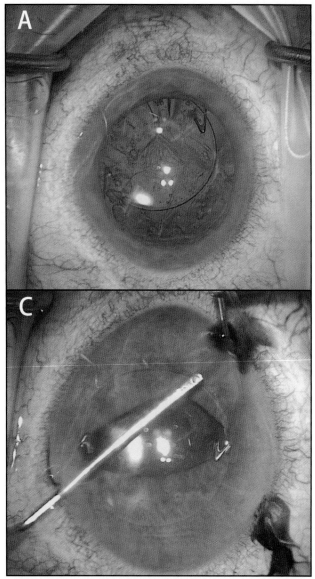

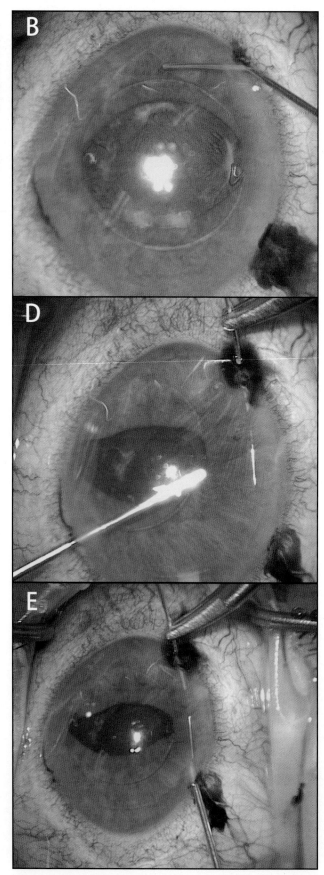

Figure 28-7. Case 6. (A) Although the posterior capsule is still intact, this patient has been referred for symptomatic IOL subluxation despite placement of a longer AQ-2010 IOL (STAAR Surgical) in the ciliary sulcus. Nd:YAG capsulotomy is being deferred until the IOL can be repositioned and stabilized with a single McCannel iris suture. (B) The first step is to center the IOL and then to prolapse the optic anteriorly through the pupil. Miochol-E is injected to further constrict the pupil and to make the iris stroma more taut. (C) As the long CIF 10-0 Prolene needle is held in position, a Lester hook is used to decenter and tilt the optic anteriorly so that the haptic imprints the iris stroma from below. (D) The Prolene needle takes a bite of iris that incorporates the haptic as far peripherally as possible. (E, F) The needle is docked into the OVD cannula tip, which will guide its exit through a preplaced paracentesis.

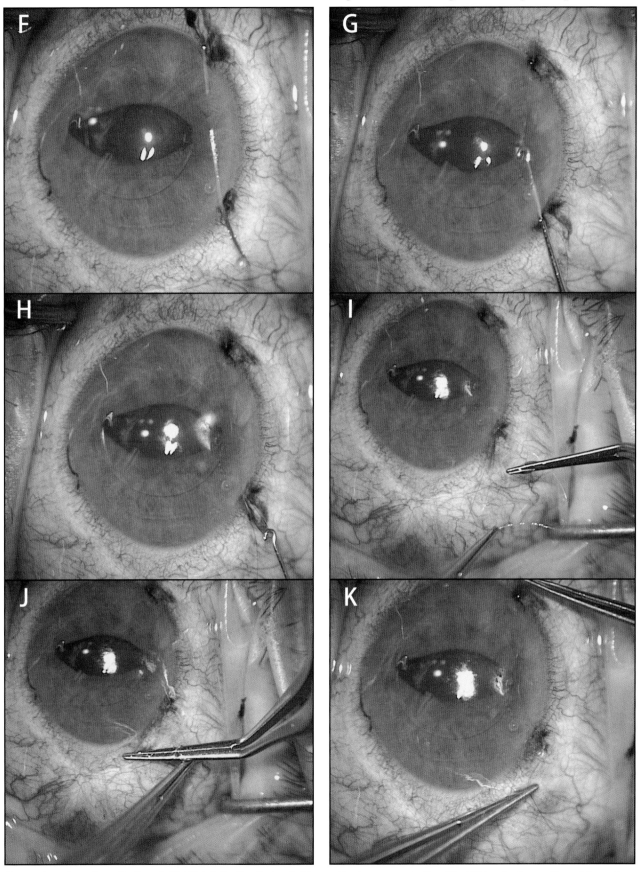

Figure 28-7 (continued). Case 6. (G, H) A Jaffe-Knolle hook (Katena Eye Instruments, Denville, NJ) hooks the section of the suture that is distal to the haptic and withdraws it through the paracentesis. (I-K) The Siepser sliding slip knot is initiated with 3 throws that allow the knot to slide into place by pulling on each opposite end of the suture.

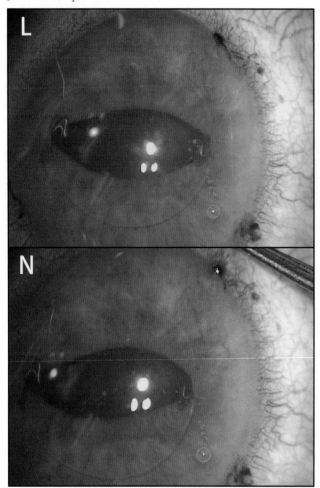

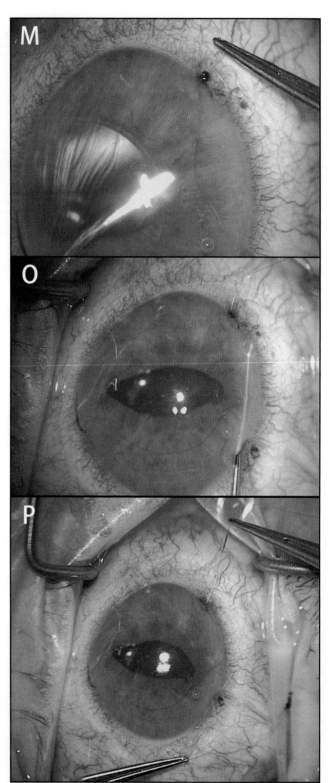

Figure 28-7 (continued). Case 6. (L) The advantage of this knot is that the peripheral iris and the haptic are not displaced from their desired anatomic positions. (M) To prevent too much iris from getting ensnared by the knot, the Lester hook is used to pull and free up any bunched up iris (N) before final tightening of the slip knot. (O, P) The second and locking slip knot is placed in a similar fashion.

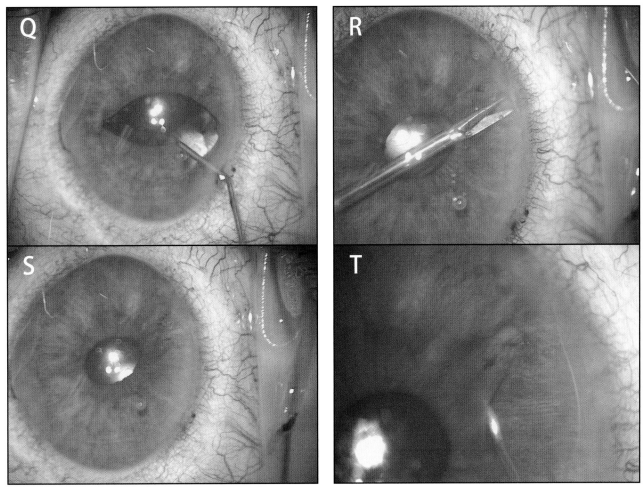

Figure 28-7 (continued). Case 6. (Q) After the third and final throw, the optic is pushed back into the posterior chamber (R) and the knot is cut with MST intraocular microscissors. (S, T) If peripherally enough, the knot will not noticeably peak the pupil.

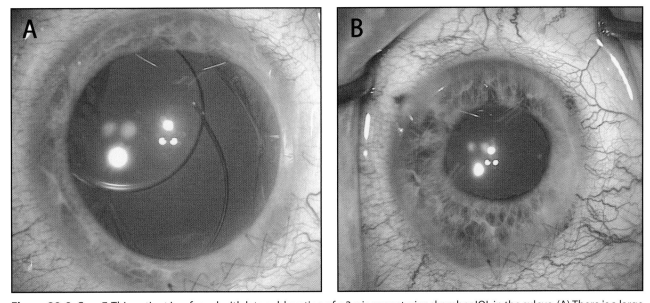

Figure 28-8. Case 7. This patient is referred with late subluxation of a 3-piece posterior chamber IOL in the sulcus. (A) There is a large capsular defect, with 2 peripheral capsular ledges. (B) Two McCannel sutures were used to fixate both haptics to the iris.

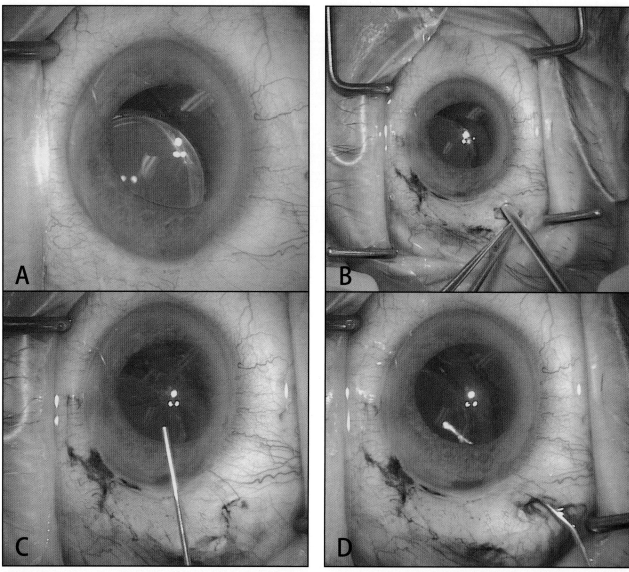

Figure 28-9. Case 8. (A) Late posterior bag-IOL dislocation in a patient with pseudoexfoliation. (B) Because the IOL is posterior and sliding over the inferior pars plana, a pars plana sclerotomy is performed to permit a posterior assisted levitation approach. (C) Dispersive OVD is injected first anterior (D) and then posterior to the IOL through the pars plana incision.

location against the iris and facilitates the needle pass (see Figures 27-12N, 28-7C, and 28-7D).

The American Academy of Ophthalmology (AAO) Technology Assessment study did not find a significant difference in published outcomes when comparing iris or scleral sutured posterior chamber IOLs or open loop anterior chamber IOLs.[39] Subsequent retrospective studies suggest that flexible, open-loop anterior chamber IOLs have outcomes at least equal to or better than those with trans-scleral suture fixated posterior chamber IOLs.[40,41] Based on the published evidence, all of these options are acceptable and it therefore becomes a decision based on each surgeon's individual preference and experience. Amidst the stress of unanticipated posterior capsular rupture and vitreous loss, one important consideration is the prolonged surgical time necessary to suture fixate an IOL. Although faster to implant, an anterior chamber IOL may require a larger incision to be made.

LATE BAG-INTRAOCULAR LENS DISLOCATION

The options for managing late postoperative bag-IOL dislocation due to pseudoexfoliation or other zonulopathy include IOL exchange (Figure 28-9) or suture refixation of the malpositioned IOL[42-48] (Figure 28-10). IOL suture fixation generally requires the presence of either a capsular tension ring (CTR) or a 3-piece IOL.[44] This option may

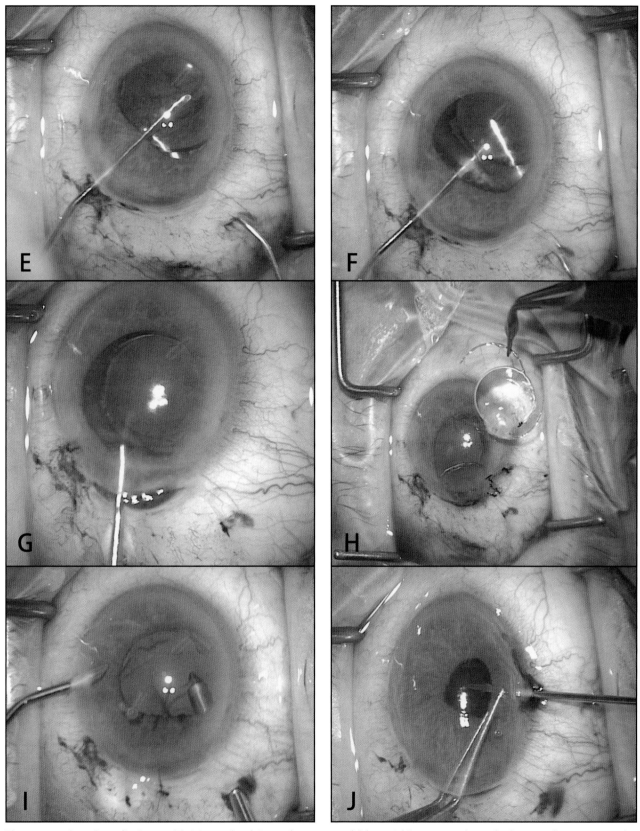

Figure 28-9 (continued). Case 8. (E) A Lester hook is used as a second "chopstick" to center the wide diameter bag-IOL complex (F) and to then prop the temporal pole upward. (G) Additional dispersive OVD is injected beneath the proximal edge of the IOL to facilitate its removal. (H) As the IOL is removed, the surrounding capsule is sheared off by the friction of the incision to reveal a severely crimped haptic caused by capsular contraction. (I) Following temporary partial closure of the incision, a pars plana anterior vitrectomy is performed (J) and a peripheral iridotomy is made superiorly by puncturing the iris with a disposable 25-gauge needle.

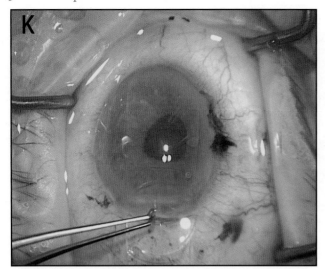

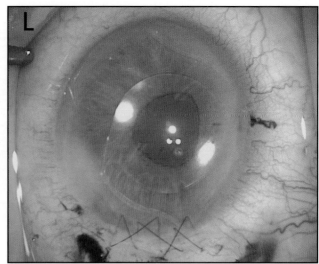

Figure 28-9 (continued). Case 8. (K) The anterior chamber IOL is inserted over a Sheet's glide (L) and the incision is closed with a running 10-0 nylon suture. There is no iris tuck and the pupil is round.

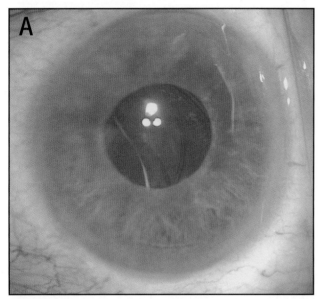

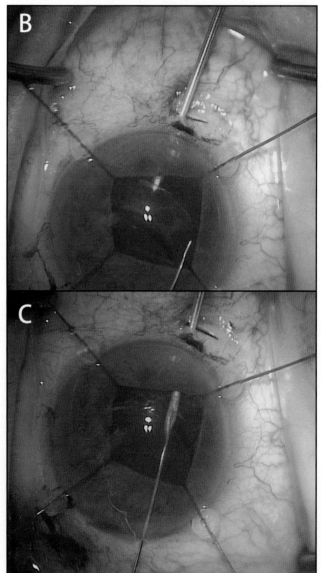

Figure 28-10. Case 9. Scleral suture fixation of CTR following late bag-IOL subluxation in a patient with pseudoexfoliation. (A) The bag is not dislocated posteriorly but there is gross pseudophakodonesis and the IOL haptic and CTR are visible through the pupil. (B) After inserting iris retractors, a disposable 25-gauge guide needle is introduced ab externo through a half-thickness scleral groove located approximately 1.5 mm behind the limbus. (C) It will pass beneath the CTR and through the peripheral capsular bag. A double armed 9-0 Prolene needle is docked into the guide needle lumen so that it will emerge through the base of the half-thickness scleral groove.

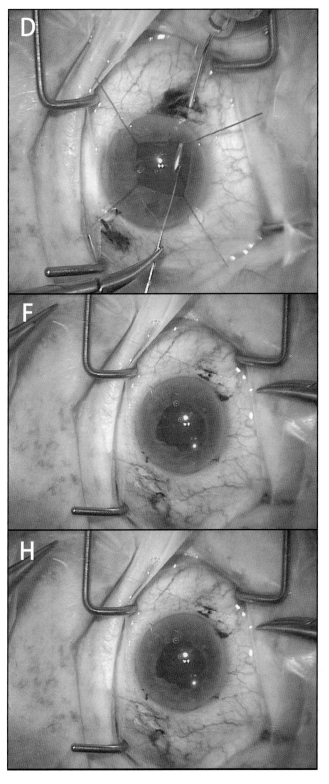

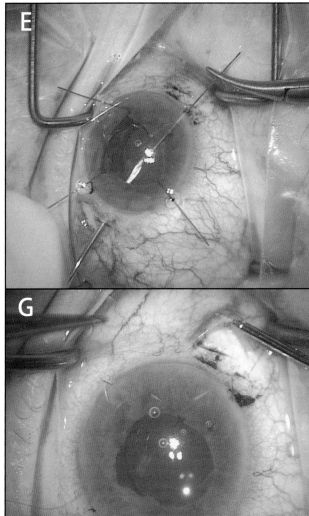

Figure 28-10 (continued). Case 9. Scleral suture fixation of CTR following late bag-IOL subluxation in a patient with pseudo-exfoliation. (D) The same steps are repeated with the second Prolene needle, except that this time the guide needle passes above the CTR. The guide needle is seen to enter the scleral groove approximately 1.5 mm adjacent to the first Prolene suture. (E) To suture fixate the opposite end of the CTR, the same steps are repeated with a half-thickness scleral groove located 180 degrees across from the first suture fixation site. (F) The Prolene sutures are tied, resulting in scleral fixation and recentering of the CTR-bag-IOL complex. (G) After trimming the suture tips, the knot retracts within the base of the half thickness scleral groove so that it is not exposed. The CTR-bag-IOL complex is centered and stable following scleral suture fixation without requiring an anterior vitrectomy. (H) The torn iris sphincter has been repaired with a single interrupted 9-0 Prolene suture.

avoid the need for an anterior vitrectomy if the hyaloid face is intact, such as when the patient presents with pseudopha-kodonesis without frank lens dislocation (Figure 28-10A). Potential drawbacks to suture refixation of any subluxated or dislocated IOL include lens tilt or decentration, IOL refractive power surprise, and vitreous incarceration.

If severe capsular contraction has permanently bent or crimped a haptic, then proper centration and alignment will be difficult to achieve (Figure 28-9H).

Posterior dislocation of the bag-IOL complex is particularly challenging to manage (Figure 28-9). The surgeon is often surprised by how far the IOL drops posteriorly when the patient is supine in the operating room (Figure 28-9A). Approaching the floating bag-IOL complex with instruments from a superiorly placed incision may not allow the proper angle of approach, and the IOL may instead tend to get pushed further away. The author has described using the posterior-assisted levitation (PAL) technique for levitating the large IOL-bag complex into the anterior chamber in this situation[43] (see Figure 28-9B-F). If this can be achieved, extracting the IOL and performing an anterior vitrectomy prior to anterior chamber IOL implantation is an excellent option[43] (see Figure 28-9H-L). In addition to the difficulties of working through a small pupil, the surgeon must be sure to excise all adherent and prolapsing vitreous prior to any attempt to scleral suture a posteriorly dislocated IOL to the ciliary sulcus.

TRIAMCINOLONE STAINING OF THE VITREOUS

As initially described by Scott E. Burk, MD, PhD, triamcinolone staining provides excellent visualization of prolapsing vitreous.[49] Although this technique can be used in any situation where there is vitreous prolapse, it is particularly helpful when there may be persistent vitreous prolapse through a zonular dialysis (see Figure 27-12B) or following IOL placement (see Figures 28-6G and 28-6H). Vitreous strands prolapsing alongside of or around the edge of an IOL are more likely to become entrapped, making it difficult to perform a complete "clean-up" of the anterior segment. In addition, performing the vitrectomy through a limbal incision tends to repeatedly draw more vitreous forward, where strands can become ensnared alongside the IOL. Therefore, if an IOL is already in place, performing a pars plana anterior vitrectomy is better able to sever any forward prolapsing vitreous strands, particularly if they are visually highlighted by triamcinolone staining (see Figure 28-6I-J).

REFERENCES

1. Gimbel HV, Sun R, Ferensowicz M, Anderson Penno E, Kamal A. Intraoperative management of posterior capsule tears in phacoemulsification and intraocular lens implantation. *Ophthalmology.* 2001;108:2186-2189.
2. Little BC, Smith JH, Packer M. Little capsulorhexis tear-out rescue. *J Cataract Refract Surg.* 2006;32:1420-1422.
3. Gimbel HV, DeBroff BM. Intraocular lens optic capture. *J Cataract Refract Surg.* 2004;30:200-206.
4. Suto C, Hori S, Fukuyama E, Akura J. Adjusting intraocular lens power for sulcus fixation. *J Cataract Refract Surg.* 2003;29:1913-1917.
5. Suto C. Sliding scale of IOL power for sulcus fixation using computer simulation. *J Cataract Refract Surg.* 2004;30:2452-2454.
6. Bayramlar H, Hepsen IF, Yilmaz H. Myopic shift from the predicted refraction after sulcus fixation of PMMA posterior chamber intraocular lenses. *Can J Ophthalmol.* 2006;41:78-82.
7. Werner L, Izak AM, Pandey SK, Apple DJ, Trivedi RH, Schmidbauer JM. Correlation between different measurements within the eye relative to phakic intraocular lens implantation. *J Cataract Refract Surg.* 2004;30:1982-1988.
8. Fea AM, Annetta F, Cirillo S, et al. Magnetic resonance imaging and Orbscan assessment of the anterior chamber. *J Cataract Refract Surg.* 2005;31:1713-1718.
9. Oh J, Shin HH, Kim JH, Kim HM, Song JS. Direct measurement of the ciliary sulcus diameter by 35-megahertz ultrasound biomicroscopy. *Ophthalmology.* 2007;114:1685-1688.
10. Kim KH, Shin HH, Kim HM, Song JS. Correlation between ciliary sulcus diameter measured by 35 MHz ultrasound biomicroscopy and other ocular measurements. *J Cataract Refract Surg.* 2008;34:632-637.
11. Chang DF, Masket S, Miller K, et al; ASCRS Cataract Clinical Committee. ASCRS White Paper: Complications of sulcus placement of single piece acrylic IOLs. Recommendations for backup IOL implantation following posterior capsule rupture. *J Cataract Refract Surg.* 2009;35:1445-1458.
12. LeBoyer RM, Werner L, Snyder ME, Mamalis N, Riemann CD, Augsberger JJ. Acute haptic-induced ciliary sulcus irritation associated with single-piece AcrySof intraocular lenses. *J Cataract Refract Surg.* 2005;31:1422-1427.
13. Uy HS, Chan PS. Pigment release and secondary glaucoma after implantation of a single-piece acrylic intraocular lens in the ciliary sulcus. *Am J Ophthalmol.* 2006;142:330-332.
14. Toma HS, Dibernardo C, Schein OD, Adams NA. Recurrent vitreous hemorrhage secondary to haptic-induced chafing. *Can J Ophthalmol.* 2007;42:312-313.
15. Boutboul S, Letaief I, Lalloum F, Puech M, Borderie V, LaRoch L. Pigment glaucoma secondary to in-the-bag intraocular lens implantation. *J Cataract Refract Surg.* 2008;34:1595-1597.
16. Kusaka S, Kodama T, Ohashi Y. Condensation of silicone oil on the posterior surface of a silicone intraocular lens during vitrectomy. *Am J Ophthalmol.* 1996;121:574-575.
17. Porter RG, Peters JD, Bourke RD. De-misting condensation on intraocular lenses. *Ophthalmology* 2000;107:778-782.
18. Wintle R, Austin M. Pigment dispersion with elevated intraocular pressure after AcrySof intraocular lens implantation in the ciliary sulcus. *J Cataract Refract Surg.* 2001;27:642-644.
19. Chang SH, Lim G. Secondary pigmentary glaucoma associated with piggyback intraocular lens implantation. *J Cataract Refract Surg.* 2004;30(10):2219-2222.
20. Iwase T, Tanaka N. Elevated intraocular pressure in secondary piggyback intraocular lens implantation. *J Cataract Refract Surg.* 2005;31:1821-1823.
21. Masket S. Cataract surgical problem. *J Cataract Refract Surg.* 2007;33(12):2013-2017.
22. Chang WH, Werner L, Fry LL, Johnson JT, Kamae K, Mamalis N. Pigmentary dispersion syndrome with a secondary piggyback 3-piece hydrophobic acrylic lens. Case report with clinicopathological correlation. *J Cataract Refract Surg.* 2007;33:1106-1109.
23. Altmann GE, Nichamin LD, Lane SS, Pepose JS. Optical performance of 3 intraocular lens designs in the presence of decentration. *J Cataract Refract Surg.* 2005;31:574-585.
24. Wang L, Koch DD. Effect of decentration of wavefront-corrected intraocular lenses on higher-order aberrations of the eye. *Arch Ophthalmol.* 2005;123(9):1226-1230.

25. Piers PA, Weeber HA, Artal P, Norrby S. Theoretical comparison of aberration-correcting customized and aspheric intraocular lenses. *J Refract Surg.* 2007;23(4):374-384.

26. Chang DF. Siepser slipknot for McCannel iris-suture fixation of subluxated intraocular lenses. *J Cataract Refract Surg.* 2004;30(6):1170-1176.

27. Hannush SB. Sutured posterior chamber intraocular lenses: indications and procedure. *Curr Opin Ophthalmol.* 2000;11(4):233-240.

28. Gabor SG, Pavilidis MM. Sutureless intrascleral posterior chamber intraocular lens fixation. *J Cataract Refract Surg.* 2007;33(11):1851-1854.

29. Hoffman RS, Fine IH, Packer M. Scleral fixation without conjunctival dissection. *J Cataract Refract Surg.* 2006;32:1907-1912.

30. Holt DG, Young J, Stagg B, Ambati BK. Anterior chamber intraocular lens, sutured posterior chamber intraocular lens, or glued intraocular lens: where do we stand? *Curr Opin Ophthalmol.* 2012;23(1):62-67. Review.

31. Price MO, Price FW Jr, Werner L, Berlie C, Mamalis N. Late dislocation of scleral-sutured posterior chamber intraocular lenses. *J Cataract Refract Surg.* 2005;31(7):1320-1326.

32. Hayashi K, Hayashi H, Nakao F, Hayashi F. Intraocular lens tilt and decentration, anterior chamber depth, and refractive error after trans-scleral suture fixation surgery. *Ophthalmology.* 1999;106(5):878-882.

33. Agarwal A, Kumar DA, Jacob S, Baid C, Agarwal A, Srinivasan S. Fibrin glue–assisted sutureless posterior chamber intraocular lens implantation in eyes with deficient posterior capsules. *J Cataract Refract Surg.* 2008;34:1433–1438.

34. McCannel MA. A retrievable suture idea for anterior uveal problems. *Ophthalmic Surg.* 1976;7:98–103.

35. Stark WJ, Gottsch JD, Goodman DF, Goodman GL, Pratzer K. Posterior chamber intraocular lens implantation in the absence of capsular support. *Arch Ophthalmol.* 1989;107(7):1078-1083.

36. Condon GP, Masket S, Kranemann C, Crandall AS, Ahmed II. Small-incision iris fixation of foldable intraocular lenses in the absence of capsule support. *Ophthalmology.* 2007;114(7):1311-1318.

37. Mura JJ, Pavlin CJ, Condon GP, et al. Ultrasound biomicroscopic analysis of iris-sutured foldable posterior chamber intraocular lenses. *Am J Ophthalmol.* 2010;149:245-252.

38. Siepser SB. The closed chamber slipping suture technique for iris repair. *Ann Ophthalmol.* 1994;26(3):71-72.

39. Wagoner MD, Cox TA, Ariyasu RG, Jacobs DS, Karp CL; American Academy of Ophthalmology. Intraocular lens implantation in the absence of capsular support: a report by the American Academy of Ophthalmology. *Ophthalmology.* 2003;110(4):840-859.

40. Donaldson KE, Gorscak JJ, Budenz DL, Feuer WJ, Benz MS, Forster RK. Anterior chamber and sutured posterior chamber intraocular lenses in eyes with poor capsular support. *J Cataract Refract Surg.* 2005;31:903-909.

41. Kwong YY, Yuen HK, Lam RF, Lee VY, Rao SK, Lam DS. Comparison of outcomes of primary scleral-fixated versus primary anterior chamber intraocular lens implantation in complicated cataract surgeries. *Ophthalmology.* 2007;114:80-85.

42. Jahan FS, Mamalis N, Crandall AS. Spontaneous late dislocation of intraocular lens within the capsular bag in psuedoexfoliation patients. *Ophthalmology.* 2001;108:1727-1731.

43. Chang DF. Viscoelastic levitation of posteriorly dislocated IOLs from the anterior vitreous. *J Cataract Refract Surg.* 2002;28:1515-1519.

44. Ahmed II, Chen SH, Kranemann C, Wong DT. Surgical repositioning of dislocated capsular tension rings. *Ophthalmology.* 2005;112:1725-1733.

45. Hayashi K, Hirata A, Hayashi H. Possible predisposing factors for in-the-bag and out-of-the-bag intraocular lens dislocation and outcomes of intraocular lens exchange surgery. *Ophthalmology.* 2007;114:969-975.

46. Davis D, Brubaker J, Espandar L, et al. Late in-the-bag spontaneous intraocular lens dislocation: evaluation of 86 consecutive cases. *Ophthalmology.* 2009;116:664-670.

47. Shingleton BJ, Crandall AS, Ahmed K. Pseudoexfoliation and the cataract surgeon: preoperative, intraoperative, and postoperative issues related to intraocular pressure, cataract, and intraocular lenses. *J Cataract Refract Surg.* 2009;35:1101-1120.

48. Jakobsson G, Zetterberg M, Lundström M, Stenevi U, Grenmark R, Sundelin K. Late dislocation of in-the-bag and out-of-the-bag intraocular lenses: ocular and surgical characteristics and time to lens repositioning. *J Cataract Refract Surg.* 2010;36:1637-1644.

49. Burk SE, Da Mata AP, Snyder ME, Schneider S, Osher RH, Cionni RJ. Visualizing vitreous using Kenalog suspension. *J Cataract Refract Surg.* 2003;29:645-651.

Please see companion narrated videos on the accompanying Web site at
www.Healio.com/phacochopvideos

29

Strategies for Unplanned Anterior Vitrectomy

Lisa B. Arbisser, MD

PREOPERATIVE EVALUATION OF PROBLEMATIC EYES

- Consider peribulbar anesthesia
- Keep vitrectomy instrumentation on standby
- Book additional time for difficult/complex cases
- Have back-up implants available
- Classify cases per level of difficulty

As all cataract surgeons know, certain cases present a red flag. Any type of zonular issue is problematic. Surgeons should anticipate compromised zonular integrity after ocular trauma, with very asymmetric cataracts, in eyes with pseudoexfoliation or an asymmetric anterior chamber, and in those that have undergone pars plana vitrectomy or peripheral iridectomy. Very dense brunescence, intumescence, small pupils, and floppy irides can raise the chances of a capsular rent. We as surgeons should diligently prepare for such complications.

Although most cataract surgeons use topical anesthesia the majority of the time (the author uses topical and intracameral lidocaine in 95% of eyes), surgeons can consider a peribulbar approach for patients who cannot cooperate for an indirect examination or tolerate light. Certainly, the peribulbar method works well for challenging cases, such as when zonules are missing or when a surgeon might need to sew the iris.

It is important to keep vitrectomy instrumentation on standby and plan for additional case time for compromised eyes. The author grades cataract surgeries on Levels 1 through 4 (routine to challenging), and allows time in each surgical day for as many Level 1 and Level 2 cases as need be. Level 3 cases include very small pupils, extremely brunescent lenses, and pseudoexfoliation—eyes that may be a little unpredictable. These cases are limited in the surgical schedule for the end of the morning and the end of the afternoon. A Level 4 case is one that will require modified tension rings, iris suturing, etc, such as subluxated crystalline lenses or implants. These surgeries are reserved for the end of the day and only one is scheduled per day. This allows the author to pace herself and not feel pressured by waiting patients.

Chang DF.
Phaco Chop and Advanced Phaco Techniques: Strategies for Complicated Cataracts, Second Edition (pp 331-350).
© 2013 SLACK Incorporated.

Preventing Complications

Recognize Zonular Laxity

Learn to recognize zonular laxity by the pin cushion effect (Figure 29-1). Difficulty opening the capsule or a dimple-down action with striae going out to the periphery indicate the likelihood of zonular issues. The sooner the potential problem is recognized the sooner the surgeon can act to prevent a complication. Always have expander hooks available.

Avoid Convexity of the Lens Dome

To avoid convexity of the lens dome, especially if the anterior chamber is crowded, the author recommends using mannitol (0.25 g per kilogram of IV push) 15 minutes preoperatively to soften the eye and create a little more space. This tactic often avoids the need for a dry vitreous tap in shallow-chambered eyes. In eyes with shallow chambers or posterior pressure, such as pediatric cases or intumescence, use a more viscous-cohesive viscoelastic, such as sodium hyaluronate 1.4% (Healon GV) or sodium chondroitin sulfate 4%, sodium hyaluronate 1.65% (DisCoVisc OVD), or a viscoadaptive agent such as sodium hyaluronate 2.3% (Healon 5). These OVDs will help prevent the capsulorrhexis from running downhill.

Burp the Bag to Prevent Tamponade of the Continuous Curvilinear Capsulorrhexis

During hydrodissection, you may burp the capsular bag by rocking the nucleus slightly as the fluid wave progresses. This maneuver will prevent the edge of the capsule from adhering to the anterior cortex, which can cause the posterior capsule to blow out. Be careful not to create a vigorous fluid wave in a crowded chamber.

Mobilize the Nucleus; Beware of Fibrosis

Do not hydrodissect capsular cortical adhesions, particularly in the presence of posterior cortical adhesions (also known as posterior polar cataracts). Only hydrodeliniate these eyes or the capsule may tear in those areas. Eyes with significant peripheral cortical fibrosis require thorough hydrodissection. Watch the whitish cortical change on the surface; it will change clock hours when the lens is rotated and it will not bounce back. If the nucleus bounces back when the surgeon tries to turn it, it is likely that the zonules are just being stretched and that the lens has not really been freed from its attachments to the capsular bag. It is always best to start phacoemulsification with the nucleus free, particularly with dense lenses.

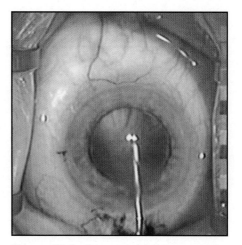

Figure 29-1. An eye with loose zonules shows significant striae (the dimple-down or pin cushion effect) when pressure is placed on the cornea.

Respect the Zonules During Nuclear Rotation

When rotating the nucleus, the author recommends using a 2-handed technique to avoid applying downward pressure, although one instrument may be used with appropriate vector force to avoid stretching or breaking the zonules (particularly subincisional zonules).

Keep the Phaco Tip in the "Safe Zone"

The beauty of the vertical phaco chop technique for nuclear disassembly, as opposed to a divide-and-conquer or a horizontal chop, is that it keeps the instruments inside the anterior capsulorrhexis. When the surgeon engages foot pedal position 3 (FP3) in ultrasound, it is beneficial for the phaco needle to be within the safe zone where it remains visible. The surgeon should only engage ultrasound when he or she can visualize the phaco tip; this will make it less likely for the surgeon to inadvertently engage the peripheral capsule.

Know Where the Edge Is and Protect the Vector

When making the capsulorrhexis, know where the edge of the continuous curvilinear capsulorrhexis (CCC) is at all times. The surgeon can control the vector of the tear by regrasping the edge of it. If the vector is appropriate and the patient moves, the capsulorrhexis will not tear out to the periphery but simply come into the center and end early. Try not to blink while making the capsulorrhexis, because if the vector shifts in an unpredictable direction from the tear, it is best to catch it within 0.50 to 1.00 mm. If the capsulorrhexis tears out to the equator, it will be difficult to recover.

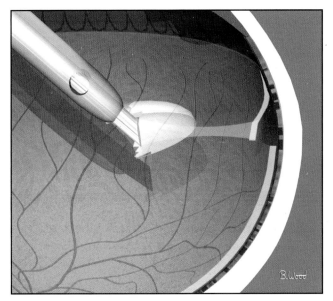

Figure 29-4. To avoid tearing the retina, do not allow the phaco tip to go behind the posterior capsule. (Reprinted from Charles S, Calzada J, Wood B. *Vitreous Microsurgery.* 5th ed. Baltimore, MD: Lippincott, Williams, & Wilkins; 2011.)

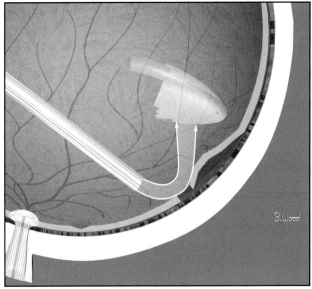

Figure 29-5. Irrigating into the vitreous to cause lens fragments to float out risks a retinal tear. This was a method for creating retinal detachment for research in animal models.

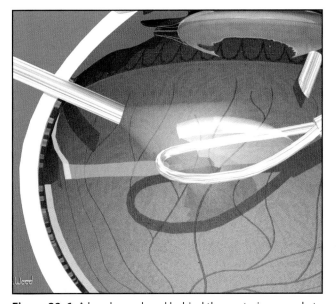

Figure 29-6. A lens loop placed behind the posterior capsule to retrieve a lens fragment risks a retinal tear.

If the author encounters a nucleus that descends below the posterior capsule, she lets it go. All ophthalmic surgeons agree that the phaco tip does not belong behind the posterior capsule unless a total vitrectomy has been done because of the risk of tearing the retina (Figures 29-4 to 29-6). The legendary Charles Kelman, MD, proposed the original PAL technique that involved inserting a spatula through the pars plana and then levitating or tire-ironing the dropped nuclear fragment into the anterior chamber.[5] Certainly, this maneuver is capable of saving a descended nucleus, but sweeping through the vitreous is dangerous.

The modification of viscolevitation—inserting a cannula of Viscoat OVD through a pars plana sclerotomy and slowly injecting the OVD to lift the nuclear fragment anterior to the posterior capsule—is controversial. Retina specialists agree that a 3-port vitrectomy using an appropriate fragmenter as needed has produced the most consistently good outcomes. Rather than place instruments through the pars plana if the nucleus is threatening to descend, nuclear spears can be used from an anterior approach. Due to the spearing of the nuclear material with the sharp points with opposing forces 180 degrees apart, the nucleus can be raised into the anterior chamber without putting any instruments into the posterior segment (see Figure 29-3).

This author personally does not perform viscolevitation. Preoperative cataract counseling should include a discussion about the rare chance of needing more than one surgery to remove the cataract for best results. Nuclear fragments can dislocate peripherally as well as posteriorly out of view behind the iris during viscolevitation. The pressure of injecting the OVD through the pars plana may promote more vitreous prolapse, and forces at the vitreous base can be significant and lead to a retinal tear or detachment. For a description of the author's experience with cadaver eyes using this technique, see the extensive article published in *Ophthalmology Clinics of North America.*[6]

PARTICULATE MARKING

- Triamcinolone acetonide binds to vitreous
- Facilitates vitreous recognition and removal
- Reduces postoperative inflammation

- Washed Kenalog (off-label use)

- Triamcinolone acetonide injectable suspension (Triesence): supplied unpreserved and is FDA approved for this purpose.

- Dilute 10:1 with BSS for particulate identification

Particulate staining was originally devised by Gholam Peyman, MD,[7] of Tucson, Arizona, and then popularized in the anterior segment by Scott E. Burk, MD, from Cincinnati.[8] Although Drs. Peyman and Burke originally used triamcinolone acetonide or washed Kenalog (an off-label use), nonpreserved Triesence is available and is an on-label, preservative-free preparation used to identify the vitreous. This technique of particulate identification can be hugely beneficial when a hyaloid break is suspected. Like throwing a sheet over a ghost, it allows the surgeon to see the invisible vitreous beautifully (Figure 29-7). Triesence must be added at the right time, when the OVD is not in the way, so that the former can bind to the surface of the vitreous. Also, the drug has the therapeutic effect of reducing postoperative inflammation. The preservatives in Kenalog are toxic to the endothelium. Triesence has essentially replaced Kenalog because it is FDA-approved for this purpose and is also billable.

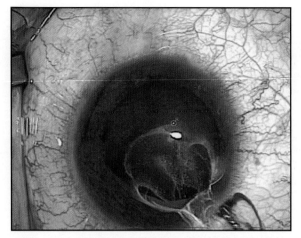

Figure 29-7. Particulate staining of vitreous with triamcinolone.

efficient and preferable. The author will only use a Trocar system when the globe is intact at the time of sclerotomy as, despite its desirable transconjunctival sutureless nature, it requires pressure to insert. These choices, and how to execute them in detail, will be further explained in the following sections.

VITRECTOMY TREATMENT OPTIONS

- Wisp around zonules: Cut with intraocular scissors to amputate and reposit with OVD

- Small prolapse or no view through pupil: Automated vitrectomy, anterior incision

- Vitreous loss or sheet around zonules: Automated approach, direct pars plana incision

- Intact globe, planned vitrectomy: Sutureless Trocar system incision

To serve the goal of vitreous traction avoidance, surgeons must consider the best approach based on the particular condition of the eye. Surgeons need not always use an automated vitrector if there is a small presentation around zonules which can be amputated with a scissor and reposited to the posterior segment with OVD. There will rarely be only a wisp that can be controlled when vitreous prolapses through a broken posterior capsule and the surgeon must decide which approach is best with the automated vitrector. In all cases the clear corneal paracentesis will be used for the irrigation cannula. When there is a small amount of prolapse without vitreous loss through incisions, vitrectomy can be nicely handled with the vitrector inserted through an anterior incision. This is always the right choice when there is no view through the pupil. In the author's experience, when there is vitreous loss through incisions or a copious amount herniated around the bag equator, a pars plana direct sclerotomy approach to vitrectomy is most

THE ANTERIOR INCISION

- Biaxial (separate sleeve from the vitrector shaft)

- Never use the primary coaxial incision site

- Make a new paracentesis to fit the bare vitrector shaft using the original sideport incision for irrigation

- Advance toward the vitreous while cutting but not vacuuming

- Hold the eye steady; tilt the vitrector below the posterior capsule

- Anticipate a repeat presentation of vitreous

Although anterior vitrectomy can be performed through an anterior or a pars plana approach, there are some absolute criteria we must follow. Regardless of the incision selected, the instruments should be biaxial with the irrigation separated from the vitrector. Although vitrectomy packs traditionally came in a coaxial configuration, interestingly, Dr. Steve Charles—for whom the coaxial irrigation sleeve is named—has said he never intended it for use in unplanned vitrectomy but designed it for pediatric surgery.[9] Surgeons must remember that vitreous always follows a gradient from high to low pressure. If the surgeon wants it to flow into the vitrector, irrigating at the tip will be counterproductive. The fluid tends to displace the vitreous body, necessitating more to be removed. The goal is to preserve as much of the vitreous structure as possible while removing any strands that have prolapsed into the anterior segment.

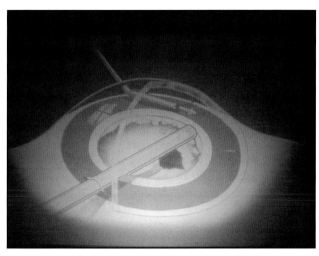

Figure 29-8. The biaxial paracentesis incisions for the vitrector.

Irrigating through the sideport incision is ideal for encouraging vitreous to remain posteriorly and keeping higher pressure in the front of the eye. Although pars plana irrigation is optimal for our retinal surgeon colleagues, the author does not recommend it in the cataract setting because it requires posterior focusing lenses or indentation to ensure complete penetration of the choroid. Furthermore, do not insert a bare vitrector through the main clear corneal incision. It will not fill the wound and will allow vitreous to flow out around it. Make a new incision that is just the right size for the bare vitrector. A standard keratome will be too large; use an MVR blade or your choice of instrument to create the paracentesis. Make this incision just the right size to maintain a closed chamber.

Regardless of which incision is selected, do not move the vitrector through the vitreous without cutting. Stay in FP2; vitreous can flow into the port while in FP1 and create traction. If using an anterior approach, tilt the vitrector down below the posterior capsule in order to pull vitreous back to the posterior segment. Removing or amputating anterior/posterior connections of any prolapsed vitreous can be difficult from this approach if there is a flat sheet or strand to the incision that is adherent to the iris.

Also, there is a tendency to call more vitreous forward while trying to remove the vitreous that is already forward. Once an endpoint is reached with this maneuver, the pressure is lowest in the anterior segment which encourages vitreous to present again on subsequent maneuvers. Figure 29-8 shows the biaxial paracentesis incisions for the vitrector. For all these reasons, a corneal incision may not be the optimal choice, but it is mandatory when there is no view available through the pupil.

RATIONALE FOR A PARS PLANA INCISION

- Vitreous follows a gradient from high to low pressure; leaves lowest pressure posteriorly
- Minimizes traction with proximity to vitreous base
- Most efficient, as it calls vitreous home
- Allows subsequent maneuvers with less representation of vitreous
- Will not unzip zonules
- Facilitates amputation of vitreous within incisions without sweeping

If a surgeon has not been trained to make a pars plana incision, he or she can go to a skills transfer lab or ask the retinal surgeon in his or her area to sit in and learn how to do it properly. Practice this incision ahead of time with eye bank or animal eyes, not in the heat of battle.

Again, the rationale for using the pars plana for vitrectomy is that, because vitreous follows a pressure gradient from high to low, it is best to leave the lowest pressure posteriorly. Traction will also be minimized by removing the vitreous closer to its base. If any vitreous follows the instrument to the incision, it will be right near the vitreous base at the pars plana, rather than up at the corneal incision. This technique is the most efficient because it calls the vitreous home. The pars plana technique also allows subsequent maneuvers while minimizing representation of the vitreous. It will not unzip the zonules when vitreous presents around the lens equator by calling more vitreous forward through the defect. Finally, the pars plana approach facilitates amputation of the vitreous within incisions. Although surgeons were taught to use a sweep from the sideport incision to drag entrapped vitreous away, this actually creates more traction on the connection through the pupil rather than efficiently freeing the vitreous from incarceration in the wound. The author strongly discourages this practice.

VITRECTOMY GOALS AND PARAMETERS

- Use Triesence to identify the presence of vitreous rather than "weck" the incision to test for vitreous loss
- Do not sweep the incision (traction), but rather amputate posterior attachments
- Confirm vitrectomy mode: irrigation, then cutting, then aspiration in foot pedal positions 1, 2, and 3

Summary of Vitrectomy Parameters*

- Less flow = less traction
- Select settings to reduce vitreoretinal traction
  - Highest cut rate available
  - Flow rate: 20 cc/min for 20-gauge vitrectomy; 15 cc/min for 23-gauge
  - Lowest vacuum to remove vitreous: 200 to 250 mm Hg for 20-gauge or 350 to 500 for 23-gauge; use panel setting, not linear
  - Irrigation bottle with 23-gauge cannula to balance for normotension, about 80 cm

Note: These settings are for the Alcon system; settings may vary on different machines.

- Maximize the cut rate to minimize traction
- Minimize the flow rate (peristaltic pump machine) to slow the action
- Balance the lowest effective vacuum with the lowest bottle height to maintain normotension
- Remove all vitreous from the anterior chamber to below the capsular plane
- Minimally disrupt the posterior-segment vitreous structure

Vitrectomy Mode: Irrigation/Cut/Aspiration

The best machine parameters for performing vitrectomy are those settings that most effectively reduce vitreoretinal traction and prevent followability. In FP1, surgeons will only be irrigating. In FP2, surgeons will be irrigating and cutting. Not until FP3 will surgeons be irrigating, cutting, and sucking, because no vacuum should be applied to the vitreous unless the surgeon is cutting it at the same time. Surgeons must always follow the sequence of irrigation, cutting, and then aspiration (I/Cut/A) when removing vitreous. Be certain not to use the "I/A Cut" setting, where FP1 is irrigation, FP2 is sucking, and FP3 is cutting. This setting will prove useful when followability is desired during removal of the residual cortex, once vitreous is likely out of the way. Most machines toggle between "Cut/IA" and "IA/Cut." Therefore, surgeons must ask for either one of those settings to get either "Cut primary" or "Aspiration primary," with the cut primary for vitreous removal.

The WhiteStar Signature Vitrectomy System

The WhiteStar Signature System (Abbott Medical Optics) has advanced capabilities for anterior vitrectomy. The surgeon has a choice of 2 high-speed guillotine vitrectomy handpieces, the 20-gauge and the 23-gauge vitrector, the latter of which can be paired with a separate irrigator for bimanual clear cornea or pars plana vitrectomy through sutureless incisions as small as 1.0 mm. Either vitrector may be used with cut rates as high as 2500 cuts per minute for cutting vitreous.

The Signature phaco system offers dual-pump technology whereby the surgeon may choose to use either a peristaltic or a venturi pump system during the anterior vitrectomy. Venturi pump systems are the industry standard for posterior segment surgeons and may offer advantages over peristaltic pumps during an anterior vitrectomy. Additionally, all the system's vitrectomy parameters are fully programmable (ASP, VAC, and CPM) for either linear or panel control. Practitioners may use 2 vitrectomy submodes: I/Cut/A, which is used in the presence of vitreous; and I/A/Cut, in the case of residual cortex or nuclear fragments that need to be engaged by the vitrector prior to cutting.

Finally, setup for the Signature vitrector is simple and quick. The scrub technician performs an automated, 5-second prime cycle to prime and test the cutter before the surgeon enters the eye.

Cutting Rate and Flow

Dr. Charles has coined the term *port-based flow limiting*, which describes the goal of achieving the highest cut rate possible, the lowest effective flow rate, and the lowest vacuum that generates the removal of vitreous.[10] As the vitreous is engaged, the faster the machine cuts, the more he or she reduces traction. The highest cut rate possible on some older phaco machines is 400 cuts per minute, but newer models can go as high as 5,000 cuts per minute. Faster cutting leads to less traction and a smoother removal of vitreous. Use the fastest cut rate your machine provides. The aspiration rate generally should be 15 to 20 cc/min (this is not independently set on venturi machines, only peristaltic pumps; see sidebar titled, *Summary of Vitrectomy Parameters*. Also see sidebars from the 3 major phacoemulsification and anterior vitrectomy manufacturers specifying features on currently available equipment: *The WhiteStar Signature Vitrectomy System, The Alcon UltraVit Vitrectomy Probe, and The Stellaris PC Vitrectomy System*).

THE ALCON ULTRAVIT VITRECTOMY PROBE

The Infiniti Vision System has an anterior segment vitrectomy kit that serves the surgeon and staff during complications. The set-up includes the new UltraVit 23 disposable vitrectomy probes that are designed specifically for the anterior segment. These probes are tapered and sized to fit 1-mm sideport incisions with minimal trauma (thus enabling a closed system). This size of probe also allows surgeons to perform sutureless biaxial vitrectomy if they prefer.

A unique pneumatic dual-drive guillotine cutter allows the UltraVit 23 probe to produce 2500 cuts per minute. Standard vitrectomy probes have single-pressure drive actuation and therefore a much lower cutting rate (a maximum of approximately 800 cuts per minute). A higher cutting rate reduces traction on the vitreous base and thereby makes vitrectomy safer.

The UltraVit 23 probe is available on Infiniti Vision Systems that were shipped prior to September 1, 2009 as a software and hardware upgrade. The UltraVit 23 kit does not require additional training for OR staff; its use is intuitive for anyone who has a basic understanding of the principles of anterior vitrectomy.

THE STELLARIS PC VITRECTOMY SYSTEM

The Stellaris PC Vision Enhancement System (Bausch + Lomb) features next-generation vitreoretinal surgical technology in the form of an ultra-high-speed cutter and the familiar lightweight microvit-style handpiece. With an optimized duty cycle, the port of the handpiece is open at least 50% of the time, even at 5000 cpm. This allows surgeons to effectively remove vitreous at even the highest cut rates. Using the lightweight pneumatic cutter and 5000 cpm with an optimized duty cycle, surgeons may control the flow intuitively via the foot pedal. The programmable foot pedal is wireless and has dual-linear control, which enables the surgeon to vary the vacuum and cut rate. The vacuum on the Stellaris PC is controlled by an advanced algorithm that produces accurate, smooth, and linear aspiration that remains predictable at vacuum as low as 2 mm Hg. If the vitrectomy technique involves a pars plana approach, the Trocar tip's long taper provides sufficient cutting surface. This tip is designed to permit a shallow angle of entry during tunnel incisions. The Trocar's needle has been redesigned to be solid instead of hollow, which reduces the force of the insertion and displaces less tissue.

Linear Versus Fixed Vacuum Setting

Vitreoretinal surgeons who work in the posterior segment every day prefer to use linear vacuum for vitrectomy because they can control the intraoperative environment. Familiarity leads to facility, so that some physicians can use a graduated FP3 with ease. Anterior segment surgeons who perform vitrectomy rarely, however, are not as adept at these maneuvers and often get nowhere because they are too timid to even venture into FP3. Staying in FP2 will accomplish nothing because there will be continuous cutting and no suction. The author believes that anterior segment surgeons should use a panel/fixed setting for vacuum instead of a linear vacuum setting for vitrectomy. We want to find and maintain the lowest level of vacuum that moves the vitreous; there is no reason to use higher or lower vacuum once the vitreous is moving. Such nonlinearity allows the surgeon to either go pedal-to-the-metal in FP3 with suction, or come up into FP2 without suction. The vacuum default settings on today's phaco machines are usually set at 150 mm Hg, ideal for primary 3-port vitrectomy. In unplanned vitrectomy, however, the anterior segment surgeon is almost always removing vitreous in a sea of dispersive OVD. The author finds 150 mm Hg to be inadequate in a viscoelastic-filled environment; the author generally uses 250 mm Hg for 20-gauge and 350 mm Hg for 23-gauge vitrectomy.

Irrigation

Surgeons must keep the irrigation bottle moderately high in order to maintain a normotensive eye. Again, the phaco machine's default setting places the bottle low. The appropriate bottle height depends on the size of cannula used. Most anterior segment surgeons opt for a 23-gauge cannula. To control the IOP, the author has a scrub nurse stand with one hand on the bottle's button, ready to raise it as needed, and one hand on the vacuum button. The author starts the vacuum for 20-gauge vitrectomy at around 200 mm Hg, and asks the scrub nurse to progress by 10-mm increments to 250 mm Hg or stop once the vitreous begins to move. As soon as movement is seen toward the vitrector port, the author has the scrub nurse raise the bottle to prevent a soft eye. The author continues in this manner until homeostatic normotension is achieved.

GETTING STARTED: VITRECTOMY MODE AND INCISIONS

The first step is to confirm initial vitrectomy mode settings and then irrigate any bubbles out of the irrigation line while the vitrector is outside of the eye. If choosing an anterior approach, make a second paracentesis a little less

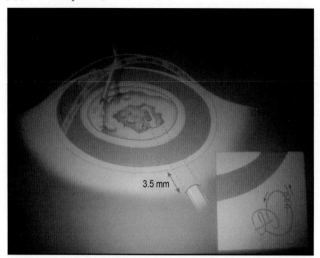

Figure 29-9. This image shows the biaxial vitrectomy approach, with irrigation through a clear corneal incision and the vitrector entering through a pars plana sclerotomy 3.5 mm posterior to the limbus. A double-bite mattress or X suture with an 8–0 Vicryl is used to close the direct-approach sclerotomy.

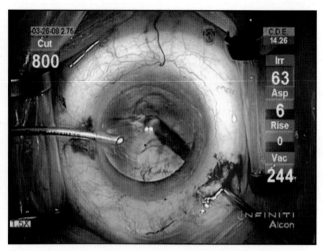

Figure 29-10. Example of 20-gauge pars plana vitrectomy in progress with anterior irrigation, port forward facing and settings correct.

than 180 degrees away from the original sideport incision, large enough to fit the bare vitrector needle. If the surgeon is planning to make a pars plana incision under topical anesthesia, make sure to first place a bleb of lidocaine with epinephrine sub-Tenon's over the intended area of the incision for the patient's comfort. This step permits a small, fornix-based peritomy to bare the sclera without cautery (Figure 29-9).

Next, secure the primary wound if there is no vitreous loss. If vitreous is incarcerated in the incision, blocking a watertight closure, then fill the anterior chamber with OVD to approximate normal pressure. Avoid making the scleral incision at 3, 6, 9, and 12 o'clock so as to miss the ciliary vessels and nerves. Use a caliper to measure 3.5 mm posterior to the limbus in the quadrant most convenient to your dominant hand, and avoid perforating vessels. Enter the pars plana with an MVR blade directed toward the optic nerve or the center of the eye until you can visualize the blade in the pupil and withdraw the blade. Insert the irrigating 23-gauge chamber maintainer or a cannula through the original clear corneal paracentesis.

Vitrectomy

Insert the vitrector through the sclerotomy and view it in the center of the iris through the pupil. Always make sure the port can be seen during vitrectomy; the only exception is when performing a dry vitrectomy to make space in a crowded anterior chamber. In this scenario, make sure the port is sideways or backward to avoid engaging the posterior capsule while removing a small amount of vitreous.

Remain in FP0 to this point. The moment the vitrector's port can be seen, go to FP2, which will cause irrigation and activate the cutter without allowing vacuum to build. The cutter can now be advanced to the center of the pupil below the broken posterior capsule and start aspirating vitreous by engaging FP3. Watch for any small bubble or particle to confirm that the vacuum is high enough to move vitreous, and raise the vacuum slowly until the movement of vitreous into the vitrector port can be visually confirmed. If the surgeon sets the vacuum on panel or fixed rather than linear, he or she can put the pedal to the metal and ask the scrub nurse to raise the vacuum slowly until it effectively begins to aspirate vitreous, usually at approximately 250 mm Hg for 20-gauge or 350 mm Hg for 23-gauge vitrectomy. As soon as effective aspiration takes place, the surgeon must raise the bottle to achieve homeostasis for a normotensive globe. The scrub nurse will also adjust this parameter on the fly and usually will find homeostasis at about 70 to 80 cm, depending on where the patient's head is relative to the machine's cassette. As noted, the flow rate on machines with a peristaltic pump usually stays at 20 cc/min for 20-gauge and 15 cc/min for 23-gauge vitrectomy, and it need not be adjusted (Figure 29-10).

Completing Vitrectomy

Keep the pedal to the metal until it is evident that there is no more prolapsed vitreous flowing to the port. If you must move the position of the vitrector, change from FP3 to FP2 in order to cut with no suction and then readjust the location of the port to address any other areas of vitreous prolapse. Do not move the vitrector around through vitreous without being in FP2 to avoid inadvertent traction.

When the surgeon thinks he or she has reached the endpoint, hold the vitrector still and come to FP0. Remove the irrigation cannula and irrigate some diluted Triesence into the anterior chamber. Again place the irrigator through the paracentesis to disperse the Triesence, thereby confirming

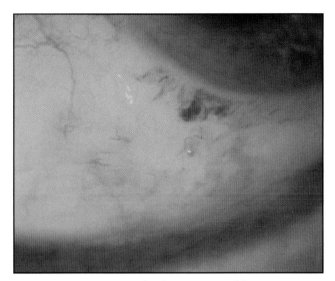

Figure 29-11. A suture under the conjunctival flap.

the complete absence of prolapsed vitreous. When extracting the vitrector from the eye, remain in cutting mode (FP2) until visualization is lost under the iris. Come up into FP1 for the brief interval that the vitrector is between the edge of the iris and when it exits the sclera, but go to FP0 right before exiting the incision, so as not to blow vitreous out of the incision. Retinal surgeons will continue irrigating until they are out of the eye, but that is because they have done a total vitrectomy. When cleaning the sclerotomy of any prolapsed vitreous, turn the cutter down toward the external lips of the wound while irrigating externally onto the incision, and sharply cut away any external strands before suturing. Never use a Weck-Cel sponge due to the capillary action which can cause some vitreous traction especially if the sponge, with vitreous adherent is lifted without the vitreous being cut.

Immediately place a scleral plug or a temporary tie suture to close the sclerotomy. If an anterior approach was used, confirm that the clear corneal incision closes and that no strand of vitreous has followed the withdrawal of the vitrector needle. The eye is now closed and ready for further maneuvers, and the vitrectomy site is available in case vitreous presents again.

Wecking and Sweeping Incisions

For generations, ophthalmic residents were told to use a cyclodialysis spatula to sweep from the paracentesis to just inside the main incision to identify, release, and remove incarcerated vitreous. This practice causes significant traction on the posterior vitreous and should be abandoned, in this author's opinion. The preferred technique is particulate identification with Triesence and sharp cutting or, ideally, using a vitrector to amputate connections posteriorly at the pupil margin (thus obviating traction). Once the vitreous

sheet either retracts to the posterior segment or is severed from the vitreous within the wound, it is safe to remove residual vitreous from the incision with a Weck-Cel sponge. Sponges should never be used to remove vitreous that is still attached posteriorly, however, because they absorb vitreous strands and lead to traction and cause inflammation upon contact with iris tissue. Any time a surgeon touches a sponge to the incision, he or she should have scissors ready in the other hand so that, should he or she discover vitreous, it can be cut without lifting or stretching the strands. Immediately cut off the vitreous at the plane of the sclera so that it is not pulled forward out of the wound. Then, the surgeon may address the vitreous in the optimal manner.

SUTURING OF DIRECT SCLEROTOMY (20- OR 23-GAUGE)

Older-style vitrectors had a flat tip that required an opening slightly larger than their gauge. The vitrector the author uses on the Infiniti Vision System (Alcon Laboratories, Fort Worth, TX) has a rounded tip that makes the incision requirement true to size and its entry less traumatic.

Closing a 20-gauge sclerotomy requires a 2-bite incision. A 23-gauge direct MVR incision may require only one bite to be watertight. Once any prolapsed vitreous at the sclerotomy lip is lysed, the author prefers to make an "X" or a mattress suture of 8-0 Vicryl (Ethicon, San Angelo, TX). It may be best to orient the needle from a posterior to anterior position when taking the half thickness bite to ensure that the needle's point does not come out too far posteriorly. It is not necessary to bury the sclerotomy knot, as it will be covered by the Tenons and conjunctival fornix-based flap that you will suture in place with the same absorbable suture. Tie the conjunctival knot on the inside of the flap for the patient's comfort (Figure 29-11). The sclerotomy should be watertight, and no bleb should form from pressurizing the globe.

SUTURELESS VITRECTOMY (23- OR 25-GAUGE TROCAR CANNULA SYSTEM)

Because we want a noncoincident incision in the conjunctiva and the sclera, it is difficult to make a sutureless incision without the help of a cannula to keep the 2 openings lined up. Finding the openings with the vitrector via an MVR blade-created shelved entry is very challenging. The cannula is a hollow tube that often encases a sharp MVR blade. The surgeon withdraws the blade once he or she has completed the incision, but the tube remains as a conduit for the vitrector needle, which can be repeatedly inserted as needed until the case is completed.

A Trocar cannula system offers another advantage. Because it protrudes into the vitreous cavity, the vitrector probe never gets close to the retinal surface, as it does when inserted through a bare sclerotomy. This design provides a margin of safety upon entry and exit and there is some evidence that it decreases the risk of retinal tears. As they become sharper and require less pressure for entry, Trocars will be the entry method of choice in all cases.

Using a Trocar cannula system requires a firm, intact eye with closed incisions to handle the pressure applied to the globe upon entry. If incisions are already present, do not simply close them with hydration. Incisions should be sutured closed because the force of inserting the trocar will likely cause iris prolapse if they are not entirely secure. A soft eye will risk choroidal detachment or hemorrhage with this procedure. If vitreous has been lost, the surgeon will not be able to close the incisions, even with sutures, so a direct MVR entry with suturing would be safest.

With a reliably firm eye, pull the conjunctiva away from the site of puncture 3.5 mm back from the limbus and initiate a partial-thickness scleral tunnel with the Trocar parallel to the limbus. Travel 1 to 2 mm, then turn the device perpendicular to the sclera and puncture the sclera in the direction of the optic nerve, driving the Trocar cannula system through the eye wall. Once the Trocar is in place, remove the MVR blade and leave the seated cannula for the vitrector's insertion.

Dr. Charles does not recommend a 25-gauge vitrector for anterior vitrectomy, because he says it is too flexible to use without akinesia (topical anesthesia).[11] The author's experience is with 20- and 23-gauge vitrectors only (see the sidebar titled, *Pars Plana Instrumentation*).

RESIDUAL CORTEX REMOVAL

- Perform a "dry technique" under OVD without irrigation
- Bimanual I/A imparts a small risk of incarcerating vitreous
- Use the vitrector on I/A/Cut mode (not the I/Cut/A default) for followability
- Coaxial I/A not recommended unless IOL optic is captured
- Prevent chamber collapse during removal of instruments: vitreous will follow the path of lowest pressure and present again

Once the vitreous and lens particles are removed, the surgeon is left with cortex. It is incumbent upon us to clean the capsular fornix thoroughly to avoid inflammation, prevent a poor-quality view with fluffed cortex in the

PARS PLANA INSTRUMENTATION

- Standard 20-gauge: direct sclerotomy entry
  - Readily available
  - Conjunctival flap
  - Sutured incision
- 25-gauge
  - Too flexible for topical anesthesia
- 23-gauge
  - Requires upgrade to standard Alcon Infinity machine
  - Direct sclerotomy entry requires suture
  - Trocar cannula system allows sutureless transconjunctival entry with excellent sealing

A Trocar requires more pressure to insert than a direct MVR blade and should only be used when corneal incisions can be closed with a normotensive or firm eye. For a sutureless incision, a limbal parallel circumferential scleral tunnel precedes the perpendicular entry into the vitreous cavity. The conjunctiva is pulled aside so the conjunctival entry wound is not coincidental with the scleral entry.

postoperative period, and ultimately to reduce the risk of CME. A laboratory study has also shown that cortex is a better breeding medium for the growth of bacteria than aqueous and residual cortex may be partially to blame for the increased incidence of endophthalmitis in complicated cataract surgeries.[12] Surgeons have 3 viable options to accomplish this goal.

The safest way to clean the capsular bag (albeit, not the most efficient) is to empty it with a dry technique. This means maintaining and expanding the chamber and the capsular fornix with cohesive viscoelastic and packing in the dispersive agent to cover the capsule or the zonular defect. Without irrigation, use a 3- or 5-mL syringe with a 26-gauge cannula (or a Simcoe cannula system) to suction out residual cortex. There should be just enough BSS in the syringe to be able to reflux in case the capsule or vitreous becomes incarcerated. When the tip is occluded with cortex, a manual application of suction strips it cleanly away if the anterior leaflet leads. A 23-gauge cannula is useful for dense cortical or epinuclear material, but surgeons must be careful not to attract the capsule into the port's opening where it will rip. Replace the cohesive OVD as needed to keep the capsular fornix expanded and the eye normotensive as cortex removal proceeds. This technique avoids the risk of displacing more vitreous with irrigation and inviting it forward, or pushing fragments to the back of the eye.

Another way to remove residual cortex is via bimanual I/A. Some surgeons prefer this strategy because of its efficiency. Bimanual I/A is a much better approach for removing residual cortex than coaxial I/A, which involves irrigating in the same area from which you are trying to remove the cortex. The biaxial approach conducts the irrigation anteriorly, which continues to encourage vitreous to stay back. You can direct the separate aspiration into the cortex and keep it fully occluded. Use a second sideport paracentesis with this technique so the chamber remains watertight with a closed main clear corneal incision. Although unlikely, if vitreous is encountered, there will be a tractional event that surgeons can mitigate by immediately stopping aspiration while holding the aspiration handpiece steady, exchanging the irrigation handpiece for an intraocular scissors, and cutting the incarcerated vitreous strand. This strategy will relieve the traction before the aspiration handpiece is withdrawn. The prolapsed vitreous must then be dealt with by reinserting the vitrector.

A safer technique than bimanual I/A is to use the vitrector on a different setting. Every phaco machine has a different way to switch from I/Cut/A, which must always be used for vitreous, to I/A/Cut. The point is to discourage followability when removing vitreous, although followability is necessary for removing cortex. Using the vitrector on I/Cut/A mode does not work for removing cortex, because it continually chops it off and never allows the cortex to flow into the port. Because the surgeon cannot strip it out of the sulcus, he or she ends up following the cortex into the sulcus and eating capsule. If the surgeon switches to I/A/Cut mode, then the cortex can be removed in FP2 when the vitreous is out of the way. If the surgeon thinks vitreous has emerged, he or she can immediately go down to FP3 and cut it off. This approach is safer than I/A in that it relieves a tractional event instantly. Finally, make sure to prevent the chamber from collapsing while the instruments are removed after a vitreous prolapse, an open hyaloid, or even just an open capsule. Because the vitrector port is larger than the usual 0.3 mm of an aspiration port, it will not efficiently remove small wisps of cortex that will not occlude the port and allow vacuum to build if a peristaltic pump is employed.

Implanting an Intraocular Lens

Inspect Prior to Implantation

To make sure the anterior segment is cleaned of all cortex, the surgeon may need to retract the iris to fully view the bag fornix. Reinstill Triesence and then rinse it away to be sure there is no vitreous present. Check that the pupil is round and that incisions are sealed. Verify the status and size of the capsulorrhexis and evaluate the

extent of the posterior capsular tear and whether there is a true continuous curvilinear tear. Be aware of any retained nuclear fragment below the posterior capsule, and make certain no fragments are hiding anteriorly under the iris or subincisionally.

Intraocular Lens Selection and Placement

When there is an uncontrolled break in the posterior capsule but the anterior CCC is intact, the author advocates implanting a 3-piece lens in the sulcus and capturing the optic through the anterior capsulorrhexis into the bag. Only when the posterior tear is converted to a true posterior continuous curvilinear capsulorrhexis (PCCC) will the author place any IOL (ideally, a single-piece one) in the capsular bag. Regardless of its location, shape, or size, an unconverted rent may extend in response to even minor pressure. If the PCCC is 4 to 5 mm and centrally located, then the surgeon can place a 3-piece lens in the bag and perform an optic capture through the PCCC into Berger's space. This is the ideal outcome.

If there was a zonular break in the presence of an intact posterior capsule and an intact anterior capsulorrhexis with a stable and centered bag, the author will use a standard capsular tension ring (CTR). If the bag is decentered then a modified Cionni CTR or segment sutured to sclera is needed. Any implant can then be placed in the stabilized bag.

If the posterior capsule is intact but there is a break in the anterior capsulorrhexis, the author will place a single-piece IOL in the bag (as long as the haptics will stay sequestered in the bag and not pop out into the sulcus). See the sidebar titled, *IOL Implantation Choices Following a Posterior Capsular Rupture*.

The Optic Capture Technique

Whenever possible, surgeons should choose an optic-capture strategy that always produces a centered, stable lens. This is the reason the author advocates making a CCC smaller than the intended optic in every case, and why she works so hard to maintain the anterior capsulorrhexis after breaking the posterior capsule. The author uses the well-known optic-capture technique described by Howard V. Gimbel, MD, MPH, FRCSC, FACS,[13] in which the sulcus is defined with OVD and the capsular bag is left uninflated. The author injects the 3-piece lens with the leading haptic clearly placed in the sulcus (Figure 29-12) and pronates the trailing haptic into place with a 2-handed technique (dialing can be risky) that minimizes displacement of the optic and stress on zonules. The author places mild pressure on the optic 90 degrees away from the haptic-optic junction to dunk the edge under the capsulorrhexis on one side and then the other, allowing the capsulorrhexis to become ovoid. With very loose zonules, this may require a 2-handed

IOL IMPLANTATION CHOICES FOLLOWING A POSTERIOR CAPSULAR RUPTURE

- Three-piece IOL in the bag, optic-captured through the posterior CCC into Berger's space
- Single-piece IOL in the bag
- Three-piece IOL in the sulcus, optic-captured through the anterior CCC
- STAAR AQ sulcus-supported 3-piece IOL, free-standing in the sulcus
- Foldable 3-piece posterior chamber-IOLs must be sutured to the iris and not left free-standing in the sulcus (a personal practice technique)
- Scleral-sutured IOL (the author's least preferred option)
- Anterior chamber 4-point fixation, open-looped, modern IOL with peripheral iridectomy
- Aphakia

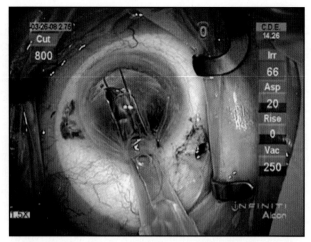

Figure 29-12. In the optic capture technique, the author directs the IOL's leading haptic into the sulcus.

technique of lifting the bag gently while sweeping under the edge of the capsulorrhexis and simultaneously applying downward pressure to the optic. The end result leaves the haptics secured in the sulcus and the optic in the bag.

If the capsule breaks after the IOL is in the bag, a less traumatic but not widely tested alternative to IOL exchange is the forward optic capture technique. A surgeon may use the optic-capture concept to his or her advantage by forward-capturing the optic in front of the intact capsulorrhexis while leaving the haptics in the bag (a personal practice technique also described by Dr. Howard V. Gimbel).[13]

If neither the anterior capsulorrhexis nor the posterior capsule is intact, the surgeon must decide between implanting a stand-alone, sutured, or scleral fixated glued sulcus IOL or a modern anterior chamber implant. In this author's opinion, it is important to secure any IOL that is not a true sulcus-supported lens (the only such lens that currently has FDA approval is the AQ series from STAAR Surgical Company). Single-piece IOLs are incompatible with sulcus fixation. The clinical study of the AcrySof natural single-piece lens was conducted with the lens implantation in the capsular bag only.[14] There are no clinical data to demonstrate its safety and effectiveness for placement in the ciliary sulcus, and plenty of evidence that it will cause pigmentary dispersion glaucoma by chaffing the posterior iris.[15] Standard 3-piece IOLs are too small for the sulcus.

They will move around and cause inflammation, CME, and pigment dispersion in a significant number of eyes. Liliana Werner, MD, PhD, has shown that the size of the sulcus varies.[16] It is not proportional to axial length or white-to-white measurements, and it is often larger than 12.5 or 13.0 mm, which is the haptic diameter of a standard 3-piece lens. Furthermore, if there is a little hole in the posterior capsule or particularly in the zonules, the sulcus-implanted lens will eventually find its way through. Having practiced for almost 30 years, the author has seen this complication on referral many times. Surgeons can purchase the STAAR lens (available in the United States) for inventory. It is made of biocompatible silicone with a rounded edge. The lens' stiff elastimide haptics are 13.5 mm apart, making it the only reliable choice for unsupported sulcus implantation.

It is a personal choice whether to anchor a standard 3-piece IOL in the sulcus with 1 or 2 iris sutures or place a PMMA lens with eyelets as a scleral-sutured lens. There is now enough data that the scleral fixated glued IOL may be another viable option.[17] In the presence of no intact anterior or posterior capsule, especially after a long case, the simplest option may be to place an anterior chamber lens through a scleral tunnel, having closed the clear corneal incision. In this scenario, the author makes a peripheral iridectomy with the vitrector. After instilling acetylcholine chloride intraocular solution (Miochol-E), the author uses the I/A/Cut mode with raised vacuum and a lowered cut rate to produce a neat peripheral hole in the iris before placing the IOL (taking care to not tuck the iris). "White-to-white plus one" is still the standard for sizing the IOL in this maneuver. A review of the ophthalmic literature shows that there is no evidence of a decrease in the quality of long-term outcomes with implanting IOLs in the anterior chamber versus suturing them in the posterior chamber.

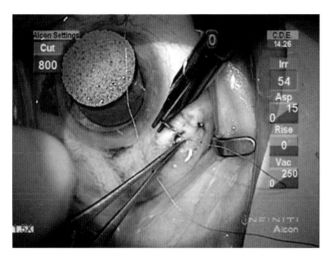

Figure 29-13. A suture is always placed in the direct entry sclerotomy. Plan to also suture the cataract incision if there is the possibility of retained lens material that may necessitate a secondary retinal procedure.

REMOVING OPHTHALMIC VISCOSURGICAL DEVICE AND CLOSING THE EYE

If the surgeon does not capture the optic in an eye that has lost vitreous, he or she should be very cautious in removing the viscoelastic at the end of the case. The author usually does this manually in these eyes by irrigating and then slightly burping the incision to let out some of the OVD. The author irrigates some more, and then uses a manual push/pull technique through the paracenteses to remove all of the viscoelastic that she reasonably can. Be careful not to lower the pressure in the anterior chamber by overzealously removing the viscoelastic, thereby allowing vitreous to present again. Of course, you can remove the viscoelastic more aggressively if you have used an optic-capture technique. The author prefers not to use Healon 5 in complicated cases, because even a little of this OVD left behind can cause a severe rise in IOP in the postoperative period. Viscoat OVD is the most forgiving agent, since it is of a smaller molecular weight. Any OVD that remains behind a properly captured optic is of no intraocular pressure concern, as it will not have access to the trabecular meshwork and will slowly be absorbed without incident.

Miochol-E will provide miosis, protect the IOL's position, and ensure a round pupil with no peak, which would indicate a vitreous wick (see sidebar titled, *Pharmacology*).

A final minim of Triesence and rigorously closed incisions with dry tunnels will confirm that no incarcerated vitreous is lurking. Even if the clear corneal incision seals flawlessly, a suture is indicated (Figure 29-13) if a follow-up retinal procedure may be needed due to retained lens material.

Then, because a break in the vitreous face significantly increases the risk of endophthalmitis, the author always prophylaxes the eye with intracameral moxifloxacin (an off-label use).[18] Immediately postoperatively, the author provides one dose of moxifloxacin hydrochloride (Avelox), a systemic form of moxifloxacin (400 mg PO), that crosses the blood-retinal barrier.

Furthermore, patients with open posterior capsules need to use a longer taper of topical steroid than routine patients and remain on topical nonsteroidal anti-inflammatory drugs (NSAIDs) for a longer period (off label) to prevent CME. Hypotensive medications are also a good idea because surgeons often leave some viscoelastic behind; these eyes often experience a postoperative rise in IOP. The author prescribes acetazolamide (Diamox) if there is no history of sulfa allergy (10% of people who have sulfa allergy are allergic to Diamox), and then the author carefully follows the patient postoperatively.

CONCLUSION

Warn vitrectomy patients to expect floaters postoperatively and to call and identify themselves as surgical patients if they are experiencing pain or decreasing vision at any time (see sidebar titled, *Postoperative Follow-Up*). Treat any IOP spikes aggressively and follow them closely, especially over the first 48 hours. Teach patients to check peripheral vision at home. The author highly recommends performing a scleral indented retinal examination and/or a retinal subspecialty consultation within 1 to 2 weeks after surgery to be absolutely sure there are no holes or tears in the peripheral retina that need to be treated. Closely monitor these patients for CME with an Amsler grid at home. Also, optical coherence tomography is indicated. Often, vitrectomy patients can achieve 20/20 uncorrected visual acuity (UCVA) on the first postoperative day, and any floaters will disappear with time. It is critical to inform these patients of their increased risk of developing a retinal tear or detachment in the future, in addition to the increased risk of glaucoma and CME. Educate patients about the signs of a retinal tear or detachment so that they may be vigilant for them, and inform patients of the need for periodic testing for glaucoma. Finally, if an eye has retained lens material, then the patient must be referred to a retinal specialist in a timely fashion for a possible definitive treatment. A recent meta-analysis of the literature shows patients fare best if the intervention is from 3 days to 7 days after surgery that was complicated by retained lens material.[19]

When surgeons prepare in advance for a loss of vitreous with a comprehensive strategy and treat patients with logic and care, surgeons can often achieve optimal outcomes, even in complicated cataract cases.

SUGGESTED READINGS

Arbisser LB. Anterior vitrectomy for the anterior segment surgeon. Focal points. The American Academy of Ophthalmology; March 2009.

Arbisser LB, Charles S, Howcroft M, Werner L. Management of vitreous loss and dropped nucleus during cataract surgery. *Ophthalmol Clin North Am.* 2006;19(4):495-506.

REFERENCES

1. Richard Mackool, MD, e-mail communication, April 14, 2011
2. Lincoff H, Zweifach P, Brodie S, et al. Intraocular injection of lidocaine. *Ophthalmology.* 1985;92(11):1587-1591.
3. Personal communication with Michael Snyder, MD.
4. Osher RH. Slow motion phacoemulsification approach. *J Cataract Refract Surg.* 1993;19(5):667.
5. Kelman CD. New PAL method may save difficult cataract cases. *Ophthalmology Times.* 1994;19:51.
6. Arbisser LB, Charles S, Howcroft M, Werner L. Management of vitreous loss and dropped nucleus during cataract surgery. *Ophthalmol Clin North Am.* 2006;19(4):495-506.
7. Spence DJ, Peyman GA. A new technique for the vital staining of the corneal endothelium. *Invest Ophthalmol.* 1976;15(12):1000-1002.
8. Burk SE, Da Mata AP, Snyder ME, Schneider S. Visualizing vitreous using kenalog suspension. *J Cataract Refract Surg.* 2003;29(4):645-651.
9. Personal communication with Dr. Steve Charles.
10. Charles S. The History of Vitrectomy: Innovation and Evolution. Retina Today. 2008;9(suppl):27-29.
11. Personal communication.
12. Lou B, Lin X, Luo L, Yang Y, Chen Y, Liu Y. Residual lens cortex material: Potential risk factor for endophthalmitis after phacoemulsification cataract surgery. J Cataract Refract Surg. 2013;39(2):250-257.
13. Gimbel HV, DeBroff BM. Intraocular lens optic capture. *J Cataract Refract Surg.* 2004;30(1):200-206.
14. Lane SS. The Acrysof Toric IOL's FDA Trial Results: A look at the clinical data. *Cataract Refract Surg Today.* 2006;5:66-68.
15. Chang DF, Masket S, Miller KM, et al; ASCRS Cataract Clinical Committee. Complications of sulcus placement of single-piece acrylic intraocular lenses: recommendations for backup IOL implantation following posterior capsule rupture. *J Cataract Refract Surg.* 2009;35(8):1445-1458.
16. Werner L, Izak AM, Pandey SK, Apple DJ, Trivedi RH, Schmidbauer JM. Correlation between different measurements within the eye relative to phakic intraocular lens implantation. *J Cataract Refract Surg.* 2004 Sep;30(9):1982-1988.
17. Kumar DA, Agarwal A, Jacob S, et al. Sutureless scleral-fixated posterior chamber intraocular lens. *J Cataract Refract Surg.* 2011;37(11):2089-2090.
18. Arbisser LB. Safety of intracameral moxifloxacin for prophylaxis of endophthalmitis after cataract surgery. *J Cataract Refract Surg.* 2008;34(7):1114-1120.
19. Vanner EA, Stewart MW. Vitrectomy timing for retained lens fragments after surgery for age-related cataracts: a systematic review and meta-analysis. *Am J Ophthalmology.* 2011:152(3):345-357.

Chapter 29 has been reprinted with permission from Arbisser LB. Comprehensive strategies for unplanned vitrectomy for the anterior segment surgeon. *Cataract Refract Surg Today.* 2012:1(suppl):3-19.

30

Posterior Capsule Rupture and Vitreous Loss
Advanced Approaches

Louis D. "Skip" Nichamin, MD

Modern phaco surgery has come to offer unprecedented patient benefits, having attained a level where it is now in large part viewed as a refractive operation. It is important to recognize, however, that the greatest benefit derived from contemporary small incision surgery is the enhanced safety of the procedure. Specifically, advances in surgical equipment and technique—including phaco chop—offer a level of control over the intraocular environment that, despite rupture of the posterior capsule, may allow for an anatomic and visual result that should rival an uncomplicated case.[1-3]

Admittedly, each case and anatomic scenario involving a broken posterior capsule is unique; however, several fundamental surgical principles apply universally and, when observed, will allow surgeons to achieve the following goals: (1) safely and thoroughly remove all lens material; (2) as needed, remove presenting vitreous without imparting unnecessary retinal traction forces; and (3) avoid further enlargement of the posterior capsular tear, with preservation of capsular tissue for implant support.[4]

The first step in managing this complication is recognition of its occurrence. Classic teaching has stressed the importance of a sudden deepening of the anterior chamber, and indeed this finding is likely to herald a breach in capsular integrity. A more subtle and perhaps earlier sign is deepening of the posterior chamber; in many cases the first sign of trouble may be a slight increase in space between the anterior lens capsule and posterior surface of the iris. In general, any increase in space or depth of the anterior segment should elicit a high index of suspicion that a problem is at hand.

Another important finding is a change in the fluidic environment. For example, either a change in the holding power at the phaco tip or in the followability of the lens material may indicate the presence of a capsular complication. In addition, a normal capsule and zonular membrane exhibit a certain tactile sense of rebound. If this elasticity is lost or diminished, it is likely that damage has occurred to these structures. Similarly, if one suddenly is unable to rotate a previously well-hydrodissected lens, zonular injury must be suspected. A final recognition concept concerns small pupil cases. Not only is surgery in general made more difficult but the early detection of trouble may be visually obscured. Pupillary stretch, hooks, and various expanders are all viable means to aid in visualization and may prevent a small problem from spiraling into a more serious situation.

Chang DF.
*Phaco Chop and Advanced Phaco Techniques: Strategies for
Complicated Cataracts, Second Edition* (pp 351-354).
© 2013 SLACK Incorporated.

Once a problem is suspected, one must have the discipline to stop working as soon as it is sensed. This does not equate, however, with removal of instruments from within the eye, because abrupt shallowing of the anterior chamber may extend the potential capsular tear. Rather, filling of the anterior chamber with an ophthalmic viscosurgical device (OVD) through the sideport incision may then permit removal of the phaco or irrigation and aspiration (I/A) instrument without incurring sudden hypotony. At the same time, the OVD is used to tamponade the anterior hyaloid face and stabilize any remaining lens material. Time then exists for careful assessment of the anatomy, which should then dictate subsequent surgical strategy. Knowledge of the various physical characteristics of different OVDs is never more important than when faced with a complication, and an OVD other than that which is normally used for routine surgery may be required. It should be noted that a low-viscosity, less cohesive, and highly dispersive agent helps to form a better plug over a capsular break and tamponade the anterior hyaloid face, particularly at higher shear rates. The more cohesive agents may be employed at other times when space maintenance is the goal. Newer viscoadaptive agents such as sodium hyaluronate 2.3% (Healon 5) may be helpful under certain circumstances, such as when dealing with a very shallow anterior chamber or small pupil, but may present new challenges as in achieving complete removal of the agent.

In order to avoid enlarging the capsular tear, the surgeon must be dedicated to the maintenance of a truly closed chamber environment. Although aided by small, self-sealing incisions, further maneuvers must utilize truly watertight incisions. This condition helps permit the next surgical principle to take place, and that is minimizing (or, in limited cases, completely avoiding) infusion. These 2 factors are the essence of avoiding extension of the capsular tear.

If significant nuclear material remains, a decision must be made regarding further phacoemulsification. This, of course, depends on the surgeon's experience and the anatomic particulars of the case. However, if conversion is felt to be necessary, generously enlarge the incision—astigmatic concerns may be addressed at a later time. Care should also be taken to avoid pressure on the globe when removing lens material; viscodissection and instrument-aided removal is preferable. A modified lens glide such as Visitec (Beaver-Visitec International, Waltham, MA) may be called into use to both support and aid in removal. Alternatively, the lens glide may be used as a pseudoposterior capsule, as described by Marc A. Michelson, MD allowing further phacoemulsification to be performed.[5] This must, however, be carried out in a low-flow state aided by the generous use of OVDs.

For residual cortex, the author strongly advocates a low-flow or manual technique of removal (or at least mobilization) with automated I/A only being performed after the

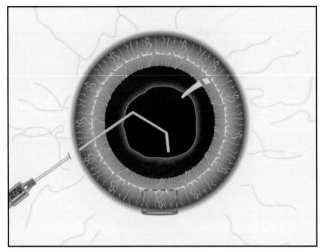

Figure 30-1. A double-bent 27-gauge cannula attached to a TB syringe filled with BSS yields exquisite sensitivity for removing recalcitrant subincisional cortex, particularly when faced with positive vitreous pressure, a torn posterior capsule, or loose/dehisced zonules.

implant has been placed and the pupil constricted. If the I/A handpiece is used in a routine fashion, the associated high flow will undoubtedly cause extension of the tear. Alternatively, if the anterior hyaloid face has been broken, cortex may be removed utilizing the vitrectomy instrument. Bimanual, separated infusion, and aspiration instruments placed through watertight paracenteses affords enhanced control and better access to residual lens material. A unimanual, nonautomated technique may offer even greater control. First, viscodissection is performed between residual cortex and the posterior capsule. An aspirating device such as a double-angled 27-gauge cannula is then placed upon a tuberculin (TB) syringe filled with balanced salt solution (BSS), which may then be inserted through various paracentesis incisions to gain 360-degree access to lens material (Figure 30-1). Gentle infusion first loosens the cortex; then, with the exquisite sensitivity afforded by this manual technique, cortical strands may be stripped from the capsular fornix and brought up into the anterior chamber. Complete removal may again be deferred until after the IOL is positioned and the pupil is made miotic.

If vitreous is present, a vitrectomy is mandated. Other authors have expounded the virtues of a bimanual, 2-port vitrectomy, yet most cataract surgeons still rely on what is familiar and seemingly easier to use—a unimanual, coaxial vitrectomy instrument. Unfortunately, this approach is inefficient, potentially more dangerous, and much more likely to lead to enlargement of the capsular rent. By simply separating the infusion line from the vitrectomy instrument, a more controlled and effective vitrectomy may be carried out. Various anterior chamber maintainers are available. Self-maintaining cannulas have the advantage of freeing up one hand, but the author prefers to maintain

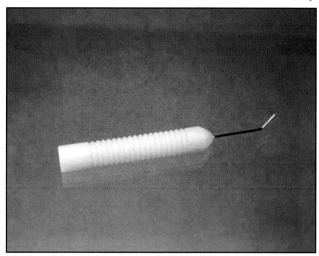

Figure 30-2. A 21-gauge blunt-tipped anterior chamber infusion cannula facilitates bimanual 2-port anterior chamber vitrectomies.

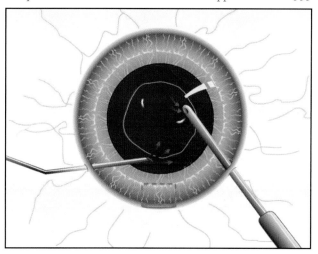

Figure 30-3. Maximal control during anterior chamber vitrectomy is obtained through the use of a closed-chamber system. Stab incisions are placed at the limbus for the separated infusion cannula and vitrectomy probe. If not self-sealing, the main cataract incision must be secured.

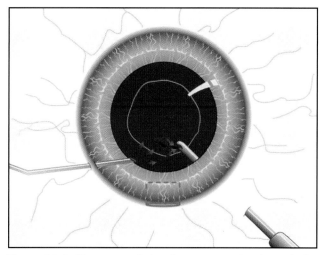

Figure 30-4. Placement of the vitrectomy probe through the pars plana may be useful in removing subincisional lens material or drawing back vitreous from the main incision.

bimanual control over the eye and have found that a blunt-ended 21-gauge infusion cannula (Storz #E4421-S21, Bausch + Lomb, Rochester, NY; Figure 30-2) is ideal. The standard infusion line connects easily to this simple instrument and is then placed through the sideport incision. The infusion rate is lowered to a level that simply maintains volume as material is removed. A microvitreoretinal (MVR) blade is then used to make a separate stab incision at the limbus to permit placement of a 20-gauge vitrectomy cutter (Figure 30-3). The incisions must be snug and watertight. If not self-sealing, the phaco incision must be sutured. Vitreous removal should be performed at low (50 to 100 mm Hg) vacuum settings with high (750 to 5000 cpm) cutting rates. If lens material is to be removed, the cutting rate is

reduced in a titrated fashion as the vacuum is carefully and gradually increased. Care must be directed toward not aspirating vitreous without simultaneous cutting. Aspiration should only be applied as necessary; for example, aspiration should be off when repositioning the vitrectomy probe. Despite the unavoidable duress that is encountered in this situation, a slow and methodical pace should be adopted. Careful visualization of the cutting port and intraocular structures will help to avoid inadvertent damage to the iris and remaining capsular tissue.

Alternatively, the cutting instrument may be placed through the pars plana (Figure 30-4). This allows the surgeon to pull down prolapsed vitreous from the anterior chamber, markedly reducing the amount of vitreous that is removed from the eye. When working from the limbus and bringing vitreous up, it is much more difficult to find an end point and one often unintentionally removes a considerable portion of the vitreous body and must then deal with a hypotonous eye.

Another significant advantage to working through a pars plana incision is the enhanced access one has to residual lens material. Cortex, epinucleus, and even medium-density nuclear material may be removed with the vitrector by gradually increasing vacuum and reducing the cutting rate. Once again, when addressing vitreous, the highest cut rate is used with the lowest possible vacuum that will permit vitreous aspiration. In this way, a more complete clean-up may be achieved, reducing secondary complications such as increased intraocular pressure (IOP), inflammation, and cystoid macular edema (CME).

It goes without saying that care and effort must be directed toward the learning and acquisition of any new surgical technique, but in reality the pars plana approach is quite straightforward. Typically, one first takes down the conjunctiva and applies light cautery at the site of the intended sclerotomy, although some surgeons will incise directly through the conjunctiva. The cardinal meridia should be avoided due to increased vascularity. Given that the posterior capsule is open, infusion may be placed through a limbal paracentesis incision or through a second pars incision. The clock hour of the vitrectomy incision should be selected to best access remaining lens material.

The pars plana is anatomically located between 3.0 and 4.0 mm posterior to the limbus, so most commonly the incision is placed 3.5 mm from the limbus, though an adjustment may be made for unusual axial lengths. Depending on surgeon preference, wounds are created to accommodate either 19- or 20-gauge instruments. A dedicated disposable MVR blade should be used to create properly sized and therefore watertight incisions for both pars plana and limbal incisions. In creating the pars incision, the MVR blade is held perpendicular to the scleral surface and usually oriented in a limbal–parallel fashion. The blade is directed toward the center of the globe with a simple in-and-out motion.

Attention is paid to preserving as much capsule as possible, especially the anterior capsular rim in order to facilitate implant placement. Infusion is kept at a minimum—just enough to maintain adequate IOP. Generous use of appropriate (often several different) viscoelastic agents will aid in volume maintenance, further decreasing the need for infusion. A dispersive agent works best to tamponade the hyaloid face, and a more cohesive viscoelastic is used to maintain space.

Care should be taken in both cleaning and closing the pars plana incision. Choices for suture closure would include 9-0 nylon or 8-0 Vicryl. Recently, 25-gauge instrumentation has become available that, in some settings, may allow for sutureless surgery. Insertion, however, requires a firm globe. These instruments can still be used in a complicated setting by first creating small incisions with a sharp blade as opposed to the usual Trocar system. One downside is their lack of tensile rigidity and, therefore, an ability to manipulate the position of the globe.

Following IOL placement, a miotic is gradually instilled. Viscoelastic is removed with the vitrectomy instrument with meticulous attention directed toward the pupil and wounds to be sure that all vitreous has been removed.

Shallowing of the anterior chamber must be avoided to prevent further vitreous prolapse: temporary air injection followed by a gradual fluid–air exchange may be useful. Rapid stromal hydration of limbal incisions is also helpful. Watertight wounds should, as always, be confirmed. Postoperatively, vigorous steroid and nonsteroidal anti-inflammatory drugs should be employed, and cycloplegic and anti-hypertensive agents should be strongly considered. Finally, although awkward, a forthright discussion with the patient should take place. Reticence on the surgeon's part will only lead to further patient doubt and potential problems.

CONCLUSION

Although increasingly rare given recent advances in phaco technique and technology, the inexorable truth is that the complication of a broken posterior capsule with vitreous loss will, eventually, be encountered. Surgeons may take solace, however, in the knowledge that by being prepared for this situation, holding to the principles and techniques of closed-chamber surgery, and maintaining their patience, the vast majority of these challenging cases will enjoy a final outcome that is as propitious as that of a routine case. The ensuing sense of equanimity that comes about from this realization is obtainable by both the young as well as experienced phaco surgeon.

REFERENCES

1. Nichamin LD. Prevention pearls and damage control. In: Fishkind WJ, ed. *Complications in Phacoemulsification*. New York, NY: Thieme; 2002:260-270.
2. Nichamin LD. Prevention and management of complications. In: Dillman DM, Maloney WF, eds. *Ophthalmology Clinics of North America*. Philadelphia, PA: W.B. Saunders; 1995:523-538.
3. Nichamin LD. Posterior capsule rupture and vitreous loss: advanced approaches. In: Chang DF, ed. *Phaco Chop: Mastering Techniques, Optimizing Technology and Avoiding Complications*. Thorofare, NJ: SLACK Incorporated; 2004:199-202.
4. Wu MC, Bhandari A. Managing the broken capsule. *Curr Opin Ophthalmol*. 2008;19(1):36-40.
5. Michelson MA. Use of a Sheets' glide as a pseudoposterior capsule in phacoemulsification complicated by a posterior capsule rupture. *Eur J Implant Surg*. 1993;570-572.

Financial Disclosures

Dr. Takayuki Akahoshi has no financial or proprietary interest in the materials presented herein.

Dr. Lisa B. Arbisser has no financial or proprietary interest in the materials presented herein.

Dr. David F. Chang is a consultant for Abbott Medical Optics, Transcend, Power Vision, and LensAR. Dr. Chang is on the speaker's bureau for Allergan, Zeiss, and Glaukos. Dr. Chang donates his consultant fees to Project Vision and the Himalayan Cataract Project.

Dr. Robert J. Cionni is a consultant for Alcon Laboratories.

Dr. Alan S. Crandall is a consultant for Alcon Laboratories.

Dr. Louis D. "Skip" Nichamin is a consultant for Bausch + Lomb and LensAR.

Dr. Randall J. Olson has no financial or proprietary interest in the materials presented herein.

Dr. Robert H. Osher has no financial or proprietary interest in the materials presented herein.

Dr. Mark Packer is a consultant for Abbott Medical Optics, Advanced Vision Science, Auris Surgical Robotics, Rayner Intraocular Lenses, and Bausch + Lomb. Dr. Packer is a consultant for and receives equity from LensAR, TrueVision Systems, and WaveTec Vision Systems.

Dr. Barry S. Seibel is a consultant and stockholder in OptiMedica and receives royalties and licenses his patent rights to Rhein Medical.

Index